DATE			

BAKER & TAYLOR

LABORATORY
INSTRUMENTATION

LABORATORY INSTRUMENTATION
Fourth Edition

Edited by

Mary C. Haven, M.S.

Gregory A. Tetrault, M.D.

Jerald R. Schenken, M.D.

VNR VAN NOSTRAND REINHOLD
I(T)P A Division of International Thomson Publishing Inc.

New York • Albany • Bonn • Boston • Detroit • London • Madrid • Melbourne
Mexico City • Paris • San Francisco • Singapore • Tokyo • Toronto

Printed in the United States of America
For more Information, contact:

Van Nostrand Reinhold
115 Fifth Avenue
New York, NY 10003

International Thomson Publishing GmbH
Königswinterer Strasse 418
53227 Bonn
Germany

International Thomson Publishing Europe
Berkshire House 168-173
High Holborn
London WCIV 7AA
England

International Thomson Publishing Asia
221 Henderson Road #05-10
Henderson Building
Singapore 0315

Thomas Nelson Australia
102 Dodds Street
South Melbourne, 3205
Victoria, Australia

International Thomson Publishing Japan
Hirakawacho Kyowa Building, 3F
2-2-1 Hirakawacho
Chiyoda-ku, 102 Tokyo
Japan

Nelson Canada
1120 Birchmount Road
Scarborough, Ontario
Canada M1K 5G4

International Thomson Editores
Campos Eliseos 385, Piso 7
Col. Polanco
11560 Mexico D.F. Mexico

    1 2 3 4 5 6 7 8 9 10 ARCFF 01 00 99 98 97 96 95 94

Library of Congress Cataloging-in-Publication Data
Laboratory instrumentation / edited by Mary C. Haven, Gregory A.
    Tetrault, Jerald R. Schenken. — 4th ed.
        p.   cm.
    Includes bibliographical references and index.
    ISBN 0-442-01520-8
    1. Medical laboratories—Equipment and supplies.   I. Haven, Mary
C. II. Tetrault, Gregory A.   III. Schenken, Jerald R.
RB36.2.L33   1994
616.07′54′028—dc20   94-13119
                                                          CIP

To two former editors of this book

Dr. Clarence A. McWhorter, 1918-1988, was chairman of the Department of Pathology when the first and second editions were printed. He had relinquished his duties as chairman but was still an active faculty member when the third edition was published. His support and encouragement were part of the impetus for us to attempt that first addition. Dr. McWhorter realized the importance of the increased emphasis on technology that was occurring in the clinical laboratory and that more information on clinical laboratory instrumentation would benefit technologists, pathologists, clinical laboratory scientists, and most importantly, patients.

M. Robert Hicks, 1934-1989, spent thousands of hours rewriting, cutting and pasting, checking references, and correcting artist drawings in the first three editions of this book. Without him the book would not exist. We missed Bob when he retired, but we always knew we could call on him for many things, including help with this fourth edition. Unfortunately, we could not. We are grateful to these kind and gentle men for guiding us through three editions and inspiring us to complete a fourth.

CONTRIBUTORS

Gene d'Allemand, M.S., M.T. (ASCP)
Assistant Chief Technologist, Pathology Center, Nebraska Methodist Hospital, Omaha, NE
Chapter 2

Judy M. Anderson, M.T. (ASCP)
Medical Technologist, Pathology Center, Nebraska Methodist Hospital, Omaha, NE
Chapter 12

Lora L. Arnold, B.A., M.T. (ASCP)
Technical Coordinator, Chemistry, Clinical Pathology Laboratory, University of Nebraska Medical Center, Omaha, NE
Chapter 19

Peggy L. Bottjen, M.T. (ASCP)
Technical Coordinator, Chemistry, Clinical Pathology Laboratory, University of Nebraska Medical Center, Omaha, NE
Chapter 14

Michaeleen M. Collins, M.S., M.T. (ASCP)
Section Manager, Immunology, Clinical Pathology Laboratory, University of Nebraska Medical Center, Omaha, NE
Chapter 17

John H. Eckfeldt, M.D., Ph.D.
Professor, University of Minnesota, Department of Laboratory Medicine and Pathology, Minneapolis, MN
Chapter 18

Robert A. Earl, Ph.D.
Director, Clinical Laboratories, Harris Laboratories, Lincoln, NE
Chapter 1

Steven M. Faynor, Ph.D.
Director of Clinical Chemistry Laboratory, Clinical Laboratories, West Virginia University Hospitals, Morgantown, WV
Chapter 11

Ronald D. Feld, Ph.D.

Director of Chemistry, Department of Pathology, University of Iowa Hospital, Iowa City, IA
Chapter 18

Linda L. Fell, M.S., M.T. (ASCP)

Clinical Coordinator, Division of Medical Technology, School of Allied Health Professions, University of Nebraska Medical Center, Omaha, NE
Chapter 20

Maximillian D. Fiore, Ph.D.

Director of Engineering, Lifescan, Inc., Milpitas, CA
Chapter 19

Vicki S. Freeman, M.S., M.T. (ASCP), S.C.

Assistant Professor, Division of Medical Technology, University of Nebraska Medical Center, Omaha, NE
Chapter 6

Ellen R. Goshorn, M.T. (ASCP), S.C.

Medical Technologist, Clinical Pathology Laboratory, University of Nebraska Medical Center, Omaha, NE
Chapter 11

David S. Hage, Ph.D.

Assistant Professor, Chemistry, University of Nebraska, Lincoln, NE
Chapter 15

Mary C. Haven, M.S.

Associate Professor, Pathology and Microbiology, University of Nebraska Medical Center, Omaha, NE
Chapters 3, 7, 10, 11

Diana L. Headley, M.A., M.T. (ASCP), S.C.

Coordinator, Clinical Laboratory, University of Nebraska Medical Center, Omaha, NE
Chapter 24

Jeffrey A. Huth, Ph.D.

Manager of Analytical Development, Roxane Laboratories, Columbus, Ohio
Chapter 9

Richard D. Juel, M.D.

Director of Laboratories, Nichols Institute, El Paso, TX
Chapter 5

Dianne M. Kelly, B.S., M.T. (ASCP), S.M.

Section Manager, Microbiology/Virology, Clinical Pathology Laboratory, University of Nebraska Medical Center, Omaha, NE
Chapter 22

James D. Landmark, M.D.

Assistant Professor, Pathology and Microbiology, University of Nebraska Medical Center, Omaha, NE
Chapter 23

Catherine Leiendecker-Foster, M.S., CLS (NCA)

Laboratory Manager, Molecular Diagnostic Laboratory, University of Minnesota Hospital and Clinic, Laboratory Medicine and Pathology, Minneapolis, MN
Chapter 18

Martin R. Lohff, M.D.
Pathologist, Pathology Center, Nebraska Methodist Hospital, Omaha, NE
Chapter 7

James H. Nichols, Ph.D.
Associate Director of Clinical Chemistry, Department of Pathology, John Hopkins Hospital, Baltimore, MD
Chapter 16

Jimmie K. Noffsinger, Ph.D.
Vice-President, Research and Development, Primus Corporation, Kansas City, MO
Chapter 18

John D. Olson, M.D., Ph.D.
Director of Laboratories, Pathology, University of Iowa Hospital and Clinics, Iowa City, IA
Chapter 21

Ulrike T. Otten, M.T. (ASCP), S.C.
Medical Technology Teaching Coordinator, Division of Medical Technology, School of Allied Health Professions, University of Nebraska Medical Center, Omaha, NE
Chapter 13

Beverly J. Pennell, M.S., M.T. (ASCP)
Supervisor, Hemostasis/Thrombosis, Pathology, University of Iowa Hospital and Clinics, Iowa City, IA
Chapter 21

Samuel J. Pirruccello, M.D.
Assistant Professor, Pathology and Microbiology, University of Nebraska Medical Center, Omaha, NE
Chapter 17

Jerald R. Schenken, M.D.
Clinical Professor, Pathology and Microbiology, University of Nebraska Medical Center, Omaha, NE

Mary A. Steinrauf, B.S., M.T. (ASCP)
Clinical Assistant Instructor, Medical Technology Division, School of Allied Health Professions, University of Nebraska Medical Center, Omaha, NE
Chapter 5

David J. Studts, B.S., M.T. (ASCP)
Technical Coordinator, Chemistry, Clinical Pathology Laboratory, University of Nebraska Medical Center, Omaha, NE
Chapter 9

Patricia K. Studts, B.S., M.T. (ASCP), NRCC-TC
Medical Technologist-Toxicology/Special Chemistry, Clinical Pathology Laboratory, Saint Joseph Hospital, Omaha, NE
Chapter 9

Gregory A. Tetrault, M.D.
Director, Clinical Chemistry, Pathology and Microbiology, University of Nebraska Medical Center, Omaha, NE
Chapters 4, 8, 12, 18, 24

Judith A. Thompson, M.S., M.B.A.
Director of Sales and Marketing, Filtron Technology Corporation, North Borough, MA
Chapter 3

CONTENTS

PREFACE

The field of laboratory medicine continues to grow even in the face of major changes in health care delivery, such as more outpatient surgery and shorter hospital stays. Both the volume and variety of laboratory tests have increased. Few laboratories operate without instrumentation. New instrumentation has improved accuracy, precision, productivity, and turnaround time in clinical laboratories. In addition, laboratory testing has expanded outside the traditional hospital and reference laboratories to physicians' offices, patients' bedsides, and even into homes.

This fourth edition of *Laboratory Instrumentation* provides an update of the new technology. All of the chapters have been completely revised. Two chapters from the third edition, Diluters and Automated Continuous Flow Chemistry Analysis, are omitted. A single chapter now covers flame emission and atomic absorption spectroscopy. Three chapters on automated chemistry analyzers are combined into a single chapter in this edition. New chapters include Nephelometry and Turbidimetry, Gas Chromatography, Mass Spectrometry, Flow Cytometry, Automated Immunoassay Systems, Automated Blood Bank Systems, and Physician's Office Laboratory Instrumentation.

The purposes of this book are (1) to explain the basic principles behind common laboratory instrumentation; (2) to describe and illustrate the component parts of representative instruments; (3) to present good quality assurance and maintenance procedures.

To this end, this book has been completely redesigned. Each chapter begins with a clear statement of objectives for the reader. Definitions and abbreviations precede the chapter introduction. A section on instrument principles and component parts usually follows the introduction. Most chapters also contain a section on quality assurance and maintenance and conclude with a summary, references, and a list of suggested readings. In addition, the first 17 chapters include problems to test reader comprehension and knowledge. Answers to problems are provided at the end of the book. The new format makes *Laboratory Instrumentation* an excellent text for a medical technology lecture course. The book will also be valuable to practicing technologists, pathologists and pathology residents, clinical chemists and microbiologists, analytical chemists, biochemists, and physical sciences students.

This book is not intended to be a compendium of all existing laboratory instrumentation. Many chapters describe instruments without referring to specific instrumentation. Reference to any specific instrument is not an endorsement by the editors or authors, and failure to mention an instrument is not an indication of disapproval.

The next edition of *Laboratory Instrumentation* most likely will have as many changes as this one. Technologies under investigation or presently used in specialized research laboratories, such as polymerase chain reaction (PCR) and $Q\beta$ replicase DNA amplification, noninvasive chemical analysis by near-infrared photometry and nuclear magnetic resonance spectroscopy, and miniaturized implantable biosensors, may be widely available by the end of the 1990s. These are truly exciting times for laboratory medicine.

GREGORY A. TETRAULT, M.D.

ACKNOWLEDGMENTS

We, the editors of *Laboratory Instrumentation,* Fourth Edition, wish to express our appreciation to our families and friends for their help, understanding, encouragement, and tolerance of our preoccupation during the preparation of this text. We also want to thank the myriad of authors who contributed their chapters and ideas to us. A special thanks is due Judy Anderson who helped us with some of the graphics. Gregory A. Tetrault was responsible for the final graphics included in the book. Mary and Dr. Schenken thank him for his creativity and expertise with computer graphics.

GLOSSARY OF ABBREVIATIONS

Word/Phrase Abbreviations

A	absorbance	ICU	intensive care unit
ac	alternating current	IRMA	immunoradiometric assay
A/D	analog to digital	ISE	ion-selective electrode
alb	albumin	HPLC	high performance liquid
bp	boiling point		chromatography
BUN	blood urea nitrogen	LC	liquid chromatography
CSF	cerebrospinal fluid	ln	natural logarithm, $\log_e$
dc	direct current	log	log to the base 10, $\log_{10}$
DVM	digital voltmeter	m	mass
e	electron	MCH	mean corpuscular hemoglobin
E	energy	MCHC	mean corpuscular hemoglobin
EDTA	ethylenediaminetetraacetate		concentration
EIA	enzyme immunoassay	MCT	mean cell threshold
ELISA	enzyme-linked immunosorbent	MCV	mean cell volume*
	assay	MCV	mean corpuscular volume*
emf	electromotive force	MIC	minimum inhibitory concentration
Eq	equivalent	mp	melting point
FPIA	fluorescence polarization	$P\mathrm{CO}_2$	partial pressure of carbon dioxide
	immunoassay	PCV	packed cell volume
GLC	gas liquid chromatography	pH	negative log of hydrogen-ion
glu	glucose		concentration
Hct	hematocrit	$P\mathrm{O}_2$	partial pressure of oxygen
Hgb	hemoglobin	R	resistance
i	current	RBC	red blood cell (erythrocyte)

*Even though the same abbreviation represents two different terms, the context in which the abbreviation is used will make its meaning clear.

RCF	relative centrifugal force	TP	total protein
RF	radiofrequency	TS	total solids
RIA	radioimmunoassay	UV	ultraviolet
SD	standard deviation	V	volt
%T	percent transmittance	W	weight
TLC	thin layer chromatography	WBC	white blood cell (leukocyte)

Unit Abbreviations

		MeV	million electron volts
A	ampere	mg	milligram
°C	degree centigrade	mL	milliliter
cpm	counts per minute	mm	millimeter
cps	cycles per second	mOsm	milliosmolar
dpm	disintegrations per minute	mV	millivolt
ev	electron volt	in^2	square inches
F	farad	μ	micro-
ft	foot	N	normal
g	gram	nm	nanometer
g	gravity	nsec	nanosecond
hr	hour	Ω	ohm
Hz	Hertz (cycles per second)	Osm	osmolar
J	joule	psi	pounds per square inch
°K	degree Kelvin	Q	coulomb
λ	wavelength	rpm	revolutions per minute
lb	pound	sec	second
mμ	millimicrometer	u	unified atomic units
M	molar	V	volt
mEq/L	milliequivalents per liter	W	watt

Prefixes for Decimal Factors

10^3	kilo	10^{-6}	micro
10^{-1}	deci	10^{-9}	nano
10^{-2}	centi	10^{-12}	pico
10^{-3}	milli		

Common Elements

Al	aluminum	Cs	cesium
Ar	argon	Cl	chloride
Ba	barium	Cr	chromium
Be	beryllium	Co	cobalt
Bi	bismuth	Cu	copper
B	boron	F	fluorine
Br	bromine	Au	gold
Cd	cadmium	He	helium
Ca	calcium	H	hydrogen
C	carbon	I	iodine

Fe	iron	K	potassium
La	lanthanum	Ra	radium
Pb	lead	Rn	radon
Li	lithium	Se	selenium
Mg	magnesium	Si	silicon
Hg	mercury	Ag	silver
Ne	neon	Na	sodium
Ni	nickel	S	sulfur
N	nitrogen	Sn	tin
O	oxygen	W	tungsten
Pd	palladium	U	uranium
P	phosphorus	Xe	xenon
Pt	platinum	Zn	zinc

1

PRINCIPLES OF ELECTRICITY AND ELECTRONICS

Robert A. Earl

Objectives

After completing this chapter, the reader will be able to:

1. Explain why some matter carries electricity and other matter does not.
2. Explain by means of an equation how current, voltage, and resistance are interrelated.
3. Calculate the total resistance of a given circuit.
4. Calculate current and potential difference for a given circuit.
5. Explain two purposes of diodes.
6. Outline how a photomultiplier tube converts radiant light energy to an electrical pulse.
7. Formulate the basic components of an electrical safety plan.

Definitions

Alternating Current: A current that is systematically changing direction and amplitude under the influence of a voltage that is similarly fluctuating.

Battery: A device constructed from solid and/or liquid chemicals whose chemical reaction will cause electrons to flow from the negative to the positive terminal.

Capacitor: An electronic circuit component that uses parallel plates to store electrical charge. Capacitor values are expressed in farads.

Circuit: The flow of charges under the influence of a difference in voltage. Although electrons are the charged elements that actually move, conventional current is thought of as the flow of positive charges. Current values are expressed in amperes.

D'Arsonval Galvanometer: An electromechanical device for measuring direct current. It consists of a wire coil that is suspended between the poles of a permanent magnet. Current through the coil creates an opposing magnetic field that causes the coil to move. A needle pointer attached to the coil measures the amount of movement, which is proportional to the current.

Diode: An electronic component that allows current to flow in only one direction.

Direct Current: A current that flows in a constant direction under the influence of a fixed voltage.

Ohm's Law: The quantitative relationship between voltage (E), current (*i*), and resistance (R). It is expressed as

$$E = i * R \qquad\qquad\qquad\qquad\qquad\text{(Eq. 1-1)}$$

Resistance: The opposition to the flow of electrons by a given conductive material. Resistance values are expressed in ohms.

Resistor: An electronic circuit component that contributes a measured resistance to a circuit.

Voltage: An electrochemical potential or force. A difference in voltage between two locations will exert a force on charged particles (such as electrons) and will cause them to move if a suitable path exists.

Introduction

Testing in clinical laboratories has increased dramatically since the 1950s. Increasing use of automated instruments has allowed us to keep up with this growth and may have even helped to fuel this increase. At first glance an automated cell counter in hematology may appear to have little in common with an automated chemistry analyzer. This is especially true if you keep the instruments at arms length and are content to consider them magic "black boxes" where you put samples in one end and answers come out the other. In reality, these two instruments share many of same electronic components. All electronic instruments need some source of electrical power. For all but the smallest portable instruments, which can operate on batteries, this comes from a power supply. This power supply converts the 110 volt (or 240 volt) alternating current into the highly stable power required by laboratory instruments. All instruments will have a mechanism for introducing the sample to be tested and a *transducer* to convert some physical or chemical property into an electrical signal. This original electrical signal is usually not strong enough for direct measurement, so instruments almost always include some sort of amplifier to boost the original signal to a measurable level. Finally, all instruments require some sort of readout device to communicate the analysis results to the operator. This may be through a meter, a strip chart recorder, a printer, or a direct interface with a central computer.

These generalized components are illustrated in Figure 1-1. They have been assembled into an amazing diversity of instruments, from the highly complex mass spectrometers to the small bedside glucose meters. A basic understanding of how these

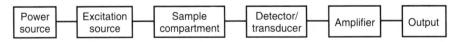

Figure 1-1.   Generalized block diagram for electronic instruments.

electrical components function should provide a better understanding of how the instruments operate. Although this knowledge will not replace the need for trained service engineers, it should provide a sound foundation for improved troubleshooting.

Principles of Electricity

All matter is made up of atoms that are composed of a positively charged nucleus of protons and neutrons surrounded by negatively charged electrons. In neutral atoms there are equal numbers of protons and electrons, and the atoms have a net charge of zero. As atoms combine with other atoms to form the various compounds, the orbiting electrons become more or less involved in the chemical bonds that hold the atoms together. When the outer electrons are not involved in bonding with neighbor atoms, they are available for carrying electrical current, and the material is called a *conductor.* The more loosely the outer electrons are held, the better conductor the material is. If the outer electrons are tightly held, they are unavailable to carry electrical current, and the material is called an *insulator.* Some materials have properties intermediate between insulators and conductors are called *semiconductors.*

Electricity involves the interaction of current or moving charges, voltage or electrochemical potential, and resistance. The basic unit of charge is called the coulomb and is designated as Q. An individual electron carries a charge of 1.6×10^{-19} coulombs, or, conversely, it takes 6.24×10^{18} electrons to equal a charge of one coulomb. *Current* is defined as the rate at which charge moves through a medium. The basic unit of current is the ampere and is designated as A. It is also sometimes shortened to amp. One ampere of current is equal to one coulomb of charge flowing past a point every second. Almost all material will offer some hindrance to the flow of charge or current. This property is called *resistance,* and the basic unit is called the ohm. It is designated by the Greek letter Ω (omega). The reciprocal of resistance is called *conductivity,* and its basic unit is the mho. The electrochemical or electromotive force that will induce the charges to move through this resistance is called *voltage* and is designated as V or v. One volt is the potential required to force one ampere of current through 1 ohm of resistance.

If the electrochemical force or voltage is applied in a constant direction, the resultant current will flow in a constant direction. This type of current is called *direct current* (dc) and is the type most often used by electronic instruments. The type of electrical power available from ordinary power sockets is called *alternating current* (ac), because the voltage swings from positive to negative and then back again. This causes the current flow to switch from one direction to the other. These sinusoidal swings in voltage are a direct result of the way electricity is produced. Electrical and magnetic radiation are very closely related. Current flowing through a conductor will induce a magnetic field around the conductor. Conversely, if a magnet is moved past a conductor so that the conductor crosses the magnetic field, current will be induced. This second property is illustrated in Figure 1-2. Once the movement of the magnet stops, the conductor no longer cuts through the magnetic field, and the current stops. If the direction of the magnet movement were to be reversed, the induced current would flow in the opposite direction. Almost all of the electrical power generated

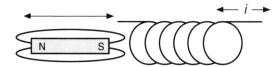

Figure 1-2. Production of alternating current (ac). As a magnet is inserted into wire coil, wires cut across a magnetic field, inducing a current. When the direction of the magnet is reversed, the direction of the current is reversed.

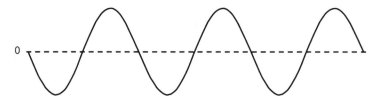

Figure 1-3. Voltage profile of ac power.

today is produced by using this very principle of magnetic fields crossing coils of conductors. The exact geometry is changed to allow the movement of the magnet (or the coils) by whatever means is available, such as steam from coal or oil fired boilers or flowing water from a dam. The voltage profile from an ac source is illustrated in Figure 1-3. As most instruments use dc power, they need to convert the ac power to dc power through a power supply or to obtain the dc power from electrochemical cells or batteries. We will cover power supplies in more detail a little later in the chapter.

BATTERIES

Many chemical reactions involve oxidation and reduction of the components of the reaction and, therefore, an exchange of electrons. If the components of the oxidation reaction are separated from the reduction components except for a conductor, the exchange of electrons can be forced to occur through this conductor. This resultant flow of electrons is the current generated by the electrochemical cell. The nature of the oxidation and reduction half cells determines the electrochemical potential or the voltage of the cell. For practical reasons this voltage is usually limited to approximately 1.5 V. If higher voltages are required, multiple cells are connected together to form batteries of cells or simply batteries. The use of liquid reaction components is messy and inconvenient, so the cells and batteries are usually constructed with paper saturated with electrolytes and electrolyte pastes. A cutaway view of such a "dry" cell is shown in Figure 1-4. Many of the electrochemical reactions are not reversible, and the battery must be discarded once the electrochemical potential has decreased to the point where it is not longer useful. However, at least two batteries employ reactions that are reversible: the nickel-cadmium battery, and

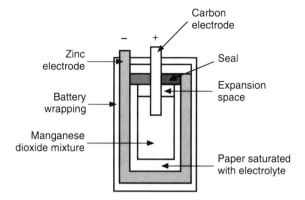

Figure 1-4. Cross section of an electrochemical cell, or "dry" cell.

the lead-acid battery. The lead-acid battery can produce a large amount of current and is an excellent source of power that can be recharged many times. This is why it has found such widespread use as the source of electricity for automobile starters. However, its size and weight as well as the corrosive nature of its contents have restricted its use in laboratory instruments. Nickel-cadmium batteries are becoming very popular in everything from flashlights to portable computers. Their relatively high cost is offset by their ability to be recharged many times. The relatively high current demand of most clinical laboratory instruments still restricts their use. With the exception of the lead-acid storage battery, all batteries have a very limited capacity to deliver current. This restricts their use as the primary power source to small, portable equipment. For the larger laboratory equipment, batteries are limited to stable voltage references.

OHM'S LAW

In the initial discussion of electricity, I mentioned that current, voltage, and resistance were all interrelated. The formula that describes this relationship is known as *Ohm's law* and is as follows:

$$E = i * R, \text{ or } V = i * R \tag{Eq. 1-2}$$

It is imperative that you become familiar and comfortable with the interrelationships of these three parameters as illustrated by this equation. A simple dc circuit is illustrated in Figure 1-5a. The set of short and long parallel lines represents a cell that is being used as a voltage source. The longer line represents the positive terminal and the shorter line the negative terminal. A battery of cells (or simply battery) would be drawn with a series of short and long lines (Fig. 1-5b). Note that the series still ends with a positive terminal on one end and a negative terminal on the other. The electromotive force or voltage supplied by the cell or battery will cause charge to move through the circuit producing a current. This current is represented by the

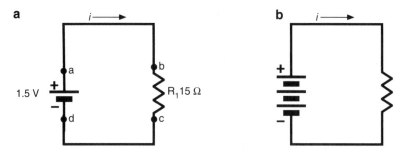

Figure 1-5.   Simple circuits illustrating Ohm's law.

arrow and the letter *i*. By convention, current is considered to flow from higher voltages toward lower voltages or from the positive to the negative battery terminals. This convention runs counter to our present understanding of current being the result of flowing electrons. Negatively charged electrons will be drawn and flow toward the positive terminal or higher voltages. However, the convention was established before this was clearly understood. To rationalize this, current can be thought of as flow of positive holes left behind when an electron moves to its new location. With this analogy, the positive holes would appear to migrate in the opposite direction as the electrons.

The amount of current that will flow in the circuit is determined by the voltage of the battery and the resistance of the circuit. However, a complete path for the electrons must exist before any current will flow. Components that are used to contribute resistance are called resistors and are represented by the sawtooth symbol. Connecting wire has a small, yet finite, resistance, but it is generally not considered, and only the resistors are shown in diagrams. Figure 1-5a contains a 15 Ω resistor, and we can use Ohm's law to calculate the current in the circuit:

$$i = E/R = 1.5\,V/15\,\Omega = 0.1 \text{ amperes, or } 0.1A \qquad \text{(Eq. 1-3)}$$

Figure 1-5 also illustrates several other important points. Because there is no resistance between points a and b, the voltage difference between these two points must be 0, even though there is a current flow of 0.1 amps between them:

$$E = i * R = 0.1\,A * 0\,\Omega = 0\,V \qquad \text{(Eq. 1-4)}$$

The same is true of points c and d. Therefore, all of the 1.5 V from the battery must be dissipated, or "dropped," across resistor R_1.

Resistors can have fixed resistances as illustrated in previous figures, or they can have variable resistances. Variable resistors are usually constructed of a length of resistive material and of a movable contact point called a wiper (Fig. 1-6). The length of the resistive material that the current has to pass through before reaching the wiper determines the effective resistance at that setting. The resistive material is usually arranged in a circular configuration so that the wiper setting can be adjusted by turning a dial.

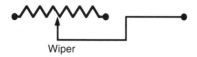

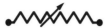

Figure 1-6. Schematic symbols used for variable resistors.

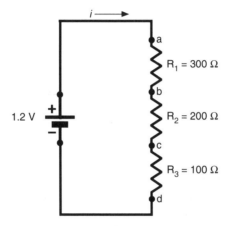

Figure 1-7. Series circuit.

SERIES CIRCUIT

When components are connected end to end to form a single pathway, the components are said to be connected *in series* (Fig. 1-7). The current in any part of a series circuit must be equal. You can think of this like water flowing in a garden hose. If there are no leaks in the hose, whatever amount of water flows in one end must flow out the other. If you put a flow restricter, such as a spray nozzle, on the end, the flow at all points in the hose slows down. Resistances in series total by simple addition. The total resistance in Figure 1-7 can be calculated as:

$$R_T = R_1 + R_2 + R_3 = 300\ \Omega + 200\ \Omega + 100\ \Omega = 600\ \Omega \qquad \text{(Eq. 1-5)}$$

Once the total resistance has been calculated, the current can be determined using Ohm's law:

$$i = E/R = 1.2\ \text{V}/600\ \Omega = 0.002\ \text{A, or 2 mA} \qquad \text{(Eq. 1-6)}$$

Figure 1-7 also illustrates a very useful application of resistors in a series circuit known as a voltage divider. The voltage at point a is 1.2 V, because the current of 2 mA has not passed through any resistors and there has been no iR drop. Point b must be at a lower potential than point a because of the voltage drop over R_1:

$$b = 1.2 \text{ V} - 0.002 * 300 \; \Omega = 1.2 \text{ V} - 0.6 \text{ V} = 0.6 \text{ V} \qquad \text{(Eq. 1-7)}$$

Similarly, point c must be at a lower voltage than point a because of the iR drop through R_2:

$$c = 0.6 \text{ V} - 0.002 * 200 \; \Omega = 0.6 \text{ V} - 0.4 \text{ V} = 0.2 \text{ V} \qquad \text{(Eq. 1-8)}$$

The voltage at d must be 0 V because it is directly connected to the negative terminal of the battery. This can be verified by using the same calculation as the other two points:

$$d = 0.2 \text{ V} - 0.002 * 100 \; \Omega = 0.2 \text{ V} - 0.2 \text{ V} = 0 \text{ V} \qquad \text{(Eq. 1-9)}$$

This series of resistors successively lowered the voltage from the starting potential of the positive terminal to the potential of the negative terminal. The exact increment of the steps can be manipulated by careful selection of the resistance values. The voltages at the intermediate points (b and c) can be drawn off and used in other parts of the circuit or other parts of the instrument. Voltage dividers such as this are very useful for creating several different voltage sources from a single power supply.

PARALLEL CIRCUITS

When the components are connected head to head to form several different current pathways, the components are said to form a *parallel circuit* (Fig. 1-8). The sum of the current in each of the parallel branches must equal the current prior to the split. The total effective resistance of a parallel network is the sum of the reciprocals of the individual resistances:

$$1/R_T = 1/R_1 + 1/R_2 = 1/100 \; \Omega + 1/300 \; \Omega = (3 + 1)/300 \; \Omega \qquad \text{(Eq. 1-10)}$$

$$R_T = 300/4 \; \Omega = 75 \; \Omega \qquad \text{(Eq. 1-11)}$$

From this calculation we can see that the total resistance for a parallel circuit is lower than the resistance in any single branch. This makes sense as the current has several

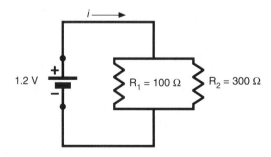

Figure 1-8.   Parallel circuit.

different paths from which to choose. The total current for Figure 1-8 can then be calculated as:

$$i_T = E/R_T = 1.2 \text{ V}/75 \text{ }\Omega = 0.016 \text{ A, or } 16 \text{ mA} \qquad \text{(Eq. 1-12)}$$

The current in the individual branches can then be calculated:

$$i_1 = E/R_1 = 1.2 \text{ V}/100 \text{ }\Omega = 0.012 \text{ A, or } 12 \text{ mA} \qquad \text{(Eq. 1-13)}$$

$$i_2 = E/R_2 = 1.2 \text{ V}/300 \text{ }\Omega = 0.004 \text{ A, or } 4 \text{ mA} \qquad \text{(Eq. 1-14)}$$

Note that these currents add up to the i_T of 16 mA.

Most real-world circuits will be composed of combinations of series and parallel sections. These can usually be broken down and systematically analyzed to determine the desired current, voltage, or resistances. This will be illustrated by using the circuit shown in Figure 1-9. Resistors (R_3 and R_4) are in series, so their resistances add for an effective resistance of 30 Ω and the circuit can be simplified as shown in Figure

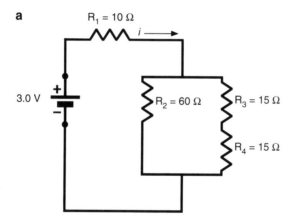

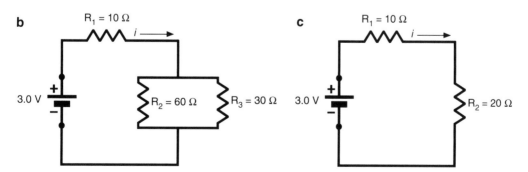

Figure 1-9. Combination series and parallel circuits. Progression from a to c illustrates the simplification of the circuit as resistances are added appropriately.

1-9a. The 60 Ω R_2 is now in parallel with the 30 Ω equivalent resistance. The effective resistance of this portion of the circuit is:

$$1/R_T = 1/60 + 1/30 = 3/60 \text{ and } R_T = 20 \ \Omega \qquad \text{(Eq. 1-15)}$$

This effective 20 Ω resistance is in series with the 10 Ω R_1. The total resistance of the circuit is $R_T = 10 \ \Omega + 20 \ \Omega = 30 \ \Omega$. The total current, i_T, would be:

$$i_T = E/R = 3 \text{ V}/30 \ \Omega = 0.1 \text{ A, or 100mA} \qquad \text{(Eq. 1-16)}$$

As i_5 also represents the total current, it would also be equal to 0.1 A. To calculate i_2 and i_3, we need to calculate the voltage drop across the parallel network portion of the circuit. The voltage drop across R_1 is:

$$\Delta E = i * R = 0.1 \text{ A} * 10 \ \Omega = 1 \text{ V} \qquad \text{(Eq. 1-17)}$$

Because the voltage at the negative terminal is 0 V, the other 2 V drop must occur across the parallel network. The current through R_2 is:

$$i_2 = E/R_2 = 2 \text{ V}/60 \ \Omega = 0.033 \text{ A, or 33 mA} \qquad \text{(Eq. 1-18)}$$

The current through R_3 and R_4 is:

$$i_3 = E/(R_3 + R_4) = 2 \text{ V}/30 \ \Omega = 0.067 \text{ A, or 67 mA} \qquad \text{(Eq. 1-19)}$$

Not all circuits will simplify to this extent, and you may not be able to rigorously analyze every portion of the circuit diagrams of your laboratory equipment; however, practice on problems of this nature helps to develop a deeper understanding of the relationship between voltage, current, and resistance.

POWER

A concept that has not been discussed yet is electrical power. *Power* is the amount of energy that is delivered or consumed per unit of time. The basic unit of energy is the joule, and the basic unit of power is the watt or joules/second. As a volt = 1 joule/coulomb and an ampere = 1 coulomb/second, we can see that a watt is also equal to:

$$\text{watt} = \frac{\text{joule}}{\text{coulomb}} \text{ (volt)} \times \frac{\text{coulomb}}{\text{second}} \text{ (amp)} = 1 \text{ volt amp} \qquad \text{(Eq. 1-20)}$$

From (Eq. 1-20) we can also see that electrical power can be calculated as:

$$P = V * i, \text{ or } P = (i * R) * i = i^2 * R \qquad \text{(Eq. 1-21)}$$

When current is forced through a resistance by a voltage, this power is dissipated in the form of heat. Resistors have varying abilities to dissipate this heat depending on their size. Resistors of the proper power capacity need to be used in the circuit depending on the anticipated current. If too much current is forced through a resistor and it exceeds its power capacity, the resistor may fail suddenly and cause damage to other parts of the circuit.

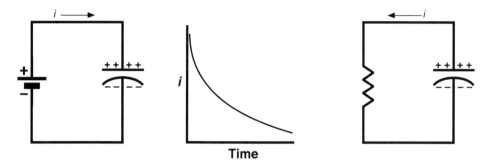

Figure 1-10. Capacitors. These figures illustrate the current profile as a capacitor charges in a dc circuit and how the stored charge can be reclaimed by removing the voltage source and providing a current path.

CAPACITORS

Capacitors are another type of component that is frequently seen in instrument circuits. They are composed of two parallel plates with nonconductive material in between. If a voltage is applied to a set of parallel plates as shown in Figure 1-10, current will begin to flow. Positive charges will accumulate on the first plate, and these will repel positive charges on the opposite plate. As positive charges accumulate on the first plate, the current will decrease as the approaching positive charges are also repelled. The buildup of positive charges on one plate and negative charges on the other develops a potential difference or voltage that is in direct opposition to the battery. As this voltage approaches the voltage of the battery, the current will drop to zero. The charges stored on the plates of the capacitors are stored electrical energy that is available for use. For example, if the battery in Figure 1-10 were replaced by a resistor, current would flow in the opposite direction until the voltage across the capacitor decreased to zero. The unit of capacitance is the farad, which is equal to 1 coulomb/volt. The farad is actually quite large, and most capacitors used in circuits would range from picofarads (10^{-12} farads) to microfarads (10^{-6} farads). In circuit diagrams, capacitors are represented by a single set of parallel lines or by a straight line and an arc. Like resistors, capacitors can have fixed capacitances or can be variable. A variable capacitor is frequently constructed with sets of parallel plates on two parallel shafts. As one of the shafts is turned, one of the sets of plates is merged with the other so that the overlapping area (and therefore the capacitance) is increased. In ac circuits, capacitors perform a variety of functions, such as tuners in radios. In dc circuits, they are used primarily to filter noise out of signals and to help to provide stable voltages from power supplies.

MEASUREMENT

A critical part of every instrument is the ability to measure currents, voltages, and resistances. The heart of most analog meters is the *d'Arsonval movement* (Fig. 1-11). This is basically a wire coil suspended in a magnetic field. When current passes

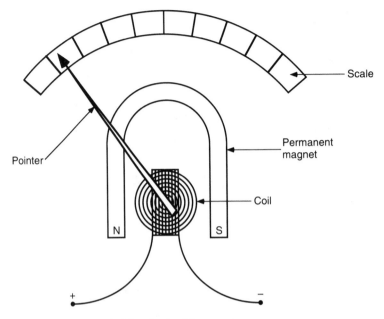

Figure 1-11.   Basic d'Arsonval meter movement.

through the coil, a magnetic field is induced in the coil. This induced field interacts with the permanent magnetic field and causes the coil to swivel on its jeweled bearings. The movement of the coil is countered by a spring. When the force of the spring equals the force generated by the induced magnetic field, the coil stops. The greater the current through the coil, the greater the induced magnetic field and the further the coil moves. When the current stops, the induced magnetic field dissipates and the spring returns the coil to its starting position. If a pointer is attached to the coil and a marked scale placed behind it, you have a basic meter.

Even through all d'Arsonval-based meters respond to and detect current, they can be used to measure current, voltage, or resistance depending on how they are connected to the circuit. If they are placed in series with the circuit as shown in Figure 1-12a, they will measure current and are called *ammeters*. When the meter is used as an ammeter, it is very important to keep the inherent internal resistance of the meter as low as possible to keep from perturbing the system during the measurement. Without the meter, the current in Figure 1-12a would be:

$$i = E/R = 10 \, V/100 \, \Omega = 0.1 \, A, \text{ or } 100 \, mA \qquad \text{(Eq. 1-22)}$$

But, when a meter with an internal resistance of 10 Ω is placed in the circuit, the total resistance changes and becomes 100 Ω. The current would then decrease to 10 V/110 Ω = 0.091 A, or 91 mA. Therefore, the current has decreased by almost 10% in our attempt to measure it. A meter with a smaller internal resistance is needed to accurately measure the current in this example.

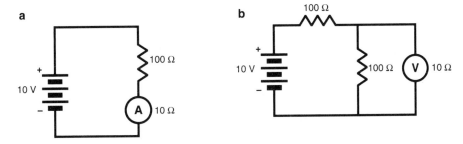

Figure 1-12. D'Arsonval meter. (a) Used an an ammeter. (b) Used as a voltmeter.

If the meter is placed in parallel with a portion of the circuit as shown in Figure 1-12b, the meter will measure the voltage drop of that portion of the circuit, and it is called a *voltmeter*. The difference in voltage between the two meter connection points causes a current to flow through the meter. The higher the voltage difference, the higher the current and the higher the meter reading. When a d'Arsonval meter is used as a voltmeter, the internal resistance should be as high as possible to avoid perturbing the circuit. Without the meter, the circuit in Fig. 1-12b would have a total resistance $R_T = 100\ \Omega + 100\ \Omega = 200\ \Omega$ and a current $i = 10\ V/200\ \Omega = 50\ mA$. The voltage drop across the resistor in question is $\Delta E = i * R = 0.05\ A * 100\ \Omega = 5\ V$. However, if the same meter from the previous circuit were used, the system would change to:

$$1/R_T = 1/100\ \Omega + 1/10\ \Omega = 1/100 + 10/100 = 11/100\ \Omega \qquad \text{(Eq. 1-23)}$$

$$R_T = 100/11 + 100 = 109\ \Omega \qquad \text{(Eq. 1-24)}$$

$$i = 10\ V/109\ \Omega = 0.092\ A, \text{ or } 92\ mA \qquad \text{(Eq. 1-25)}$$

The voltage drop across R_1 would be $100\ \Omega * 0.092\ A = 9.2\ V$. The voltage measured by the voltmeter would be the balance of the 10 V supplied by the battery, or $10\ V - 9.2\ V = 0.8\ V$. The reason that 5 V is not measured across this resistor is that 90% of the total current would actually flow through the meter and not through R_2! This is obviously highly undesirable, and a meter with much higher resistance is required. If the meter had a resistance of $10,000\ \Omega$, the situation would be much better:

$$R_T = 100\ \Omega + 10,000/101\ \Omega = 199\ \Omega \qquad \text{(Eq. 1-26)}$$

$$i = 10\ V/199\ \Omega = 50.2\ mA \qquad \text{(Eq. 1-27)}$$

And the measured voltage would be:

$$10\ V - 100 * 0.0502 = 4.98\ V \qquad \text{(Eq. 1-28)}$$

This represents a perturbation of less than 1%.

If the meter is equipped with a known voltage source and hooked up in series with an unknown resistance, it can measure resistance as $R = E/i$ and is called an *ohmmeter*. Because the meter is actually measuring current that is inversely related

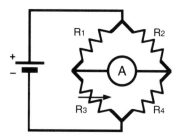

Figure 1-13. Wheatstone bridge circuit.

to resistance, the response is not linear, and the scale of the meter has to be drawn appropriately. Although it is useful for finding breaks in circuits due to blown fuses, and so on, an ohmmeter does not usually measure resistances very precisely. When very accurate and precise resistance measurement is required, a circuit called a *Wheatstone bridge* is used (Fig. 1-13). With the unknown resistance (R_x) placed as shown, the variable resistor (R_3) is adjusted until the ammeter indicates no current flow. At zero current, the potential on both sides of the ammeter must be equal, and the voltage drop to these two points must be equal:

$$i_1 * R_1 = i_2 * R_3, \text{ and } i_1 * R_2 = i_2 * R_x \qquad \text{(Eq. 1-29)}$$

$$R_x = (R_2 * R_3)/R_1 \qquad \text{(Eq. 1-30)}$$

This type of circuit is used extensively in laboratory instruments when the signal transducer produces a change in resistance in response to a change in the measured parameter.

DIODES

Up to now we have limited the discussion to components whose response to current is independent of the direction. There are many useful components where this is not the case. *Diodes* represent the simplest example of this type. Diodes and their extensions, triodes, tetrodes, and so on, were developed by using vacuum tube technology. These have been almost totally replaced by semiconductor components. However, my initial discussion will focus on vacuum tubes (Fig. 1-14), because it is conceptually easier to visualize how they work. The major parts are a heated wire, a cathode, and a plate that serves to collect electrons. Sometimes the cathode is directly heated by passing current through it and there is no need for a separate heater wire. All of the components are encased in a glass envelope that has been evacuated. This allows electron travel between the electrodes without interfering collisions with air molecules. As current is passed through the heater wire, its temperature rises and it heats the cathode. As the temperature of the cathode increases, some of its electrons pick up enough energy to escape the surface and form an electron cloud. This rise in temperature, which is required to "boil" electrons from

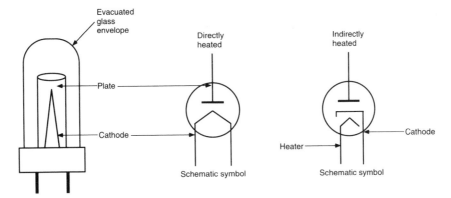

Figure 1-14. Vacuum tube diode.

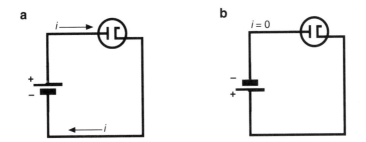

Figure 1-15. Vacuum tube diode (a) Forward biased. (b) Reverse biased.

the cathode, accounts for the warm-up time required for all tube-based equipment such as radios and TVs. In the absence of an electric field, these electrons remain in the immediate vicinity of the cathode. If the plate is placed at a higher voltage than the cathode, the negatively charged electrons will be attracted to the positively charged plate and will migrate toward it. This flow of electrons from the cathode to the plate will result in an electrical current. Because of the convention of considering current to be the flow of positive charges, conventional current will flow from the plate to the cathode. In this arrangement the diode is said to be forward biased. If the plate is placed at a voltage lower than that of the cathode, the negatively charged electrons will not migrate toward the plate and no current will flow (Fig. 1-15). In this arrangement the diode is said to be reverse biased. This property of allowing current to flow in one direction but not in the other is useful for converting ac into dc in a process called rectifying. This will be covered a little later in the chapter.

A diode can also be constructed using semiconductors. Because there is no large evacuated tube, components built from semiconductors are often referred to as *solid-state* components. Solid-state semiconductor components are constructed from crystalline silicon or germanium, both of which have four valence electrons. The conductive properties of these crystals can be enhanced by adding very small amounts of other elements. These other elements, or *doping agents,* must have chemical properties that are similar enough to the major element that it can be incorporated into the crystal lattice. If the element that is added has more valence electrons than the rest of the crystal, as in the case of arsenic, the crystal will have a relative excess of electrons and is called an n-*type semiconductor.* These "excess" electrons are relatively free to move in response to an electrical field and promote better current conduction in the semiconductor. If the doping element has fewer valence electrons than silicon or germanium, as in the case of aluminum, which has three, the crystal will have a relative deficit of electrons at the site of the doping element and is called a p-*type semiconductor.* This relative electron deficit can be thought of as a positive hole that can accept an electron from an outside source. These positive holes also promote current conduction by providing a pathway for electron flow.

A solid-state diode (Fig. 1-16) can be constructed by chemically fusing *p*-type and *n*-type semiconductor materials. If the solid-state diode is placed in a circuit with the *p*-type material at a higher voltage than the *n*-type material, it is said to be *forward biased* and current will flow (Fig. 1-17). The positive holes are repelled by the positive voltage and are attracted across the junction by the lower voltage. The excess electrons in the *n*-type material are repelled by the negative voltage and are attracted across the junction by the positive voltage. The net effect is movement of charge or current across the junction and through the diode. Conventional current will flow from the *p*- to the *n*-type material. If the diode is reversed so that the positive voltage

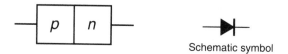

Schematic symbol

Figure 1-16.   Schematic of a solid-state diode.

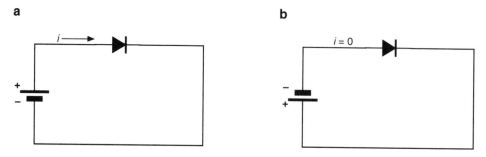

Figure 1-17.   Solid-state diode. (a) Forward biased. (b) Reverse biased.

is applied to the *n*-type material and the negative voltage is applied to the *p*-type material, the diode is *reverse biased* and no current will flow. The positive holes in the *p*-type material are attracted away from the junction toward the negative terminal. The electrons in the *n*-type material are attracted away from the junction toward the positive terminal. This separation of charge at the junction sets up an induced voltage that stops the flow of charges.

POWER SUPPLIES

Most laboratory instruments require dc to operate, but the power most readily available from wall outlets is ac. Fortunately, this ac power can be converted to dc power. Along with this conversion, the voltage also needs to be lowered from the usual 220 V or 110 V. Power supplies perform both of these functions and are a vital component of most laboratory instruments.

Dropping the voltage down to the level required is easily accomplished while the power is still in its ac state by using a *transformer.* If the ac power is directed through coils, a magnetic field will be induced in a process that is the reverse of the one used to generate the ac power. The magnetic field induced by the current in the primary coils can induce another ac electrical signal in a nearby set of secondary coils. If both sets of coils are wrapped around a metallic core, this effect is enhanced (Fig. 1-18). The number of windings in the respective coils will determine the voltage of the induced ac signal. If there are half as many windings in the secondary coils as in the

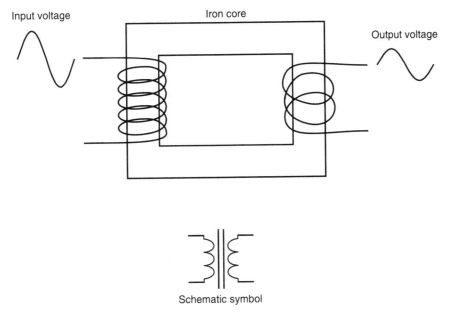

Figure 1-18. Transformer.

primary coils, the induced voltage will be half the size of the primary voltage. If there are twice as many windings, the voltage will be twice as large. Therefore, by selecting a transformer with the appropriate number of windings on the primary and secondary coils, it is possible to reduce the incoming voltage from 110 V (or 220 V) to any voltage required.

When a diode is placed in a circuit with alternating voltage and current, the diode will allow current to pass only when it is forward biased. When the voltage swings and reverse-biases the diode, the current stops. This is illustrated in Figure 1-19. This is the second step performed by a power supply, and it is called *rectification*. This signal is called half-wave rectified because only the forward biased half of the signal is passed through. If a second diode is added and a center-tapped transformer is used, the bottom half of the input signal can be flipped over and passed through (Fig. 1-20). This arrangement is much more energy efficient and makes the next step in the ac to dc conversion easier. Most power supplies use an arrangement of four diodes called a bridge rectifier (Fig. 1-21) to transform the incoming ac power. The

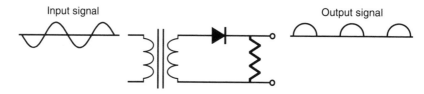

Figure 1-19. Half-wave rectifier.

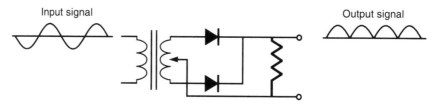

Figure 1-20. Full-wave rectifier.

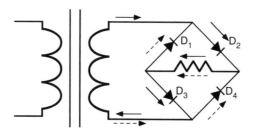

Figure 1-21. Bridge rectifier. Resistor represents the circuit using power from bridge rectifier.

instrument or circuit using this power is symbolized as a resistor in this diagram. During the positive half of the input voltage, diodes D_2 and D_3 are forward biased and current flows from right to left through the resistor representing the circuit. During the negative half of the input voltage, diodes D_4 and D_1 are forward biased and current again flows from right to left through the resistor. So, in both halves of the input signal, current flows in the same direction in our circuit. It has been full-wave rectified. Although this arrangement requires twice as many diodes, it does not require a center-tapped transformer and, because two diodes are used in series in each half, the demands on the diodes are much lower.

Once the ac voltage has been rectified, the next step is to filter the pulsating voltage so that very stable output voltage can be delivered. *Capacitors* (Fig. 1-22) fill this need very well. During the positive portion of the input voltage, current passes though the diode and charges the capacitor. As the voltage reaches the peak and then declines, the capacitor will start discharging and will attempt to make up for the declining voltage. Eventually, the capacitor will lose its charge and the voltage will start to drop. When the ac voltage swings again, the capacitor will start to charge again and the process will be repeated. The larger the capacitor, the more charge it can store and the better it is able to bridge the low-voltage periods. The demands on the capacitor are decreased when the input signal is full-wave rectified. In this case, the gaps between the voltage surges are much smaller and not as much charge is needed to bridge them. If a sufficiently large capacitor is used, essentially constant output voltage can be obtained. More efficient filtering schemes are also possible, but they are beyond the scope of this chapter.

Diodes can serve one other purpose in our power supply, that of voltage regulation. The input line voltage may vary slightly because of line surges and drops. This could have very serious consequences on the instrument fed by our power supply. The output must be stabilized or regulated to provide constant output even in the face of minor input fluctuations. One way to accomplish this is with zener diodes. Ordinarily,

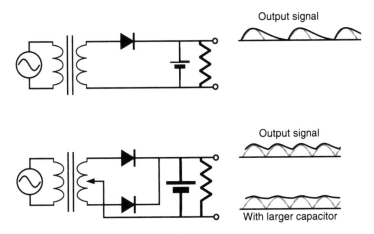

Figure 1-22. Effect of filtering capacitor on rectified ac.

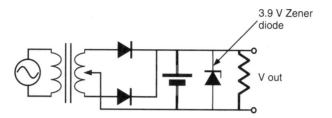

Figure 1-23. Zener diode–regulated power supply.

no current will flow through a reverse-biased diode. However, if the reverse-biasing voltage is increased, at some point the diode will break down and allow current flow. In ordinary diodes, this happens at unpredictable voltages and the diodes are permanently damaged. *Zener diodes* are specifically constructed to break down at very reproducible voltages and are not destroyed in the process. A zener diode-regulated power supply is shown in Figure 1-23. The zener diode shown has a breakdown voltage of 3.9 V. If the output from the transformer is 4.2 V, the voltage out exceeds the zener voltage and the diode will become a conductor. Because some of the current is passing through the diode, the current through the resistor decreases and the voltage out decreases. When it reaches 3.9 V, the zener diode shuts off and the voltage out is maintained at 3.9 V. If there is a surge in the input voltage, the zener diode increases the current it carries to maintain V_{out} at 3.9 V. If the input voltage decreases to the point that the voltage in the transformer decreases below 3.9 V, the zener diode will stop conducting and all of the current will pass through the resistor maximizing the output voltage. However, it will drop below 3.9 V. Therefore, zener diodes are effective at regulating output voltage as long as the input voltage exceeds their potential.

AMPLIFICATION

As mentioned in the introduction, all scientific instruments employ some type of transducer to convert a physical or chemical property into an electrical signal. Almost without exception, this electrical signal must be amplified before it can be measured and converted to an output. Transistors and vacuum tubes called triodes are common ways of accomplishing this. As in the case of vacuum tube diodes, solid-state transistors have replaced vacuum tube triodes. However, they will be used to start our discussion because they clearly illustrate the principles involved.

A *vacuum tube triode* (Fig. 1-24) is essentially a diode that has an extra grid placed between the cathode and the plate. As you will recall from our earlier discussion, electrons are emitted from the electrically heated cathode. If the plate is held at a positive voltage, these electrons will migrate toward the plate and a current will flow. If the control grid is held at a negative voltage, the electrons will be partially shielded from the positive voltage and the current will be diminished or stopped

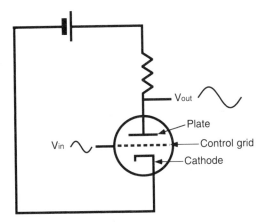

Figure 1-24. Vacuum tube triode amplifier.

depending on the size of the negative voltage applied. If the control grid is held at a slightly positive potential, the electrons are attracted toward it and end up at the plate. The control grid is actually a wire wrapped around the cathode, so the electrons have no problem getting past it to the plate when the voltage on the control grid is favorable. In use, the plate is held at a positive potential and small voltage fluctuations on the control grid produce relatively large changes in the cathode to plate electron flow (or plate-to-cathode current flow). As the plate-to-cathode current rises, the voltage drop across the resistor increases and the voltage out decreases. So, the output signal is inverted as well as amplified.

Transistors are solid-state amplifiers that work in a similar fashion. Transistors are constructed using the same *p*-type and *n*-type semiconductors used to make diodes. In a junction transistor there are two *np* junctions formed by sandwiching one type of material between two pieces of the other. Therefore, there are *pnp* and *npn junction transistors* (Fig. 1-25). The section in the middle is called the *base* and performs a function very similar to the control grid in the vacuum tube. The other two sections are called the *emitter* and the *collector* and perform functions similar to the cathode and plate in the vacuum tube. The operation of this type of transistor can be explained by examination of the circuit in Figure 1-25. The emitter-base *pn* junction is forward biased as the *p*-type material is connected to the positive terminal and the *n*-type material is connected to the negative terminal. This positive bias allows conventional current flow from the emitter toward the base. Because the base layer is very thin (approximately 0.001 inches), most of the charge carriers pass through this region. Once through the base they will see the even more negative collector and move toward it, giving rise to an emitter-collector current. A *npn* junction transistor operates in a similar fashion except it is helpful to think in terms of electron flow. In order for the emitter-base *np* junction to be forward biased, the base must be more

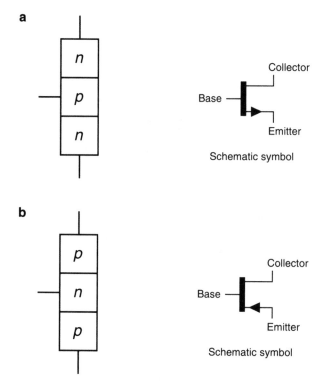

Figure 1-25. Junction transistors.

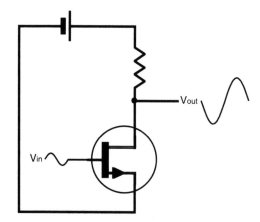

Figure 1-26. Junction transistor amplifier.

positive than the emitter. The electrons are attracted from the emitter to the base. Most of them overshoot the thin base section and are attracted to the even more positive collector, giving rise to an emitter-to-collector flow of electrons or a collector-to-emitter conventional current. In either case the direction of the arrow in the schematic symbol shows the direction of conventional (positive) current. Figure 1-26 shows the transistor equivalent circuit of the vacuum tube amplifier circuit shown in Figure 1-24. Small fluctuations in the base voltage produce relatively large changes in collector-to-emitter currents. Large currents produce large iR drops in the resistor and result in low output voltages. Therefore, this circuit also inverts the signal as it amplifies it. Amplifier circuits can and do get much more complicated than that shown in Figures 1-24 and 1-26; however, the principles remain the same.

INTERGRATED CIRCUITS

The trend since the 1970s has been to incorporate more and more transistors in sophisticated circuits on a single silicon chip. These *integrated circuits* in the form of a single chip or component are able to carry out complex functions that required entire circuit boards in the past. The *operational amplifier,* or op amp, is a good example of this. Op amps are full multistage amplifiers integrated into a single silicon chip and are widely used in scientific equipment. A typical op amp circuit is shown in Figure 1-27. A simple triangle is used to represent the op amp rather than draw all of the individual transistors that comprise it. The points marked with the $-$ and $+$ are the inverting and noninverting inputs, and the point on the right is the output. In this type of circuit the op amp will produce a voltage output that is sufficient to keep the input current at the inverting input equal to zero. The input current through R_1 is:

$$V = i * R_1, \text{ or } i = V/R_1 \tag{Eq. 1-31}$$

The output current has to be equal in magnitude and opposite in sign:

$$-V_0/R_2 = V_i/R_1, \text{ or } V_0 = -V_i(R_2/R_1) \tag{Eq. 1-32}$$

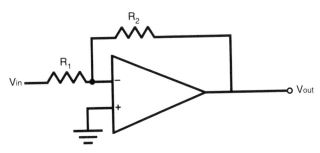

Figure 1-27.   Operational amplifier circuit.

Thus, the gain of this amplifier is easily controlled by varying the size of the resistor in the feedback loop. If this resistor (R_2) is increased at the same input voltage, the output voltage must increase proportionately in order to keep the input current equal to zero.

If the resistor in the feedback circuit is replaced by a capacitor, the circuit will become an *integrator*. If a constant voltage is applied to the inverting input, constantly increasing voltage must be produced at the output to continue to cause current to pass through the capacitor and neutralize the incoming current. If the incoming voltage were to decrease to zero, the output voltage could stop rising but would remain constant in order to keep the capacitor charged. This type of circuit is very useful as an electronic integrator. Many other useful circuits can be built using op amps as the fundamental component, and they are frequently seen in the circuit diagrams of electronic instruments.

SIGNAL TRANSDUCERS

All electronic instruments need a *transducer* to convert the physical or chemical property that the instrument measures into a measurable electrical signal. These can take a wide variety of shapes and sizes. We will discuss a few briefly to illustrate the points presented so far.

Many instruments rely on the measurement of the optical properties of a sample to perform this function. All of these instruments require a transducer to convert radiant light energy to an electrical signal. Phototubes (Fig. 1-28a) and photomultipliers (Fig. 1-28b) are common ways of accomplishing this. Both of these start with a photocathode coated with a photoemissive material. As photons strike this material, atoms absorb enough energy to eject an electron. If a positive electrical potential is applied to a collecting anode, these ejected electrons will migrate toward it, giving rise to a photocurrent. The entire process takes place in an evacuated tube so that collisions with air molecules do not interfere with the electron's migration. The resultant current will be small but proportional to the amount of light striking the photocathode.

The photomultiplier amplifies this photocurrent through a series of dynodes (Fig. 1-28b). A very large voltage difference is maintained between the photocathode and the terminal collecting anode. This can be as high as several hundred volts. A voltage divider network breaks this voltage into a series of smaller steps. The first dynode is physically arranged so that the electrons emitted in response to the absorbed photon are accelerated toward it by its positive potential relative to the photocathode. By the time the electrons reach it, they have picked up enough energy so that their impact on the dynode surface ejects several electrons for every electron striking the surface. The ejected electrons from the first dynode are accelerated toward the second dynode by its more positive potential. Once again, multiple electrons are ejected for every incident electron. This process is repeated through each successive dynode until the electrons finally arrive at the anode where the current is measured. The amplification through this cascade of electrons through the dynode chain can be as high as 10^6. A very similar process is used in the electron

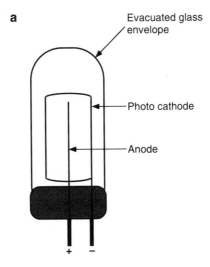

a

Evacuated glass
envelope

Photo cathode

Anode

+   −

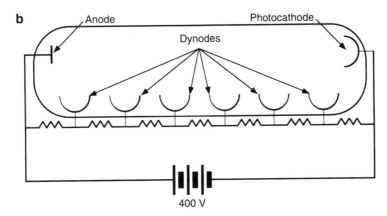

b

Anode

Photocathode

Dynodes

400 V

Figure 1-28.   (a) Phototube. (b) Photomultiplier tube.

multiplier detector in a mass spectrometer. In this transducer, the collision of a charged ion with the cathode starts the electron cascade down the dynode chain.

The basics of the circuit used in the first Coulter® (Coulter Corp., Hialeah, FL 33012) *cell counter* is shown in Figure 1-29. The cell counter is a transducer that converts number of cells to current spikes and cell size to drop in current. An applied potential between two plates causes a current to flow between them that is proportional to the resistance of the solution in accordance with Ohm's law. The solution connecting the two electrodes is forced to go through a very small constriction. If a particle such as a cell passes through this constriction, some of the surrounding electrolyte will be excluded and the resistance between the two electrodes will increase. The electrodes will sense this as a momentary decrease in the current. The

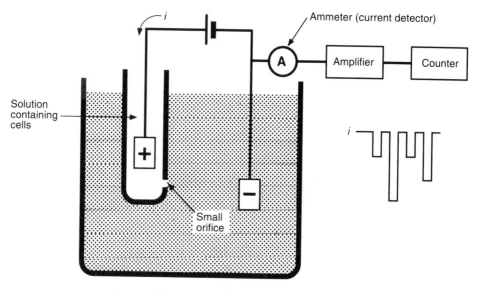

Figure 1-29.   Simplified diagram of cell counter.

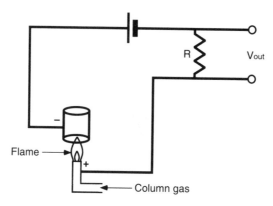

Figure 1-30.   Simplified schematic of flame ionization detector.

size of the decrease will be proportional to the size of the particle passing through the constriction. In a sufficiently dilute solution, the individual cells can be counted and sized by counting the negative current spikes and measuring their intensity. Chapter 20 also discusses cell counting.

A *flame ionization detector* in a gas chromatograph is shown schematically in Figure 1-30. The detector converts ion charges to an electric current. An electrical potential is maintained between two electrodes in close proximity to a flame at the end of a chromatographic column. As carbon- and hydrogen-containing materials elute from the column and are burned in the flame, ions are formed. These ions are collected at the electrodes and give rise to a small current. This current must be amplified many times before it can be measured and converted to an output. Gas chromatographs and their detectors are discussed in Chapter 15.

DIGITAL ELECTRONICS

In most electronic instruments today, there is a trend toward *digital electronics*. This is essential if the instrument is going to be controlled by an on-board digital computer or communicate with an outside laboratory computer. Digital electronics involves only two discrete signal levels that can be called 0 and 1, true and false, or on and off. Each binary digit that can be in one of the two states is called a bit. If more than two states need to be represented, additional bits are required. Each additional bit doubles the number that can be represented. For example, with one bit, only two different states can be represented: 0 and 1. With an additional bit, four combinations are possible: 00, 01, 10, and 11. This progression can be continued until enough bits are present to represent the desired number. It should be obvious from this discussion that more binary digits are required to represent a number than its decimal equivalent. However, the electrical demands of working with binary numbers are less because minor fluctuations around the voltages chosen to represent the two different states can be ignored. For example, if $+5$ V were selected to represent 1 and 0 V were selected to represent 0, even voltage variations of 1 V would not cause any confusion about the state of any selected bit as it is still easy to differentiate between 4 V and 1 V. However, if that same 0 to 5 V spread were divided into 10 equal segments of 0.5 V each, that same 1 V of noise would represent 2 units of uncertainty. This is one of the reasons that the somewhat foreign binary system was selected for digital electronics.

Digital circuits are ideally suited for counting and performing additions; however, we exist in an analog world where the quantities we want to measure do not always occur at discrete levels but cover a continuum. Therefore, we need a mechanism to make the transition from analog to digital and from digital to analog. Analog to digital (A/D) converters and digital to analog (D/A) converters provide these translations, which can be accomplished by a variety of methods and are usually integrated into a single component. One common method of converting an analog voltage into a digital signal is to first convert the voltage to a frequency and then count the number of pulses in a given time period. Digital numbers can be converted to an analog voltage by applying a standard voltage through a network of resistors that scales the voltage appropriately. The scaled voltage from each bit of the digital number is summed to an output voltage. The resultant analog voltage can then be used to control a function of the instrument.

Safety

Maintaining a safe work environment is a vital concern in the design and maintenance of clinical laboratory equipment. It is mostly achieved through adequate grounding. Good safety practices as well as federal regulatory bodies require that all instruments with exposed metal in their cases have their cases electrically connected to earth ground. If adhered to, this requirement will ensure that the instrument case (the part the operator is most likely to touch) is not at a significantly different voltage than the rest of the surroundings. It is not sufficient to simply isolate the case from the rest of the circuitry and assume that no voltages have been applied to the case. During use or movement of the instrument, a wire could come in contact with the case and expose the operator to a dangerous situation. If the case is properly grounded and a wire carrying an unsafe potential comes in contact with the case, the direct connection with ground will burn out a fuse in a properly protected circuit. If the instrument is not adequately protected by fuses, one or more components of the instrument might be damaged. But this is far better than the loss of life that might result if the case were not grounded. Even if an instrument was properly grounded at installation, it should be checked periodically because grounding wires may become corroded and break during use.

During the design process it is possible to predict the maximum current that will flow through the circuit under normal operating conditions. Power line surges or unexpected, catastrophic electrical component failure may cause currents higher than normal. Such increases may put other electrical components at risk of failure. To guard against this, properly designed circuits incorporate fuses at key locations throughout an instrument's circuits. Fuses are nothing more than special conductors with well-defined current-carrying capacities. When these currents are exceeded, the fuse "blows" or "burns out," the electrical connection is broken, and the current stops. Fuses are frequently made from thin wires of low melting-point metals such as lead. These wires are usually enclosed in a glass envelope for mechanical stability. Some circuits have higher current demands during startup and shutdown than during routine operation. Rather than increase the size of the fuse to handle these peak loads and put the rest of the circuit at risk during steady-state operation, vendors will frequently incorporate a fuse that can tolerate short-duration current surges above their rated capacity. These "slow blow" fuses are commonly used in circuits containing large electrical motors.

When a fuse burns out in an instrument, it means that the current at that point exceeded the predicted operating specifications. The burned-out fuse is generally a symptom of the problem, not its cause. Under no circumstances should a fuse with a higher current rating be substituted to cover the symptom of a fuse that repeatedly burns out.

Summary

This chapter explained the principles of electricity and electronics. Electricity is the movement of charged particles, usually electrons. Charge is measured in coulombs, the rate of charge flow is measured in amperes, resistance to charge flow is measured in ohms, and electrochemical potential is measured in volts.

Ohm's law describes the relationship among voltage, current, and resistance. Application of Ohm's law and the rules for calculating resistances in parallel and series circuits allow calculation of unknown current, resistance, or voltage. This is the basis of potentiometers, ohmmeters, and voltmeters.

Most laboratory instruments and computers require direct current. Diodes allow current to flow in only one direction and are often used to convert alternating current to direct current. Triodes and transistors are used to amplify weak electrical signals (such as those from photodetectors).

Transducers convert one type of energy into another. Many laboratory instruments contain photomultiplier tubes that convert light to electricity. Other detectors convert cell size or number of ions to electricity. Piezoelectric crystals convert pressure to electricity. Microphones convert sound to electricity.

Integrated circuits condense the electronics from numerous vacuum tubes or transistors to small silicon chips. Thousands of circuits can be etched onto a 1 cm^2 chip. Integrated circuits are present in all microcomputers and in many laboratory instruments.

Most electrical equipment in the laboratory can be dangerous if not handled safely. Safety is achieved by understanding hazards, inspecting equipment periodically, and following procedures for dealing with accidents or unusual situations.

Questions and Problems

1. For the following circuit, calculate

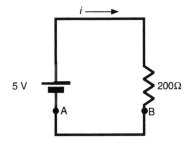

   a.   The current i
   b.   The difference in potential between point A and point B
2. For the following circuit, calculate

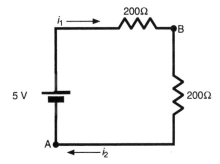

   a.   The total resistance
   b.   The current i_1

    c. The current i_2
    d. The potential at point B
3. Explain the principle of a photomultiplier tube.
4. Find the total resistance in the following circuit

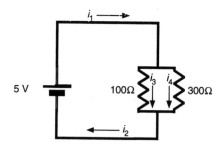

5. What is the total current in the circuit in Question #4?
6. List two important safety practices for electrical equipment

Suggested Readings

Skoog DA, Leary JJ. Principles of instrumental analysis, 4th ed. Fort Worth: Saunders College Publisher: 1992:10-45.

Willard HH, Merritt LL Jr, Dean JA, Settle FA Jr. Instrumental methods of analysis, 7th ed. Belmont, CA: Wadsworth Publishing, 1988:40-49.

2

CENTRIFUGES
Gene d'Allemand

Objectives

After completing this chapter, the reader will be able to:

1. Understand the terminology associated with the use of a centrifuge in the clinical laboratory.
2. Describe the components of a general-purpose centrifuge, and list how they affect the operation of the instrument.
3. Given variables of centrifugal speed, time, radius, or force; identify and calculate centrifugation parameters.
4. Construct and apply the procedures necessary for safe, efficient operation and proper maintenance of a centrifuge.

Definitions

Adapters: Inserts used in large shields or cups to allow the use of smaller glassware, giving the original shield or cup added versatility.

Angle Head: Another term for fixed-angle rotor.

Brushes: The graphite plates that serve as the conductor between the electrical circuit and the commutator in a centrifuge motor.

Centrifuge: A device used to apply a centrifugal force for separating substances differing significantly in their masses.

Centrifugal Force: The force that impels matter outward from a center of rotation. It depends on three variables: mass, speed, and radius. In the clinical laboratory, work usually involves aqueous solutions with a specific gravity of near 1.000; therefore, mass is not considered in calculations.

Commutator: The revolving part that collects current from the brushes in a centrifuge motor.

Cushions: Pads, usually rubber, positioned at the bottom cavity of shields, cups, or adapters. They distribute the effects of centrifugal force over a greater area and thus reduce glassware breakage.

Fixed-Angle Rotor: A rotor with drilled holes that support tubes at a fixed angle, usually 25 to 52°.

Gravity: The unit of measure for the rate of acceleration of gravity, equal to 9807 mm/s²; abbreviated *g*. For reference, the earth's force is expressed as $1 \times g$.

Horizontal Rotor: A rotor that allows tubes to swing from a vertical to a horizontal position when subjected to centrifugation; also called the horizontal head.

Relative Centrifugal Force (RCF):   A method of comparing the forces generated by various centrifuges, considering the speed of rotation and the radius of rotation. Relative centrifugal force is calculated according to the formula:[1]

$$RCF = 1.12 \times 10^{-5} (r) (rpm)^2 \qquad \text{(Eq. 2-1)}$$

where r = the radius in centimeters, rpm = the number of revolutions per minute, and 1.12×10^{-5} is a constant calculated from angular velocity. The radius is measured from the center of rotation to the bottom of the tube when measuring maximum RCF. Relative centrifugal force is expressed as some number times gravity.

Revolutions per Minute (rpm):   A unit expressing the number of complete rotations per minute in time; a measure of speed.

Rotor: The device used to hold the shields, cups, and tubes.

Shields, Cups, and Carriers: Containers used to hold the various sizes of glassware.

Stroboscope: A tachometer instrument for measuring the speed of rotation by matching rotation with the frequency of flashing light.

Swinging Bucket: Another term for horizontal rotor.

Trunnion Carrier: A metal carrier that holds tubes upright for filling and balancing before centrifugation. It can act as a stand for the tubes after processing.

Ultracentrifuge: A very high-speed centrifuge capable of obtaining extremely high RCF values.

Introduction

Centrifuges are instruments designed to accelerate the sedimentation process by applying centrifugal force. Various types of centrifuges are used in the clinical laboratory for separating suspended particles from a liquid in which the particles are not soluble. Liquids of differing specific gravity (density) also may be separated.

There are three general types of centrifuges: the horizontal-rotor, the fixed-angle rotor, and the ultracentrifuge. Many variations of horizontal- and fixed-angle rotor centrifuges are found in the clinical laboratory. These include benchtop and floor-standing units, high-speed units, and refrigerated units. Special-purpose instruments include microhematocrit, cell washer, and cytocentrifuge systems.

Principles

In the clinical laboratory, the centrifuge usually functions as a filtration or packing device. In clinical and research laboratories, the development of large-batch centrifuges that can sediment a precipitate from a solution in a short time have mostly replaced the tedious process of filtration. This development has sped up the process of separation and, when coupled with refrigeration, has also reduced sample lability to a minimum.

Usual applications include the separation of serum or plasma from red blood cells, the separation of precipitated solids from the liquid phase of a mixture, or the separation of liquids of varying density. Special-purpose units include such applications as quantitative red blood cell packing for measuring hematocrit, automatic cell washing and component preparation for immunohematology, and monolayer cell preparations for cytology. Ultracentrifuges employ very high speed and force to achieve difficult and precise quantitative separations of ultrasmall particles or macromolecules.

The *horizontal-rotor centrifuge* shields or cups are in a vertical position when the centrifuge is at rest and assume a horizontal position when the centrifuge is operating. The horizontal rotor will operate at speeds to about 3000 revolutions per minute (rpm). Because of excess heat developed by air friction, higher speeds cannot be practically attained without wind shielding. Depending upon the radius of the rotor, these units attain forces of approximately $1650 \times g$.

The *fixed-angle rotor centrifuge* shields or cups are positioned rigidly at a fixed angle, usually 25 to 52°, to the shaft around which they rotate. Angle-rotor units may attain much higher speeds because of the aerodynamic construction of the rotor. The cups of the fixed-angle rotor are enclosed by a metal case that reduces wind resistance, lowering the sample temperature increase commonly exhibited by the horizontal-rotor centrifuge. The fixed-angle units can reach speeds of about 7000 rpm and exhibit forces of over $9000 \times g$.

In the horizontal-rotor centrifuge, the particles being sedimented travel at a right angle to the shaft and the length of the column of liquid where they are distributed uniformly against the bottom of the tube. The surface of the formed sediment pellet is flat and remains so when the rotor stops and the tube assumes a vertical position. In the fixed-angle rotor centrifuge, the particles have a shorter distance to travel; that is, across the column of liquid to the side of the container. The particles pack against the side and bottom of the tube, leaving the surface sediment parallel to the shaft of the centrifuge. As a fixed-angle rotor slows and stops, gravity causes the sediment to slide down the tube leaving a somewhat poorly packed pellet. Because sedimentation of large particles (such as separation of erythrocytes from plasma) is efficient at low force, 1000 to $1200 \times g$, and because a flat sediment pellet is produced, the horizontal-rotor centrifuge offers some advantages for the clinical laboratory.

High-speed microcentrifuges are common in many laboratories. These units incorporate either a fixed-angle or horizontal rotor with a small radius. With sample volumes of 2 to 3 ml, they can achieve speeds of 15,000 to 20,000 rpm and forces around $15,000 \times g$. The StatSpin® (StatSpin Technologies, Norwood, MA 02062-4327) group of centrifuges incorporates a proprietary drive system allowing use of a variety of small self-balancing rotors with virtually no wind resistance and very quiet operation; included are disposable rotors. There are several special sample collection and preparation tubes available that facilitate use of the various rotors. The StatSpin® is employed for, among other things, very rapid separations for plasma and urine and microhematocrit determination.

Refrigerated centrifuges are available in both bench-type and floor models. They have internal refrigeration systems capable of maintaining temperatures ranging from −15 to 25°C during centrifugation; they may incorporate either fixed-angle or horizontal rotors. Refrigeration permits separation at higher speeds by protecting samples from the heat generated during the centrifugation process.

Centrifuges capable of producing speeds of 100,000 rpm with *relative centrifugal force* (RCF) values of 600,000 × *g* are called *ultracentrifuges*. Most are fixed-angle models, although occasionally horizontal rotors are used in these instruments. In addition, some have vertical rotors where the axis of the tubes is fixed parallel to the rotor's axis of rotation. Even with the high forces produced, several hours or even days are often required to achieve complex separations under controlled temperatures. Centrifugation techniques using the ultracentrifuge include differential, rate zonal, and isopyknic separations. Differential centrifugation separates particles from a mixture by sedimenting those of larger mass to the bottom, leaving a portion of the small particles in the supernatant. The rate zonal technique separates particles based on differences in sedimentation rate in a density gradient, such as sucrose. The isopyknic technique separates particles based on differences in density (composition) in a density gradient, such as cesium chloride. The large ultracentrifuge is significantly more complex than general laboratory centrifuges and has not found widespread use in the clinical laboratory. The information presented under components, operation, and maintenance does not strictly apply to the ultracentrifuge.

One variation of the ultracentrifuge used in the clinical laboratory is the *Airfuge®* (Beckman Instruments, Brea, CA 92621). This instrument is a miniature ultracentrifuge that uses a small turbine rotor driven by air pressure. It can achieve speeds of 95,000 rpm and forces of 178,000 × *g*. The rotor spins nearly friction-free on a cushion of air; temperature can be controlled by the temperature of the drive air. There are a variety of rotors available. General applications include receptor assays, protein fractionation, and drug-binding assays. The most common clinical laboratory application is the clarification of lipemic sera.[2]

Selecting a centrifuge for the laboratory should involve a careful review of several factors. The number and volume of samples being separated during a run and at what RCF value are central to the choice. Other considerations include size, noise level, timing and refrigeration needs, frequency of use, maintenance requirements, and rotor versatility. By consulting the manufacturer's literature, you can usually find a wide variety of rotors, adapters, and other accessories to increase the versatility of a particular centrifuge model.

Components

Knowledge of basic operating principles and components is important for establishing and performing proper maintenance on the centrifuge. The parts of a common centrifuge include the chamber, which encloses the internal parts, a cover with latch, the centrifuge rotor with shields or cups, and the motor-drive assembly. Most centrifuges include a power switch, a braking device, a speed control, a timer, and possibly a tachometer. Some centrifuges include a protective shield to minimize aerosol production.

Centrifuge motors are generally high-torque series-wound dc motors; they turn faster as voltage is increased. Alternating current (ac) motors, where speed adjustment is achieved through stepwise reduction of the number of poles in the magnetic field, are usually found in smaller centrifuges. Diodes and capacitors are used to rectify ac. The rotor shaft is driven directly or through a gyro; occasionally, a pulley system is used.

In centrifuge motors, electrical contact to the commutator is provided by graphite brushes; they gradually wear down as they press against the commutator turning at high speed. If the graphite is allowed to wear away completely, the retainer spring of the brush will contact the smooth surface of the commutator and will cut grooves or scratches in its surface. A rough commutator surface will cause rapid wear of new brushes. The graphite that is worn away may deposit around the contacts, causing arcing and burning, both of which decrease the efficiency of the motor and may damage it; in extreme cases, a fire may start in the motor.

The shaft of the motor turns through sleeve bearings located at the top and bottom of the motor. Most units contain sealed bearings that are permanently lubricated; others require periodic application of oil or grease. Many centrifuges contain an internal imbalance switch that turns the unit off before vibrations from load imbalance can damage bearings on the drive shaft.

The speed of the centrifuge is controlled by a potentiometer that raises and lowers the voltage supplied to the motor. The calibrations furnished on the speed control of a centrifuge are often only relative voltage increments and should never be taken as accurate indicators of speed. Because speed depends on voltage in most centrifuges, as resistance is increased, speed is lost. Sources of resistance, in addition to electrical inefficiency, include air resistance and turbulence, brush friction, and worn bearings. Those resistances can cause a centrifuge to operate at differing speeds on the same speed-control setting. Different accessories, loads, and varying states of repair also result in speed-control problems. Calibration and periodic recalibration of centrifuge speed is extremely important.

Most modern centrifuges have an interlocking safety latch that prevents the lid from being opened while the rotor is in motion. Operating a centrifuge with the lid raised is dangerous and must be avoided. In addition to being hazardous and reducing the centrifuge's speed through increased air resistance, it also causes the revolving parts of the centrifuge to vibrate. Vibrations cause extensive wear on the centrifuge and mixing of the sedimented particles.

As a centrifuge operates, it generates heat. The rise in temperature depends on ambient temperature, rotor design and speed, and the duration of centrifugation process. When samples being centrifuged are temperature labile, a refrigerated centrifuge should be used.

Tachometers are provided on many centrifuges, and they indicate the speed in rpm. With mechanical tachometers, a flexible shaft or cable attached to the motor spindle turns inside a flexible housing and is attached to a meter movement at the other end. As the cable turns, it causes the needle to move upscale. Modern centrifuges use electronic tachometers in which a magnet rotates around a coil, producing a current that may be measured. If a tachometer is not attached to the centrifuge, a stroboscope or an electronic meter can be used to determine the actual rpm at each centrifuge setting. For any given setting, the speed of the centrifuge will vary with the specimen load. The rpm determined at each centrifuge setting should be recorded and attached to the centrifuge for easy reference.

The rpm value is only one factor involved in determining centrifugal force. The true efficiency of a particular centrifuge is expressed in RCF, some number times gravity. The RCF value is calculated from the experimentally determined rpm and the radius of the rotor plus carrier (see formula under Definitions). The RCF value also can be obtained from a nomogram (Fig. 2-1). To determine the RCF value from the nomogram,[3] find the known rotating radius on the left and the known rpm on the far right graph; use a straightedge ruler to connect the two. The point at which the ruler intersects the middle graph is the RCF value. Most manufacturers include a nomogram in the instruction manual accompanying the centrifuge.

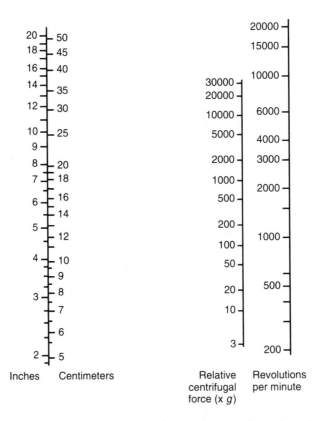

Figure 2-1.   Nomogram for determining relative centrifugal force, RCF $\times$ *g*.

The term *rpm,* when applied to a centrifuge, does not indicate the force applied to samples in the centrifuge. Comparisons made between centrifuges must be in terms of RCF. When a RCF value specified in a procedure cannot be achieved on a particular centrifuge, it is possible to adjust the length of time the samples are centrifuged to achieve equivalent centrifugal force. Time required would be calculated as follows:

$$T = \frac{T_S \times RCF_S}{RCF}$$ (Eq. 2-2)

where

T = run time needed
T_S = run time specified in a procedure
RCF = RCF obtainable
RCF_S = RCF specified in a procedure

A timer device is commonly employed in many centrifuges. Some are spring-driven clock mechanisms that turn the unit off after a preset time cycle. Others are electronic timers that perform the same function. Many units have switches that allow the units to be operated continuously without using the timer device.

Braking devices are incorporated to provide rapid deceleration of the rotor. Two general types of brake mechanisms are found on centrifuges. One type is mechanical and functions by physically applying pressure to the rotor when a lever is pressed. The other type, found on most units, is electrical and functions by reversing the polarity of the electrical current to the motor.

Maintenance and Quality Assurance

Daily inspection, periodic function verification, and proper preventive maintenance are vital to the efficiency and longevity of the centrifuge. A regular schedule for function checks must be established and followed to ensure proper operation of the instrument. Always consult the manufacturer's instruction manual for specific operating and maintenance procedures.

DAILY OPERATION

Daily operation includes observation and inspection of the following:

1. The centrifuge should not be on the same electrical circuit as sensitive electronic measuring devices (such as spectrophotometers) because of the generation of electrical noise and high-current drain at startup. The unit should not be operated near combustible fluids, because sparking brushes could cause ignition.
2. Check the cleanliness of the chamber, and immediately clean up all spills. Be aware of biohazardous materials (microbiologic, radioactive, chemical) that require specific decontamination procedures. Observe for gray or black dust buildup within the chamber; this can be a sign of sandblasting of the rotor

chamber caused by glass particles and must be removed. Refrigerated units require periodic defrosting.

3. Use the correct tube sizes and types for the particular centrifuge, and use only tubes rated to withstand the RCF value to which the tube is likely to be subjected.
4. Always balance the load of the centrifuge before operating. The load must be balanced both by equal mass and by centers of gravity across the center of rotation. Do not run the centrifuge with buckets, carriers, or shields missing from the unit.
5. Centrifuge only sealed or stoppered tubes if possible; this is particularly important when centrifuging body fluids or other potentially hazardous materials.
6. Always keep the cover closed when the unit is operating. This will help to prevent dangerous aerosolizing of biohazardous materials and scattering of physically dangerous particles into the environment.
7. Observe for unusual noises or vibrations during operation. Do not operate a centrifuge in excess of the manufacturer's recommended maximum speed for the rotor in use. At low speeds, vibration occurs naturally during acceleration and deceleration. This speed range, known as the critical speed of the rotor, and is usually 500 to 1000 rpm for most centrifuges. Avoid prolonged operation at the critical speed.
8. Use the braking device with caution; braking may cause some resuspension of the sediment. Never open the chamber until the rotor has come to a complete stop.

FUNCTION VERIFICATION

The frequency of function verification procedures should be appropriate for the application of the centrifuge. It is recommended that such procedures be performed at 3-month intervals, with more frequent checks on systems that have critical application. Checks performed and resulting data should be recorded so that the information is readily available for the operator. Correction factors for speed, timing, or temperature should be posted on the system.

Tolerance limits for function checks should be established. The limits set will depend on the application of the centrifuge. Include information for corrective action should checks exceed tolerance limits.

Function verification procedures should include the following:

1. *rpm calibration.* The *best* way to check the function of a centrifuge is to check its speed. Depending on how the unit is equipped, both the speed control and built-in tachometer should be checked with an external device. This may be accomplished with either a stroboscope or a mechanical or electronic tachometer of good accuracy. Several speeds regularly used on the unit should be checked. Values obtained with the external measuring device should agree within 5% of those from a built-in tachometer. Centrifuges that cannot be checked for speed without opening the chamber lid should only be tested by factory-trained personnel.
2. *Timer.* The timer should be set for common intervals and these intervals checked

against an accurate timing device. The timing interval includes the period of acceleration and spin, but not the brake or stopping time. General laboratory centrifuges should be accurate to 10% of the timed interval.

3. *Temperature.* The thermometer on refrigerated units should be checked against a certified thermometer, and a correction factor derived if necessary.

PREVENTIVE MAINTENANCE

Preventive maintenance should be performed on the same time schedule as function verification procedures. Preventive maintenance should be documented and include the following:

1. *Lubrication.* Depending on the type of centrifuge, bearings on the upper and lower end of the motor shaft may be permanently lubricated or sealed; if they are not sealed, follow the manufacturer's instructions for lubrication. Bearing wear may be checked by determining the amount of side play in the shaft.

2. *Motor components.* Brushes should be removed and checked for wear. Replacement is recommended if they are worn to more than one-half their original length. When reinserting used brushes, replace them in the same orientation and be certain that spring tension is adequate to maintain good contact with the commutator. New brushes should be broken in by slowly accelerating the unloaded unit to midspeed and then allowing it to operate this way for a period of time. The condition of the commutator should be examined. To avoid electrical arcing, the commutator and brush holders must be free of dirt, oil, and dust. Severe arcing of new brushes can be a sign of a bad commutator. If the commutator is scratched or scored, it will have to be removed and machined smooth by lathe or replaced. On refrigerated centrifuges, the manufacturer's instruction manual should be consulted for maintenance procedures on the refrigeration system.

3. *Electrical integrity.* Both grounding resistance and current leaking should be checked periodically. The fuse should be checked for proper rating; if the unit has a circuit breaker, it should be checked for proper operation. In addition, the line cord, plug, lamps, and wiring should be examined for defects.

4. *Mechanical integrity.* If the unit has a safety interlock, this device should be checked for proper working order. Gaskets, latches, hinges, and control knobs should be examined to determine that all are functioning and in good condition. The rotor and shields or carriers should be examined for signs of mechanical stress (cracks, corrosion) and for cleanliness and balance.

Summary

Centrifuges are widely used in the clinical laboratory to separate whole blood into cellular components and serum or plasma, to sediment, to precipitate, and to separate liquids of varying densities.

The component parts of a centrifuge are: a closed chamber that houses the rotor, shields (or cups), and samples; a motor for providing power; graphite brushes for providing electrical contact to the commutator; a potentiometer for controlling centrifugation speed; a power switch; a braking device; and a timer. When biological samples are separated, a protective shield should cover the sample to minimize aerosol production. A safety latch to keep the chamber locked while the centrifuge is spinning is another important safety feature.

The force applied to samples in the centrifuge is determined by a formula that includes rpm, as well as the radius of the sample from the shaft on which the rotor spins.

Proper maintenance of a centrifuge includes cleaning up spills immediately, balancing the sample load, centrifuging sealed or covered specimens, keeping the lid closed, checking the brushes periodically for wear, lubricating the bearings on the motor shaft if they are not permanently lubricated and sealed, and checking grounding resistance and current leakage.

Questions and Problems

1. What RCF would result from centrifuging a sample at 2500 rpm, assuming the centrifuge had a rotating radius of 20 cm?
2. A procedure calls for a 10-minute centrifugation at $1500 \times g$ in a centrifuge with a rotating radius of 25 cm. What speed setting should be used to achieve this force?
3. A procedure calls for 8 minutes of centrifugation at $3000 \times g$. What time length would be required to achieve equivalent force using a centrifuge that can achieve a maximum force of $2400 \times g$?
4. A procedure statement calls for centrifuging a sample for 10 minutes at 2500 rpm. What is wrong with the statement?

References

1. Bermes EW Jr, Young DS. General laboratory techniques and procedures. In: Tietz NW, ed. Textbook of clinical chemistry. Philadelphia: WB Saunders, 1986:25-62.
2. Creer M, Ladenson J. Analytical errors due to lipemia. Lab Med 1983, 14:351-55.
3. Lee LW, Schmidt DA. Elementary principles of laboratory instruments, 5th ed. St. Louis: CV Mosby, 1983:301.

Suggested Readings

A centrifuge primer. Palo Alto, CA: Beckman Instruments, Spinco Division, 1980.

Bishop ML, Duben-Von Laufen JL, Fody EP. Clinical chemistry principles, procedures, correlations. Philadelphia: JB Lippincott, 1985.

Kaplan LA, Pesce AP. Clinical chemistry theory, analysis, and correlation, 2nd ed. St. Louis: CV Mosby, 1989.

Laboratory instrument maintenance and function verification. Chicago: College of American Pathologists, 1982.

Strickland RD. Centrifuges and centrifugation. In: Werner M, ed. CRC Handbook of clinical chemistry, Vol. 1. Boca Raton: CRC Press, 1982.

3

ANALYTICAL BALANCES

Judith A. Thompson
Mary C. Haven

Objectives

After completing this chapter, the reader will be able to:

1. Explain the differences between mechanical balances and electronic balances.
2. Calculate the sensitivity of an analytical balance.
3. Demonstrate how to determine the accuracy of an analytical balance.
4. Design a preventive maintenance schedule for an electronic balance.
5. Discuss environmental considerations for the location of an analytical balance.

Definitions and Abbreviations

Accuracy: The agreement between the measured weight and the calibrated weight of an object. It depends on the calibration of the weight and the scale divisions of the balance. For equal-arm balances, accuracy also depends on the lever arm error and variation of sensitivity due to load placed on the pan.

ASTM: American Society for Testing and Materials.

Balance: A mechanical instrument for the comparison of weights.

Capacity: The largest load that can be weighed on a balance. The capacity of most analytical balances is 200 g.

Mass: A measure of the quantity of matter in an object; a constant, independent of gravitational force.

NIST: The National Institute of Standards and Technology, formerly the National Bureau of Standards.

Precision: The degree of agreement between repeated weighings of the same mass, expressed as one standard deviation in mass units.

Readability: The smallest fraction of the scale division that can be read. The validity of this reading depends on the precision of the instrument.

Sensitivity: The ratio of the change in scale divisions to a specific weight change, expressed as scale-division deflection per mass unit. It depends on the deflection of the beam and the optical magnification of this deflection.

Weighing: The comparison of an unknown mass to a calibrated one.

Weight: The force with which a mass is attracted by earth. It depends on gravity, which varies with location and time. The relationship is expressed as weight = mass × gravity.

Weights: Objects of known mass, made from corrosion-resistant material (brass, gold, platinum, stainless steel). NIST, with the ASTM, have established classes of weights, setting acceptable tolerance limits and specifications for material and construction. In the clinical laboratory, NIST Class S, ASTM Class 1 weights[1] are used for routine calibration and accuracy checking of the analytical balance.

Introduction

The analytical balance is one of the most basic and accurate instruments in the clinical laboratory. It is used for the preparation of standard solutions and whenever accuracy of 1 mg or less is required. Most analytical balances have a capacity of 200 g. Semimicrobalances are capable of weighing up to 100 g, and microbalances have a capacity of 20 to 50 g. There are a variety of analytical balances available. Substitution balances were standard equipment in the clinical laboratory, but electronic balances, faster and easier to operate, have now largely replaced them.

Principles and Component Parts

MECHANICAL BALANCES

Mechanical balances are based on the principle of a first-class lever.[2] The central moving part is the beam, which rests on the knife edge, acting as the fulcrum. This system allows for the direct comparison of masses rather than weights, so that correction for the effect of gravity is not necessary. There are two types of mechanical balances used for analytical work: the equal-arm balance and the single-pan substitution balance.

The *equal-arm balance* consists of a knife edge supporting the exact center of the beam (Fig. 3-1) so that the lengths of the two lever arms, L_1 and L_2, are equal. The pans are linked to the ends of the beams by stirrups, which rest on two outer knife edges. The three knife edges lie in the same plane about which motion occurs. The lengths of the two lever arms are equal; therefore, the mass supported by each arm must be equal for the system to be in equilibrium. If an unknown mass, m_x, is added to one side, the beam is deflected. The deflection is offset by adding standard weights, m_s, until the beam returns to the horizontal position so that $m_x L_1$ equals $m_s L_2$. If L_1 equals L_2, then m_x equals m_s.

The beam of the *single-pan substitution balance* is situated asymmetrically on the central knife edge (Fig. 3-2). The pan is supported by a stirrup placed on the outer knife edge. Again, both knife edges are in the same plane. A series of calibrated weights are supported from the same end of the beam from which the pan is suspended. A fixed-constant counterweight on the opposite end of the beam keeps the

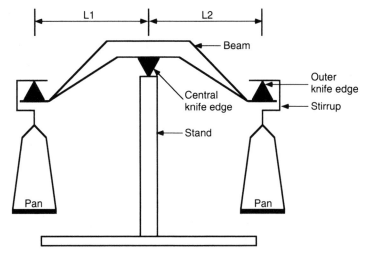

Figure 3-1. Equal-arm balance.

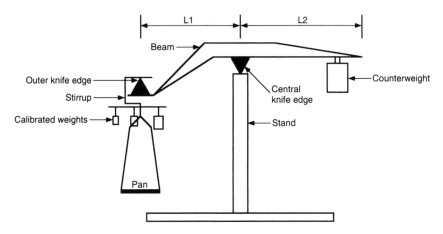

Figure 3-2. Substitution balance.

balance in equilibrium. The lengths of the lever arms, L_1 and L_2, are not equal; therefore, for the beam to remain in a horizontal position, the masses at either end of the lever arm are not equal. When an unknown weight is placed on the weighing pan, the beam deflects in the direction of the heavier side. To return the system to equilibrium, a corresponding mass of calibrated weights is removed from the front of the beam. The mass on the front of the beam is equalized by this substitution process, and the beam is restored to equilibrium. This is called weighing by substitution.

The condition of the knife edges is critical to the performance of these mechanical balances. The edges are made from an extremely hard material, such as sapphire, and must be precision-ground to minimize the area of contact and to reduce friction. There is considerable stress at the point of contact with the beam, and mechanical shock can easily damage these parts. To protect the knife edge, a beam arrest or beam support lifts the beam slightly from the knife edge. Pan arrests help to control the movement of the pans. Both beam and pan arrests should be engaged when the balance is not in use or when the pans are being loaded or unloaded.

Mechanical balances are also equipped with dampers, which oppose the movement of the beam, allowing it to come to equilibrium rapidly. Magnetic dampers are commonly used with equal-arm balances and consist of a metal plate fixed to the beam and positioned between the poles of a magnet. When the beam is set in motion, the plate moves through the magnetic field that opposes the oscillations. The air damper is used on the substitution balance. It consists of a piston attached to the beam and of a cylinder mounted on the balance case. When the beam is set in motion, the air within the cylinder expands and contracts, opposing the movement of the beam.

The substitution balance has several advantages over the equal-arm balance. The weighing procedure using an equal-arm balance is time-consuming and demands considerable skill. With an equal-arm balance, the sensitivity depends on the load placed on the balance. With increased loading there is increased friction due to mechanical imperfections in the knife edges and slight displacement of the terminal knife edges from the same plane as the central knife edge. The load is always constant on the substitution balance, and, therefore, the sensitivity is constant. Lever-arm error is eliminated because comparison of the known mass with an unknown mass takes place on the same lever arm. Two knife edges instead of three reduces friction.

ELECTRONIC BALANCES

In the *electronic balance* (Fig. 3-3), an electromagnetic force is used to counterbalance the object's weight and restore the beam to its zero position. The magnitude of the force is proportional to the load, and a microprocessor converts current to a digital display in grams. Electronic balances consist of four basic component systems: a weighing pan, a null detector, a feedback loop to control the balancing force, and a readout device.

The weighing pan is where the unknown weight is placed. The null detector senses the position of the balance beam and is used to determine the balance point at which the system is in equilibrium. This null detector is often a combination of a light-emitting diode, a detector, and a mechanical plate with a small hole through which the light passes when equilibrium is reached. To return the system to equilibrium, electromagnetic restoring forces are used in place of standard weights. The signal from the null detector is applied directly to control a current through an electromagnet to return the balance to equilibrium. When the null meter reads zero, the compensating force required to bring the balance to equilibrium is proportional to the weight of the pan. The current required to produce the compensating force is converted to a digital display of the weight.

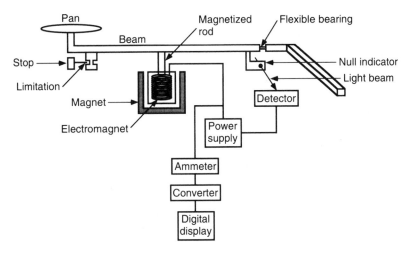

Figure 3-3. Electronic balance.

Electronic balances have several advantages over mechanical balances.[3] The precision is greatly increased with a digital display, replacing visual interpretation of a scale. Hand dialing to apply built-in weights is eliminated. In addition, electronic balances have automatic tare correction that automatically subtracts the weight of the container. Therefore, the time required to make a weighing is substantially decreased.

The disadvantages of electronic balances include: (1) variations from the true weight depending on the length of time since the "on" switch has been activated; (2) variations in weight depending on the location of the object on the balance pan; and (3) interference from other electronic sources, the cathode ray tube (CRT) from the computer screen, a radio transmitter, and so on. This interference causes erratic behavior of the digital display. Each electronic balance should be verified by checking the warm-up time needed for a particular balance and for the presence of off-center errors.

Maintenance and Quality Assurance

The performance of an analytical balance should be judged by sensitivity, precision, accuracy, and readability. The sensitivity is the ratio of the scale response change to weight change and is usually expressed as scale-division deflection per mg. If a 1-mg weight produces a displacement of three scale divisions from the rest point, then the sensitivity is expressed as three scale divisions per mg. The precision of the instrument is expressed as the standard deviation of repetitive measurements of the same mass. The accuracy can be checked using NIST Class S, ASTM Class 1 (working reference standards[4]) weights. The readability of the instrument is the smallest fraction of a division to which the index scale can be read with ease. When selecting an analytical balance for a particular weighing requirement, the capacity of the instrument should also be considered.

To ensure proper operation of an analytical balance, study the instruction manual provided by the manufacturer of the instrument. The balance must be level and should be placed near a support wall on a solid support, either marble or concrete. The balance should be located away from elevators, vibrations, vents, drafts, direct sunlight, windows, refrigerators, freezers, and drying ovens. Preferably it should be in a room of relatively constant temperature ($\approx 20°C$) and humidity (45-60%). Objects that will overload the balance and exceed its capacity should not be placed on the pan. Objects to be weighed should not be handled with fingers. Fingerprints have weight and can be corrosive to calibrated metal weights. Tongs or specially designed weighing papers should be used for transferring objects. Glass containers are preferable to plastic ones for weighing chemicals. Plastic containers can generate electrostatic forces. The balance should be cleaned after each weighing. Corrosive materials should not be placed or used near an analytical balance. The beam support and pan arrest should always be engaged whenever loading or unloading the pan. When not in use, all weights should be returned to the zero position, the beams and pan placed in the support position, and nothing should be left on the balance pan.

For optimum balance performance, preventive maintenance and calibration should be done according to the manufacturer's instructions at least once a year. For an electronic balance, calibration should be checked every time the balance is moved, the warm-up time required should be verified, and a calibrated weight (use a weight that is at least 60% of the total capacity of the balance) should be checked at various locations on the pan. The accuracy of the balance should be checked monthly using NIST Class S, ASTM Class 1 weights. If the weights show that the balance is operating outside specifications, call the manufacturer or a qualified service representative.

Summary

Analytical balances are necessary instruments in a clinical laboratory. Without a balance, primary standards, or standards for recovery studies, could not be prepared. Analytical balances are either mechanical or electronic. Mechanical balances include a beam and the use of weights to balance the load placed on the balance pan. The simplest mechanical balance, the equal-arm balance, has a knife edge in the exact center of the beam and two pans, one on each end of the beam. The load is placed on one of the pans, with known weights added to the other pan until the load is balanced.

A modification of the mechanical balance is the single-pan substitution balance in which the knife edge is situated asymmetrically. A fixed counterweight balances the pan and a series of calibrated weights. When a load is placed on the single pan, the beam is balanced by removal of calibrated weights until the system is again in equilibrium.

An electronic balance is a single pan balance without weights. The load on the pan is balanced by an electromagnetic force, and a null detector determines when the system reaches equilibrium. The magnitude of the electrical current is proportional to the sample weight and is converted through a microprocessor to a digital display of weight.

Balances are sensitive analytical instruments and need to be carefully located away from vibrations, drafts, rapid and severe changes in temperature, or humidity. The balance should be kept clean and its accuracy checked with NIST Class S weights at regular intervals, usually monthly. Yearly maintenance by a factory representative is recommended.

Questions and Problems

1. How does an electronic balance differ from a mechanical balance?
2. The following data were obtained when checking the Class S weights last month.

Class S Weight (g)	Allowable Variance (g)	Observed Weight (g)
0.001	±0.0001	0.0010
0.100	±0.0001	0.0999
1.000	±0.0002	1.0001
50.000	±0.0003	49.9998
100.000	±0.0003	99.9980

Is the balance performing satisfactorily? If no, explain and recommend action to be taken.
3. Design an evaluation of a new electronic balance. What functions should be verified?
4. Outline considerations on where this new balance should be located.
5. A 100-g weight, with tolerance limits as stated in question #2, was placed at each corner of the balance pan and weighed in that position. The following weights were obtained: 100.0001, 99.9997, 100.0002, and 100.0000. What conclusions can you draw from these data?

References

1. Standard specifications for laboratory weights and precision mass standards. E617-81. Annual book of ASTM standards. Philadelphia, PA. 1989; 14.02:353-70.
2. Schrenk GH, Hahn, RB, Hartkopf AV. Quantitative analytical chemistry: Principles and life science applications. Boston: Allyn & Bacon, 1977:54-68.
3. Coyne GS. The laboratory handbook of materials, equipment and technique. Englewood Cliffs, NJ: Prentice-Hall, 1992:113-22.
4. Jeffery GH, Bassett J, Mendham J, Denney RC. Vogel's textbook of quantitative chemical analysis, 5th ed. New York: John Wiley & Sons, 1989:72-78.

Suggested Readings

Hargis LG. Analytical chemistry: Principles and techniques. Englewood Cliffs, NJ: Prentice-Hall, 1988.
Steiner P. Basic laboratory principles. In: Kaplan LA, Pesce AJ, eds. Clinical chemistry: Theory, analysis, and correlation, 2nd ed. St Louis: CV Mosby, 1989.
Linne JJ, Ringsrud KM. Basic techniques in clinical laboratory sciences, 3rd ed. St. Louis: Mosby Year Book, 1992.

4

OSMOMETRY

Gregory A. Tetrault

Objectives

After completing this chapter, the reader will be able to:

1. Describe the colligative properties of solutions.
2. List the component parts of freezing-point osmometers.
3. Explain how the measuring system of freezing-point osmometers works.
4. Describe supercooling and seeding and how they are used in osmometry.
5. List the component parts of vapor pressure osmometers.
6. Explain how the measuring system of vapor pressure osmometers works.
7. Define dew point, and give its relation to vapor pressure osmometry.
8. List the advantages and disadvantages of vapor pressure osmometry.
9. Draw a block diagram of a colloid osmotic pressure osmometer.
10. Define oncotic pressure and its physiological importance.
11. Describe good maintenance and quality control practices for osmometry.

Definitions

Chemical Activity: The thermodynamically effective concentration of a molecule, atom, or ion.

Colligative Properties: Properties of solutions that depend on the effective number of particles in solution. The four colligative properties are boiling point, freezing point, osmotic pressure, and vapor pressure.

Colloid: A large molecule (>30,000 MW) in solution.

Colloid Osmotic Pressure: The fraction of osmotic pressure due to large molecular weight particles (>30,000 MW) in solution.

Crystalloid: An uncharged small molecule (<30,000 MW) in solution.

Dew Point: The temperature of air at which water vapor condenses to form dew.

Galvanometer: A device for measuring small changes in current.

Heat of Condensation: Thermal energy released when a substance changes phase from a gas or vapor to a liquid.

Heat of Fusion: Thermal energy released when a substance changes phase from a liquid to a solid.

Oncotic Pressure: Osmotic pressure exerted by colloids in solution.

Osmolality: 1 osmole of particles in a kilogram of water.

Osmolarity: An aqueous solution containing 1 osmole of particles in a liter of solution.

Osmole: Avogadro's number (6.023×10^{23}) of particles.

Osmotic Pressure: The pressure required to keep a solution in equilibrium with pure solvent when the two are separated by a semipermeable membrane that only allows passage of solvent molecules.

Pressure Transducer: A device that converts pressure to an electrical signal.

Seeding: The process by which a phase change is initiated in a supercooled liquid.

Supercooling: Rapidly reducing the temperature of a solution below its freezing point (or a gas below its condensation point). The stability of a supercooled substance is related to the amount of supercooling and to the propensity for seeding to occur.

Thermistor: A device whose electrical conductivity varies with temperature. Derived from the phrase *thermal resistor.*

Thermocouple: A device composed of two or more types of metals or alloys in which current is produced by a temperature difference between ends.

Vapor Pressure: The pressure over the surface of a liquid due to evaporation of solvent.

Wheatstone Bridge: An electrical device composed of multiple resistors that is used to measure an unknown resistance.

Introduction

Osmometry is the measurement of the *osmolality* of a solution. Osmolality is a measure of the *chemical activity* of dissolved solute particles. A 1 osmolal solution contains one *osmole* of solute particles in 1 kilogram of solvent (usually water).[1] Solutes in water have mathematically predictable effects on certain physical (colligative) properties of the solution. Osmometry is based on one of the four *colligative* properties of aqueous solutions. Dissolving one mole of an ideal solute in 1 kg of water causes the following changes in colligative properties:

1. Osmotic pressure increases from 0 to 17,000 mm Hg.
2. Boiling point rises to 100.52°C.
3. Freezing point falls to −1.858°C.
4. Vapor pressure drops by 0.303 mm Hg.

Most clinical laboratory osmometers measure the freezing point or vapor pressure of a solution. Osmolality is calculated from the measured value. The usual samples are serum and urine.

Freezing-Point Depression Osmometers

Measurement of the *freezing point* of a pure liquid is quite simple. As heat is removed, the temperature falls (at a rate inversely proportional to the temperature difference between the sample and the cooling device) until the freezing point is reached. At this point the temperature stays constant, because the phase change from liquid to solid uses all the negative thermal energy. Once the phase change is complete, the temperature of the frozen liquid will again fall until it reaches that of the cooling device. Therefore, measurement of the freezing point is simply a matter of recording the plateau temperature.

Unfortunately, freezing-point measurement is not as simple when there are dissolved solute particles in the liquid. Cooling proceeds as before, except that when the initial freezing temperature is reached there is no plateau. Instead, temperature continues to fall because crystallization removes pure solvent from the solution, leaving behind a smaller mass of liquid with a higher concentration of dissolved solute particles. Thus, the freezing point is lowered, and the temperature falls more until the new freezing point is reached (Fig. 4-1). The process repeats until solidifica-

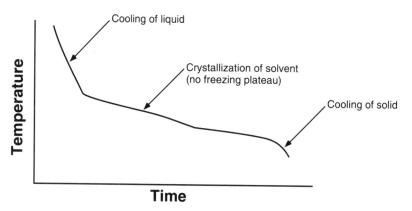

Figure 4-1.   Cooling curve for a solution containing dissolved particles.

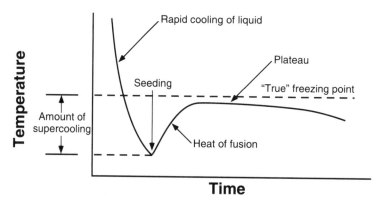

Figure 4-2.   Cooling curve for a supercooled solution containing dissolved particles.

tion finally occurs. Because there is no plateau and determination of the precise initial freezing point is nearly impossible, a different method is employed—the supercooling technique.

Supercooling is a process in which the solution is quickly chilled to a temperature below its freezing point. If done correctly, the solvent molecules will aggregate but will not crystallize spontaneously (at least for a while, as formation of pure ice crystals is a relatively slow process). Crystallization is accelerated by "seeding" the solution. (Yes, this is the same type of "seeding" that is done to form rain clouds, except that there the transition is from water vapor to liquid). Seeding, in a freezing-point depression osmometer, results from violent agitation of the stirring wire (instead of the slow, steady mixing used at other times). Once crystallization begins, the temperature of the solution rises because of the release of the *heat of fusion* (Fig. 4-2). A temperature plateau is reached (about 30-180 seconds later) that is slightly below the true freezing point of the original solution. Final measurement is made at this temperature.

COMPONENT PARTS

These are the most common types of osmometers in clinical laboratories. The components of a freezing-point depression osmometer (Fig. 4-3) are:

1. A cooling module maintained at -5 to -7°C for chilling the sample
2. An operating head with a thermistor temperature probe and a stirring wire
3. A galvanometer connected to a Wheatstone bridge for measuring resistance in the thermistor probe
4. A readout meter calibrated in milliosmols (mOsm)

Cooling Module

The cooling module is an insulated tank usually containing a mixture of ethylene glycol and water. This solution is maintained at -5 to -7°C by a refrigeration unit. The cooling module also contains an automatic bath stirrer or circulating pump to ensure uniform temperature throughout the coolant fluid. The chosen bath temperature is precisely maintained with less than 0.1°C variation.

Operating Head

The operating head contains a thermistor probe that sits in the center of the sample when the unit is operating. A stirring wire is adjacent to the thermistor probe. These two items protrude from a rectangular box that contains an electric motor or other device to vibrate the stirring wire and the electric connections from the thermistor probe. The entire operating head slides down on to the sample container. The head may be moved automatically or manually, depending on the instrument's design.

The thermistor is a metal wire with a glass bead at the end. The thermistor is often surrounded by a plastic sleeve. The electrical resistance of the thermistor varies predictably with temperature.

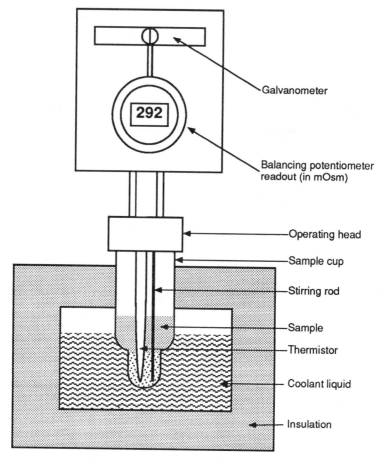

Figure 4-3.   Freezing-point depression osmometer.

Measuring System

The thermistor probe is connected to a galvanometer that in turn is connected to a Wheatstone bridge (see Chapter 1, Fig. 1-13). A galvanometer responds to small changes in current (due to changes in the electrical resistance of the thermistor as its temperature varies) and is used to measure the direction of current flow in the Wheatstone bridge. The balancing potentiometer continually adjusts the variable resistance of the Wheatstone bridge such that the galvanometer returns to the null position (no net current flow). The final adjustment of the variable resistance yields the osmolality of the solution being analyzed.

CALIBRATION

The calibration of a freezing-point depression osmometer is similar to that of a pH meter: standards above and below the osmolal range of interest are used to adjust slope and intercept. The usual standards are 100 and 1000 mOsm/kg. The variable resistance of the measurement resistor is set to the standard's osmolality, and the other two resistors in the Wheatstone bridge are adjusted to give the correct response to thermistor changes over the osmolar range of interest. Many users confirm calibration by assaying a 300 or 500 mOsm/kg standard. This is done in addition to using serum or urine controls.

Vapor Pressure Osmometers

Vapor pressure osmometry actually measures the dew point of a solution, which is related to its vapor pressure. A disk of filter paper is saturated with the solution being measured and is placed in a sealed chamber. The chamber is cooled to a temperature below the dew point by applying current to a thermocouple. Condensation of water within the sealed chamber produces a temperature rise (from the heat of condensation) that is monitored through the thermocouple. The temperature stabilizes at the dew point. Vapor pressure osmometers are less common but are still used in clinical laboratories.

COMPONENT PARTS

Vapor pressure osmometers contain the following components:

1. A sample holder
2. A sealed chamber with one thermocouple junction
3. A voltmeter to measure thermocouple potential at equilibrium

Sample Holder

The Model 5500 vapor pressure osmometer (Wescor, Inc., Logan, UT 84321, is the only maker of vapor pressure osmometers in the US) uses a metal slide with a shallow well for the sample (Fig. 4-4). A 5-mm filter paper disk is placed in the well

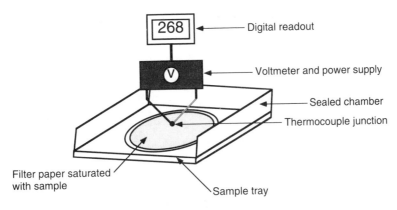

Figure 4-4. Vapor pressure osmometer.

and $10\,\mu L$ of specimen is applied to the paper. The slide is pushed into the instrument so that the sample enters into the sealed chamber.

Sealed Chamber, Thermocouple, and Voltmeter

After a short time, temperature and vapor pressure equilibrium are established within the sealed chamber. This reference temperature is measured by the thermocouple. A thermocouple consists of two different metals joined so that a temperature difference between the junctions produces a voltage difference (Fig. 4-5). Heating one end of a metal wire increases the number of electrons available for conduction. The excess of electrons will flow to the colder end of the wire, creating a negative charge. The magnitude of this charge is directly related to the temperature difference between the ends of the wire.

After the reference temperature is recorded, current is applied to the thermocouple so that the end in the sealed chamber cools, while the other end warms. Cooling progresses until the temperature falls below the dew point. At this point the current to the thermocouple is turned off. Water then condenses within the sealed chamber, and the heat of condensation raises the thermocouple temperature. Eventually, an equilibrium temperature is reached at which further rises in temperature from condensation are balanced by cooling due to evaporation. The voltmeter records the thermocouple potential, which is proportional to the dew point of the sample.

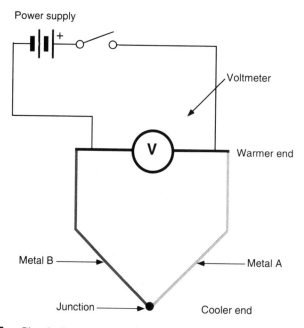

Figure 4-5.   Circuit diagram of a thermocouple with power supply and voltmeter.

CALIBRATION

The calibration of vapor pressure osmometers is similar to that of freezing-point depression osmometers, except that vapor pressure osmometers are not commonly used with samples less than 200 mOsm/kg H_2O.

Comparison of Freezing-Point Depression and Vapor Pressure Osmometry

The vast majority of clinical laboratories use freezing-point depression osmometry. The advantages of vapor pressure osmometry—lower cost, easier maintenance, smaller sample volume, and ability to handle viscous and colloidal specimens—are outweighed by its disadvantages—lower precision, nonlinear response below 200 mOsm/kg H_2O, inaccuracy below 100 mOsm/kg H_2O, and inability to measure the effects of volatiles (alcohols, ethylene glycol, dissolved gases) on total osmolality.[1]

Colloid Osmotic Pressure

Colloid osmotic pressure is the contribution of large molecules (>30,000 MW) such as proteins to total osmotic pressure. A sample is introduced into a chamber separated from a saline solution by a semipermeable membrane. Because large molecular weight substances cannot cross the semipermeable membrane, a concentration gradient results. Liquid flows from the saline side of the chamber into the sample side, resulting in a drop in pressure in the saline side. Flow continues until a balance is achieved between the concentration gradient (drawing liquid away from the saline side) and the pressure reduction. The pressure change corresponds to the colloid osmotic pressure. In hemodynamics the colloid osmotic pressure is also known as the *oncotic pressure*. There are some clinical conditions, such as administration of dextran plasma volume expanders, in which accurately measuring the oncotic pressure of serum is useful.

COMPONENT PARTS

The component parts of a colloid osmotic pressure measuring device are:

1. A chamber divided by a semipermeable membrane
2. A mercury manometer
3. A pressure transducer and meter

Chamber

The two-sided chamber is separated by a membrane impermeable to substances with molecular weights over 30,000 MW (Fig. 4-6). A saline solution fills the side of the chamber connected to the pressure transducer. The sample is introduced to the other side. Saline is used to set the zero-point of the colloid pressure osmometer.

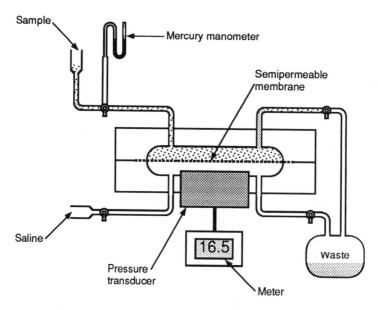

Figure 4-6.   Colloid osmotic pressure osmometer.

Mercury Manometer and Pressure Transducer

The mercury manometer is connected to the sample side of the chamber. It is used to calibrate the pressure transducer. The pressure transducer reacts to decreased pressure on the saline side of the chamber. When a sample containing proteins or other high-molecular weight substances is introduced, water and saline molecules pass through the semipermeable membrane in an attempt to equalize concentrations on both sides of the chamber. Because large molecular weight substances cannot cross the membrane, there is a net flow of liquid into the sample side. Soon an equilibrium is reached, and the pressure drop on the saline side is recorded by the transducer. If the original volumes of the two sides of the chamber are equal, then the pressure drop equals the oncotic pressure.

Maintenance and Quality Assurance

Freezing-point depression osmometers require regular maintenance. Frequent (usually daily) checks of coolant level, bath temperature, and calibration are necessary. Some manufacturers also recommend daily checks of sample repeatability (precision).[2] Other less frequent maintenance needs are checking the alignment of the operating head, adjusting the placement of the thermistor probe and stirring wire, cleaning or replacing the refrigerator air filter, defrosting the cooling module, and changing the coolant fluid.

Vapor pressure osmometers require less types of maintenance than freezing-point depression osmometers but are more difficult to maintain in good working order.[3] Frequent cleaning of the thermocouple is necessary for reproducibility, especially at lower osmolalities. Calibration and repeatability must be checked regularly. The sample holder must be scrupulously cleaned after each use.

Colloid pressure osmometers have average maintenance requirements. As with the others, frequent calibration and repeatability testing are necessary. Other maintenance tasks include cleaning the sample and saline chambers, replacing the semipermeable membrane, and calibration of the pressure transducer with a mercury manometer.

Osmometers are discrete analyzers. Samples are usually run soon after arrival in the laboratory (batching is uncommon). Therefore, the definition of a run for quality control purposes is not clear-cut. Many laboratories define a run as a day or a shift. The length of time for a run will depend on frequency of use, the specific osmometer used, and the stability of calibration. Calibration should be checked according to manufacturers' instructions or even more frequently. The standards used for calibration should bracket the range of interest. Serum specimens are usually between 250 and 350 mOsm/kg. Urine specimens can vary from less than 50 to over 1200 mOsm/kg. Most laboratories calibrate for urine testing with 100 and 1000 mOsm/kg standards.

Most laboratories purchase prepared calibration standards, but some make their own. Standards are usually composed of NaCl solutions. The osmolality of a NaCl is calculated from the following equation:

$$Osmolality = f * n * c \qquad \text{(Eq. 4-1)}$$

where

> f = osmotic coefficient
> n = number of particles when molecule dissociates in solvent
> c = concentration in moles/kg solvent (H_2O)

Nonelectrolytes such as glucose do not dissociate, so $n = 1$. A molecule of NaCl dissociates into two particles when dissolved in water, so $n = 2$. The osmotic coefficient is a measure of the effective number of particles in solution. Ideal solutes such as glucose and ethanol have osmotic coefficients of 1, but other solutes will have values between 0 and 1. For example, NaCl (remember $n = 2$) in water has an osmotic coefficient of 0.93 at 290 mOsm/kg H_2O. The value is even less at higher salt concentrations. The reason for this is that Na^+ and Cl^- are attracted to each other, and they occasionally get close enough together to act as only one particle. The frequency of these 'close encounters' is greater at higher salt concentrations, so the osmotic coefficient decreases.

Summary

Osmometry is the measurement of the *osmolality* (chemical activity of dissolved particles) of a solution. Particles dissolved in water have known effects on the four colligative properties. Osmometers measure one of the colligative properties. The commonest type of osmometer measures the freezing-point depression due to dissolved particles. Vapor pressure osmometers are also used in clinical laboratories. A third type of osmometer measures colloid osmotic pressure across a semipermeable membrane.

Osmometers in use today are manual devices for single samples. Simple, but frequent, maintenance is required. Calibration is performed with commercial or self-prepared aqueous standards. Preparation of standard must take into account the osmotic coefficient (f) of the solute at the concentrations of interest.

Questions and Problems

1. Name the four colligative properties of aqueous solutions.
2. Human urine can contain enough dissolved particles to reach 1200 mOsmol/L. Calculate the osmotic pressure of such a solution. How many atmospheres is that? (An atmosphere, 760 mm Hg, is the air pressure at sea level).
3. A manufacturer concludes that a freezing point-depression osmometer should be able to distinguish between solutions that differ by only 2 mOsmol/L (e.g., 287 and 289 mOsmol/L). How sensitive to temperature changes must the thermistor be?
4. Explain why vapor pressure osmometers are unreliable with aqueous solutions under 200 mOsmol/L.
5. Draw a diagram of a colloid osmotic pressure osmometer.
6. Calculate the weight of NaCl needed to prepare 0.5 L of a 300 mOsmol/L standard.

References

1. Freier EF. Osmometry. In: Tietz NW, ed. Textbook of clinical chemistry. Philadelphia: WB Saunders, 1986:129-35.
2. User's Guide: Advanced Digimatic® Osmometer (REV06-12-85). Needham Heights, MA: Advanced Instruments, 1985:17-25.
3. Kaplan LA. Osmolality. In: Kaplan LA, Pesce AJ, eds. Methods in clinical chemistry. St. Louis: CV Mosby, 1987:18-21.

5

REFRACTOMETRY

Richard D. Juel
Mary Ann Steinrauf

Objectives

After completing this chapter, the reader will be able to:

1. Explain the laws of refraction and reflection.
2. Define refractive index.
3. Explain the importance of critical angle and how it is used to determine refractive index.
4. List the component parts of refractometers.
5. Explain the purpose and workings of an Amici compensator.
6. Explain how Abbé, Pulfrich, and total solids refractometers work.
7. Understand the effect of temperature on refractive index.
8. Draw a schematic of an immersion refractometer.
9. List maintenance and calibration requirements for refractometers.

Definitions

Critical Angle: When light passes from one medium, such as air, into a more dense medium, such as glass or water, the angle of refraction is always less than the angle of incidence. As a result of this decrease in angle, there exists a range of angles for which no refracted light is possible. Consider the diagram for which several angles of incidence and their corresponding angles of refraction are shown (Fig. 5-1). In this diagram, angle 4 is the critical angle. One should note that in the limiting case where the incident rays approach the angle of $90°$ (where they graze along the surfaces), the refracted rays approach a certain angle c, beyond which no refracted light is possible. This limiting angle is called the critical angle. In any

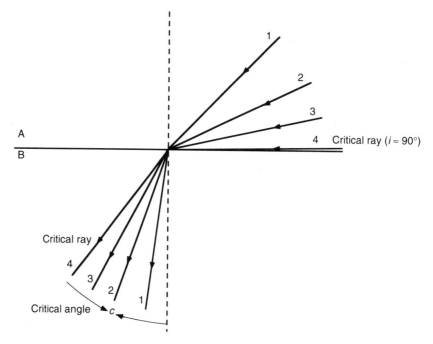

Figure 5-1.   Critical rays and corresponding critical angles.

medium, the value for the critical angle depends on the index of refraction. One can calculate the critical angle of refraction by using Snell's Law.[1]

$$\sin i / \sin r = n \qquad \text{(Eq. 5-1)}$$

where

  i = angle of incident light from normal
  r = angle of refracted light in medium B
  n = the ratio of the speed of light through medium A to that of medium B

In determining the critical angle (c), angle i equals 90° (sine of 90° = 1), and angle r equals angle c. Therefore, solving for the critical angle,

$$\sin c = 1/n \qquad \text{(Eq. 5-2)}$$

The rays formed by the refraction of the grazing rays are termed critical rays.

  Dispersion: The angular spread of the wavelengths (colors) produced by sending white light through a prism. The band of colors produced is a spectrum. A prismatic spectrum is nonlinear.

  Index of Refraction: If medium A is a vacuum (or, for practical purposes, air), the value of the constant in Equation 5-2 is called the index of refraction, n, of medium B. By experimental measurements of the angles i and r, one can determine the values of n for various transparent substances.

  Law of Reflection: The angle at which a ray of light strikes the reflecting surface is equal to the angle the reflected ray makes with the same surface (Fig. 5-2). These angles are

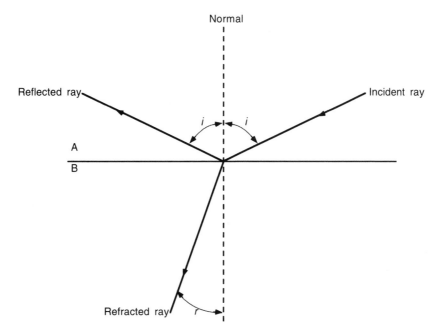

Figure 5-2. Reflection and refraction of an incident light ray passing from a low refractive index medium (A) to a high refractive index medium (B).

customarily measured from a line perpendicular to the plane of the reflective surface. This line is called the normal.

Law of Refraction: The sine of the angle of refraction (r) bears a constant ratio to the sine of the angle of incidence (i) (Eq. 5-1). This constant is the same for all angles of incidence. Again, these angles are measured in relation to the normal. This law is also referred to as Snell's law.

Reflection and Refraction: When a ray of light (incident ray) strikes any boundary between two transparent substances (A and B) that have appreciably different velocities for transmitted light, part of the ray is reflected, and the rest is refracted. The refraction (bending) is due to the change in the velocity of the light when passing from A to B. The angle of incidence (i) is the same for the incident ray and the reflected ray (Fig. 5-2).

Principles

The *refractive index,* like the melting point and the boiling point, is a constant characteristic of any homogenous substance. The refractive index is related to the number, charge, and mass of the vibrating particles in the material through which electromagnetic radiation is transmitted. Measurement of refractive index, *refractometry,* can be used to confirm a substance's identity, to analyze a mixture, to determine the specific gravity of a solution, and to estimate the size, shape, and molecular weight of a polymer.

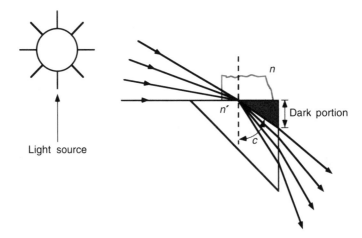

Figure 5-3.   Prism of a critical angle refractometer. The dashed line is the normal. The critical angle, *c,* is indicated. The refractive indices of the sample and the refractometer prism and *n* and *n',* respectively.

The refractive index of a substance can be precisely determined with an optical instrument that measures angles of light refraction: a *refractometer.* Many refractometers measure the critical angle of a substance. The Abbé, Pulfrich, and immersion (dipping) refractometers are examples of this type. They differ mainly in the measurable ranges of refractive indices and in the types of light source.

In critical angle refractometers, a convergent beam of light strikes the interface between the unknown sample of refractive index *n* and a prism of known refractive index *n'.* The beam of light passes from a rarer to a denser medium (Fig. 5-3). Some of the light beam's rays graze the surface of the sample at the critical angle. The non-grazing rays are refracted at angles smaller than the critical angle. A sharp boundary is formed in the refractometer prism between light and dark portions (Fig. 5-3). The angle of this boundary is the critical angle. Measuring this angle allows one to calculate the value of *n.* Because the grazing rays may enter the prism (refractive index *n'*) anywhere along the interface, an infinite number of critical rays is produced. These rays can be coalesced into a single light-dark boundary with condensing or focusing lenses between the prism and the viewing scope or eyepiece of the refractometer.

Refractometry has advantages over other types of analyses: The instruments are of simple design; measurements are quick and easy; analyses are nondestructive and work with small samples; and applications are numerous.

Components of Refractometers

A refractometer is composed of a light source, a temperature control or temperature compensation device, a refracting prism, focusing optics, and a readout device.

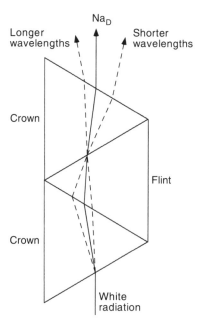

Figure 5-4. Amici prism. The D line of sodium emerges at the same angle as the incident white light beam.

LIGHT SOURCE

For operating convenience, refractive indices are commonly obtained in the visible range. In this range, most substances are nonabsorbing. The latter is an advantage, because detection would be a problem if there is significant loss of light intensity. For a precise determination of refractive index, monochromatic light must be used. A variety of electrical discharge lamps are able to produce either a suitable single spectral line or a closely spaced pair of lines. The most widely used is the intense sodium doublet (the *D line*) at 589.0 and 589.6 nm, although a mercury or hydrogen lamp can also be used. The advantage of a sodium lamp is that a filter is seldom necessary; even though other emission lines are present, their intensity is less than 1% that of the D lines. On occasion, a determination of the dispersion of the refractive index (i.e., its variation with wavelength) is helpful. For this, a mercury lamp with different filters yields four intense line spectra at 579.0 (yellow), 546.1 (green), 435.8 (blue), and 404.7 (violet) nm. A still more versatile unit is a mercury lamp to which cadmium is added so that there is also a bright red cadmium line at 643.8 nm. White light can be used for precise refractometry. However, dispersion is the deterrent to its use in critical-angle refractometry. It is imperative that there be compensation for the dispersion. Critical-angle instruments using daylight or tungsten sources use Amici prisms for this compensation, which are small, direct-vision spectroscopes. They are constructed of different varieties of glass and are designed so that the light is dispersed without deviating the wavelengths at the D line. A combination of such prisms is an *Amici compensator* (Fig. 5-4).

With the Amici compensator, the boundary appears sharp; however, the accuracy of the measurement of *n*, regardless of the type of refractometer, only approaches 0.0001 refractive index units. A disadvantage when using the Amici prisms is that the index of refraction cannot be measured at wavelengths other than the D line without making an elaborate reading correction.

TEMPERATURE CONTROL

The refractive index depends on temperature and wavelength, as is shown by the data for water (Table 5-1). Most liquids show a change in the refractive index of approximately −0.00045 units/°C. Solids are less sensitive to temperature changes: approximately −0.00001 units/°C. Thermal expansion of the solution or solid causes the observed decreases in refractive index. For a reading to be reliable to the fourth decimal place, the temperature of liquid samples must be thermoregulated to ±0.2°C. Temperature control must be tighter if greater precision is required. For very high levels of precision, the entire refractometer must be thermoregulated. This is usually accomplished by circulating fluid from a constant-temperature bath through a "jacket" surrounding the sample. Maintaining temperature uniformity of a liquid sample also requires minimization of evaporation.

REFRACTING PRISM

Refracting prisms are made of transparent solids with high refractive indices. The refractive index of the prism determines the range of refractive indices that can be measured. Substances with refractive indices higher than that of the refracting prism cannot be analyzed. Refracting prisms can be triangular, rectangular, or trapezoidal. Samples are applied directly on the refracting prism in some refractometers. Other refractometers sandwich liquid samples between refracting and illuminating prisms.

Measurement of the refractive index of a transparent solid sample requires a smooth interface between the sample and the refracting prism. This is partly achieved by cutting and polishing the sample to achieve a smooth, flat surface. However, for precise measurement of the refractive index of a solid, a drop of contacting liquid

Table 5-1

Influence of Wavelength and Temperature on Refractive Index of Water

Source Element	Wavelength	Index of Refraction				
		10°C	20°C	30°C	40°C	50°C
Hydrogen	656.3	1.3337	1.3312			
Sodium	589.3		1.3330	1.3319	1.3305	1.3289

with a high refractive index (such as 1-bromonaphthalene) is used.[2] This minimizes diffraction and reflection.

FOCUSING OPTICS

All refractometers have optics either to directly view the refracting prism or to focus the light emerging from the refracting prism. The focusing optics may also contain Amici prisms (see Light Source section) or other devices to compensate for dispersion of white light. Examples of focusing and compensating optics are shown in the Instruments section.

READOUT DEVICE

The simplest refractometer readout device is an etched or printed scale. Light from the refracting prism is focused on the scale. The reading is taken at the boundary of light and dark. The scale may display critical angle in degrees, refractive index, specific gravity, or other units. An eyepiece with magnifying optics is used to view the light-dark boundary.

Recording refractometers are also available. A mirror is rotated until the light-dark border is detected by a pair of phototubes. The pen of a strip chart recorder moves up and down as the mirror rotates. This technique can monitor changes in refractive index of a flowing stream of liquid.

Instruments

ABBÉ REFRACTOMETER

The *Abbé refractometer* (Fig. 5-5) measures the critical angle of a liquid sample. A few drops of the sample are placed between the illuminating prism and the refracting prism. Both prisms are partially hollowed to allow circulation of water (to maintain a controlled temperature). Light is reflected from a mirror and passed through the illuminating prism, which has a rough-ground upper surface. The rough surface diffracts light and provides an infinite number of rays. These rays pass through the thin layer of liquid and strike the polished surface of the refracting prism, where they are refracted. The critical angle (c) is formed within the refracting prism and cannot be measured. Instead, the critical ray's angle of emergence (a) is measured (Fig. 5-6).

The critical ray forms the border between the light and dark portions of the field when viewed with the telescope, which is attached to the scale. The sharp edge of the light-dark boundary is aligned with the cross hairs in the telescope's ocular. The reading is taken from the ruled scale. The scale is graduated in 0.001 refractive index units based on the D lines. An attached magnifier allows estimation of the next decimal, providing a readability of ±0.0002. Two measurement ranges are available (by switching prisms): 1.30-1.71 and 1.45-1.84.

A tungsten lamp is usually used as a light source. Two Amici prisms are placed in front of the objective of the telescope, one above the other (Fig. 5-5). These prisms

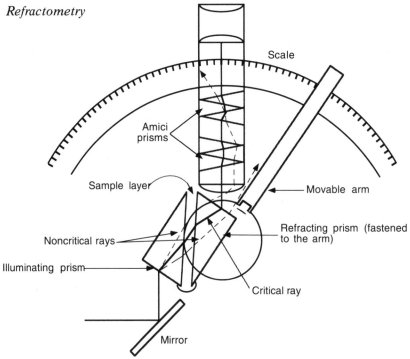

Figure 5-5. Abbé refractometer.

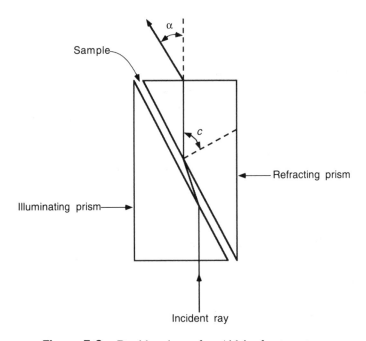

Figure 5-6. Double prisms of an Abbé refractometer.

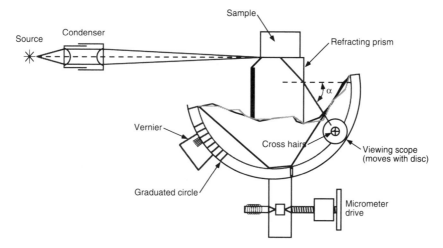

Figure 5-7. Pulfrich refractometer.

eliminate a colored, indistinct boundary between the light and dark fields that would otherwise occur (because of the variation of refractive index with the wavelength of light).

PULFRICH REFRACTOMETER

In a *Pulfrich refractometer,* the refracting prism is always beneath the sample (Fig. 5-7). A beam of monochromatic light is directed along the surface of the refracting prism at the grazing angle. A reservoir (for liquid samples) is mounted on the horizontal surface of the prism. After refraction, light rays emerge from the second face of the refracting prism. The angle of emergence (a) of the critical ray is viewed through a telescope. The telescope is connected to a rotatable scale that is ruled in degrees. The scale is also fitted with a vernier, which allows estimation of a to the nearest minute (one-sixtieth of a degree). The telescope and scale are rotated so that the light–dark boundary is focused on the cross hairs of the eyepiece. The scale and vernier are then read. Tables are used to convert a to refractive index. The conversion factor also depends on the wavelength of the incident light.

The accuracy and precision of Pulfrich refractometers are ±0.0001 units for direct measurements. The accuracy of the instrument can be increased to ±0.00005 with a micrometer drive to position the telescope cross hairs (Fig. 5-7). The measurable range of refractive indices with the standard refracting prism is 1.33 to 1.60. This may be extended to 1.84 by substituting a denser refracting prism.

IMMERSION (DIPPING) REFRACTOMETER

An *immersion refractometer* (Fig. 5-8) is the simplest to use, but it requires a 10 to 15 mL liquid sample. It is similar to the Abbé refractometer except for the lack of

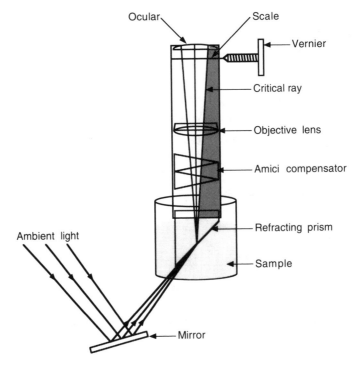

Figure 5-8.   Immersion refractometer.

an auxiliary prism. The refracting prism is rigidly mounted at the base of the telescope, which also contains Amici compensating prisms. A graduated scale (from −5 to 105) is located within the telescope at the focal plane of the eyepiece. Ambient (white) light is most often used, although a more intense light source can be positioned in front of the light-gathering mirror mounted below the telescope.

The refracting prism is immersed in a small beaker containing the sample. Light is reflected upward through the liquid and into the refracting prism. The critical ray projects as a light-dark boundary. The scale is moved with a micrometer screw until the nearest gradation coincides with the boundary. Readings are taken from both the scale and the micrometer. A table is consulted to convert these readings to refractive index units. The micrometer reading shows the decimal to be added. The smallest division, 0.01, corresponds to a 0.000037 change in refractive index at the D line (n_D). Thus, this instrument can be more accurate and precise than the Abbé or Pulfrich refractometer. However, to achieve high accuracy and precision, the refractometer and liquid must be at the same, known, temperature. This requires up to five minutes of immersion if the sample liquid is not at room temperature. Complete conversion tables are unavailable for many temperatures. Measurements must be made at one of the recommended temperatures for greatest accuracy.

Immersion refractometers cover a narrower range of refractive indices than other types. The maximum refractive index is about 1.5.

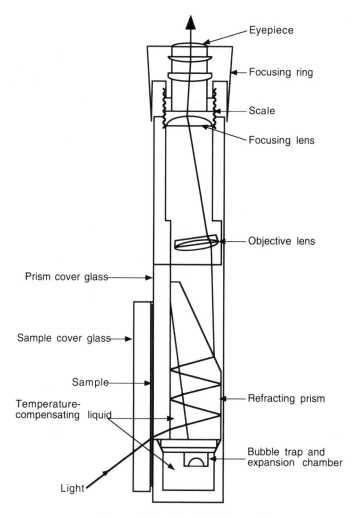

Figure 5-9. Total solids meter.

TOTAL SOLIDS METER

The *total solids* (*TS*) meter is the most commonly used refractometer in clinical laboratories. As with the other refractometers discussed, it measures the critical angle. Total solids meters can be calibrated in degrees, refractive index units, protein solids concentration, solids concentration, or specific gravity. Numerous studies have established the relationships between refractive index and these other values.

The TS meter requires only a drop of sample for ordinary use. It can also be used as a dipping refractometer. When analyzing a small sample, a drop of liquid is drawn into the space between the cover plate and the refracting prism cover glass by capillary action (Fig. 5-9). The instrument is then exposed to an external light source, which can be either natural or artificial illumination. Rotating the eyepiece brings the light-dark boundary into focus. Readings are taken from the scale visible through the eyepiece.

The TS meter incorporates a temperature-compensating liquid in a sealed chamber. This provides effective compensation for aqueous solutions at temperatures of 15 to 37°C. The liquid-filled chamber lies between the prism cover glass and the front of the measuring prism. The refractive index of this liquid varies with the temperature. This variation in refractive index with temperature changes the deflection of the light rays in such a way as to compensate for temperature changes in the refractive index of the aqueous sample. To allow for thermal expansion, an air bubble is placed in the temperature-compensating liquid. The air bubble is kept out of the optical path by a bubble trap at the base of the chamber (Fig. 5-9).

When a small sample is used, temperature equilibration between the sample and the TS meter occurs almost instantaneously. However, when it is used as a dipping refractometer, several minutes must be allowed for thermal equilibration.

Total solids meters have an accuracy of 0.0001 refractive index units. They are widely used in clinical laboratories because of their low cost, durability, precision, accuracy, and ease of operation.

Maintenance and Quality Assurance

Refractometers are precise optical instruments. All optical surfaces must be kept scrupulously clean for accurate results. External optical surfaces should be inspected for scratches and abrasions and polished or replaced when necessary.

Temperature control is important in refractometry of liquid samples. For assays done at ambient temperatures, adequate time must be given for temperature equilibration. This is especially important for immersion refractometry. To achieve high accuracy and precision, the room temperature must be accurately measured, and temperature correction tables should be consulted. The room itself should not be subject to rapid changes in temperature. Temperature measurements should be made with a liquid-in-glass thermometer that has been calibrated with a NIST-certified thermometer. Calibrated thermometers should also be used to measure the temperature of circulating fluid in refractometers with constant-temperature baths.

Refractometer calibration should be checked regularly. Weekly monitoring is suggested.[3] This is usually accomplished by measuring the refractive index of distilled water ("zero" standard) and of a liquid standard with a high refractive index. Again, temperature must be known and controlled. The scale should be adjusted based on the expected refractive indices of the two standards at the measured temperature.

Summary

Refractometry is the measurement of the refractive index of liquids or homogenous solids. The refractive index of a substance is related to the decrease in velocity of a monochromatic light beam passing through the substance. The refractive index is a fixed property of a substance if temperature and wavelength are not varied.

Most refractometry is based on measuring the critical angle of a substance. The critical angle is the angle of refraction resulting from a light ray grazing the flat surface of a substance (90° angle of incident light).

Most refractometers contain a light source, a temperature control or temperature compensation device, a refracting prism, focusing optics, and a readout device or scale. The light source for many refractometers is ambient light or an ordinary light bulb. Some refractometers have no device for controlling temperature or for compensating for different ambient temperatures. These refractometers are restricted to use at selected temperatures.

The four major types of refractometers are Abbé, Pulfrich, immersion, and total solids. All but the Pulfrich types are commonly found in clinical laboratories. If temperature is precisely controlled, immersion refractometers provide the best accuracy and precision for liquid samples. However, unlike the other refractometers, immersion types require large sample volumes.

Refractometers are precise optical instruments that require regular cleaning, inspection, and calibration.

Questions and Problems

1. A light beam strikes the surface of a solution at 30° from the perpendicular. It is bent to 22°. What is the refractive index of the solution?
2. The critical angle of a transparent solid is 47°. What is the refractive index of the solid?
3. Draw and label the components of a refractometer. Indicate the light path through the refractometer.
4. What is the purpose of an Amici compensator?
5. Why is it important to control (or at least to know) the temperature of the refractometer and the liquid sample?
6. Describe how to calibrate a refractometer.

References

1. Skoog DA, Leary JJ. Principles of instrumental analysis, 4th ed. Fort Worth: Saunders College Publishing, 1992:67-86.
2. Willard HH, Merritt LL Jr, Dean JA. Instrumental methods of analysis, 5th ed. New York: D Van Nostrand, 1974:420-27.
3. Schumann GB, Schweitzer SC. Examination of urine. In: Kaplan LA, Pesce AJ, eds. Clinical chemistry: Theory, analysis, and correlation, 2nd ed. St. Louis: CV Mosby, 1989:820-49.

Suggested Readings

Bender GT. Principles of chemical instrumentation. Philadelphia: WB Saunders, 1987:124-39.
Schumann GB, Schweitzer SC. Examination of urine. In: Henry JB, ed. Clinical diagnosis and management by laboratory methods. Philadelphia: WB Saunders, 1991:387-44.
Strasinger SK. Urinalysis and body fluids, 2nd ed. Philadelphia: FA Davis, 1989:42-53.

6

SPECTROPHOTOMETRY

Vicki S. Freeman

Objectives

After completing this chapter, the reader will be able to:

1. Discuss the relationship of electromagnetic radiation to wavelength and frequency.
2. Differentiate between light emission, light reflection, and light transmittance.
3. Discuss how Beer's law relates to Lambert's law.
4. Explain the relationship between each of the following:
   a. Color and wavelength
   b. Absorbance and concentration
   c. Transmittance and concentration
   d. Transmittance and absorbance
   e. Path length and transmittance
5. Use Beer's law to calculate the following:
   a. Molar absorptivity
   b. Absorbance
   c. Concentration
   d. Light path
   e. Transmittance
6. Calculate the concentration of a sample using the one standard method.
7. Construct graphs of calibration curves of both absorbance and transmittance using either linear or semilog paper.
8. Discuss conditions that produce deviations in Beer's law and how to correct for them.
9. Explain the functions of the light source, monochromator, sample holder, detector, and readout device in a photometric instrument.

10. Identify the appropriate use for each type of radiant energy source.
11. Compare the three monochromator systems: filter, prism, and diffraction grating.
12. Differentiate between a photocell and a photomultiplier tube.
13. Differentiate between a photometer and a spectrophotometer.
14. Compare the three categories of photometric instruments: single beam, double beam, and dual wavelength.
15. Draw a diagram of a single-beam spectrophotometer.
16. Draw a diagram of a double-beam spectrophotometer.
17. Discuss the advantages of double-beam and dual-wavelength photometers.
18. Formulate a quality assurance program for a photometric instrument.

Definitions[1]

Absorbance (A):   The amount of light retained by a solution or substance. It is equal to the base 10 logarithm of the reciprocal of the transmittance.

Absorption: Capture of a photon by an atom or molecule. The energy of the captured photon results in excitation.

Absorption band: Region of the absorption spectrum in which the absorptivity passes through a maximum or inflection.

Absorption spectrum: A plot of absorption (absorbance) as a function of wavelength.

Absorptivity (a):   The ratio of the absorbance to the product of concentration and optical path length.

Absorptivity, Molar (e):   The absorptivity expressed in units of liter/(mole-cm).

Band pass: Total wavelength range emerging from the monochromator exit slit.

Beer's Law: The relationship between absorption of a beam of parallel, monochromatic radiation in a homogeneous, isotropic medium and concentration of the absorbing substance.

Colorimetry: Determination of analyte concentration by measurement of visible light absorption.

Dispersion: Separation of a polychromatic light beam into many monochromatic beams, as with a prism.

Frequency (v):   Number of cycles of electromagnetic radiation passing a fixed point per unit time.

Light: Radiant energy in a spectral range visible to the normal human eye (380–700 nm).

Nanometer (nm):   The international unit of wavelength measurement, equal to 10^{-9}m.

Photometry: Measurement of transmitted, absorbed, or reflected light.

Radiant Energy: Energy transmitted as electromagnetic radiation.

Spectral bandwidth: The wavelength interval of the light leaving the exit slit of a monochromator at a radiant power level halfway between the background and the peak of the absorption band.

Stray light: Radiation that reaches the detector at wavelengths that do not correspond to the spectral position under consideration or from sources other than light passing through or emitted from the sample.

Transmittance: The ratio of the intensity of light transmitted (I) through the sample to the initial intensity of the light beam (I_0).

Transmittance, % (% T):   Transmittance in units of percent: $100\% \times I/I_0$.

Wavelength (λ):   The distance between two points that are in phase on adjacent waves.

Introduction

Many of the traditional clinical chemistry methods are based on the quantitative measurement of light transmitted through a colored substance. This analytical method is called *colorimetry* and the measurement *photometry*. This transmitted light is measured by instruments called *photometers* and *spectrophotometers*. In this chapter we discuss the basic principles of electromagnetic radiation, Beer's law and its derivations and conditions for validity, the components and categories of photometric instruments, and quality assurance and routine maintenance of photometric instruments. In colorimetry, a colored solution absorbs electromagnetic radiation energy from a light source. The amount of energy absorbed is related to the concentration of the absorbing substance(s).

Principles

ELECTROMAGNETIC RADIATION

To understand spectrophotometry, we must first understand the basics of *electromagnetic radiation* and the electromagnetic light spectrum. Electromagnetic radiation has dual properties. It possesses a certain amount of energy. This energy travels in sine waves in the form of small particles of energy called *photons*. The energy of each photon is not the same. The energy contained in a photon is directly proportional to the frequency of the electromagnetic wave. The total energy in a beam of electromagnetic radiation is the sum of the energies of its photons.[2]

Equation 6-1 shows the relationship of the wave's frequency and the wavelength to the amount of energy (E):

$$E = h\nu, \text{ but } \nu = c/\nu \qquad \text{(Eq. 6-1)}$$

$$E = hc/\lambda \qquad \text{(Eq. 6-2)}$$

where

h = Planck's constant $(6.62 \times 10^{-27} \text{ erg-s})$
ν = frequency (s^{-1})
c = speed of light $(3 \times 10^8 \text{ m/s})$
λ = wavelength (m)

Energy is directly related to the frequency and inversely related to the wavelength. The frequency is the number of cycles per second. Each complete cycle equals one wavelength (Fig. 6-1).

Therefore, carrying the calculations further, the relationship between wavelength and frequency is an inversely proportional one:

$$\lambda = c/\nu \qquad \text{(Eq. 6-3)}$$

The electromagnetic spectrum consists of different-size wavelengths—from short, high-energy radiation to long, low-energy radiation. This energy is related to the frequency and wavelength of the electromagnetic spectrum. Light is just one form of energy in this spectrum.

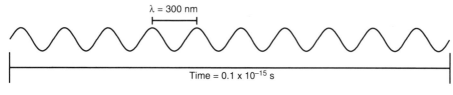

$\lambda = 300$ nm

Time = 0.1×10^{-15} s

$\nu = 10$ cycles/$(0.1 \times 10^{-15}$ s$) = 1 \times 10^{17}$

Figure 6-1. Single wave of light. Ten complete cycles occur in only 0.1×10^{-15} seconds. Therefore, the frequency is 1×10^{17} cycles/s. The length of a single cycle (wavelength) is 300 nm.

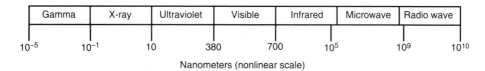

Gamma	X-ray	Ultraviolet	Visible	Infrared	Microwave	Radio wave

10^{-5} 10^{-1} 10 380 700 10^5 10^9 10^{10}

Nanometers (nonlinear scale)

Figure 6-2. Wavelengths of seven types of electromagnetic radiation. The scale is not linear. Gamma rays have the shortest wavelengths and, therefore, the highest frequencies and energies. Radio waves are longest (over 1 meter) and have the lowest frequencies and energies. Visible light includes only 320 nanometers of this displayed spectrum ranging from 10^{-5} to 10^{10} nanometers.

Figure 6-2 shows the electromagnetic spectrum in terms of approximate wavelengths. The divisions overlap because there is no sharp dividing line between each kind of wave. The international unit for wavelength measurement is the nanometer (nm), 10^{-9} meters.

The visible region (from approximately 380–700 nm) is the area seen by the human eye. The shortest wavelength corresponds to the color violet and the longest to the color red. White light is a continuous spectrum of wavelengths.

Three processes determine the color of an object or solution: light emission, light reflection, and light transmission/absorption. In light emission, a compound is excited by absorbing energy from a light source. This energy is then released as emitted photons that return the compound to its ground, unexcited state. This process is used in flame emission photometry and fluorescence.

In light reflection, a nontransparent object absorbs all the wavelengths in the spectrum except for the ones we see. The object reflects the wavelengths that we interpret as color. A black object absorbs all visible light; a white object reflects all visible light.

When white (polychromatic) light passes through a solution, the solution absorbs certain wavelengths and allows the unabsorbed wavelengths to be transmitted. This is called *light transmittance* or *absorption*. The color of the substance visible to the eye is the light that is transmitted by the solution. This color is complementary to the

Table 6-1
Complementary Colors and Their Wavelengths

Color of Solution in White Light	Color Absorbed	Wavelength Absorbed (nm)
Green-yellow	Violet	400–440
Yellow	Blue	440–475
Red	Blue-green	475–490
Purple	Green	490–570
Blue	Yellow	570–600
Green-blue	Orange	600–650
Green	Red	650–700

absorbed colors. Table 6-1 shows the relationships between solution color, absorbed color, and wavelengths in the visible spectrum.

An example of this transmittance is a solution of copper. The copper solution appears blue because it absorbs the complementary color yellow from white light and transmits the remaining blue light. Measurement of this transmitted light is called colorimetry.

LAMBERT'S LAW

Lambert in the 1700s discovered that when monochromatic light interacts with an absorbing material, the transmittance varies with the thickness of the material. Equation 6-4 predicts this interaction.

$$I = I_0 e^{-kx}$$

(Eq. 6-4)

where

I = intensity of transmitted light*
I_0 = intensity of incident light
k = absorption coefficient
x = thickness of material

As the thickness (x) increases, the transmittance decreases.

In the 1800s, Beer applied Lambert's findings to spectrophotometry. In spectrophotometry, the light that passes through the solution is monochromatic. This means that the light transmitted and measured is of only one wavelength. When this beam of light, called the *incident radiant energy* (I_0), passes through the solution, some of that light is absorbed. The rest of the light is transmitted (Fig. 6-3). The intensity of this transmittance (I) will be less than the original intensity (I_0).

---

*Intensity of light is also known as radiant power (P).

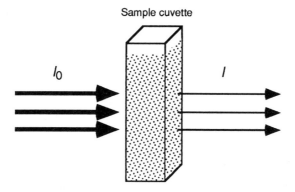

Figure 6-3.   Light from the source has initial intensity I_0. Because of absorption by the sample, the intensity of exiting light (I) is reduced.

The ratio of radiant energy transmitted by the solution to the radiant energy incident on the solution is called the *transmittance* ($T = I/I_0$). The relationship between absorbance and concentration is described in the following section.

BEER'S LAW

Beer's law states that the amount of light absorbed is proportional to the number of molecules in the absorbing substance through which the light passes. Therefore, the concentration of a substance in solution is directly proportional to the amount of light absorbed. The concentration is logarithmically and inversely proportional to the amount of light transmitted.

The amount of light absorbed, called *absorption* (A or ABS), is directly proportional to the concentration (c) of the compound in solution, as well as the molar absorptivity (a) of the solution, and path length (b) through the solution.

$$A = abc \qquad \text{(Eq. 6-5)}$$

The relationship between absorbance and transmittance is a mathematical one and is calculated as follows:

$$I = I_0\, 10^{-abc} \qquad \text{(Eq. 6-6)}$$

But I is the percentage of light transmitted after absorption, and I_0 is the incident light of 100% transmittance. Substituting these values into Equation 6-6 gives:

$$\% \, T = 100\% \, 10^{-abc} \qquad \text{(Eq. 6-7)}$$

Taking the log of both sides of the equation and rearranging Equation 6-7 yields

$$\log \% \, T = \log 100 \, (-abc) \qquad \text{(Eq. 6-8)}$$

After rearrangement, Equation 6-8 becomes

$$abc = \log 100 - \log \% \, T \qquad \text{(Eq. 6-9)}$$

or

$$abc = 2 - \log (\% \, T) = A \qquad \text{(Eq. 6-10)}$$

where

A = absorbance
a = molar absorptivity (L/gm/cm)
b = optical path length (cm) of cuvette
c = concentration (gm/L, mg/mL)

Looking at Equations 6-5 through 6-10, we see that increased concentration results in increased absorption and decreased transmittance. The decrease in percentage transmittance varies inversely and logarithmically with the concentration (Fig. 6-4a).

If the pathlength (b) and the absorptivity (a) are constant, then the concentration and absorbance are directly related. Absorptivity is a property of the chosen wavelength and the compound being measured. If the path length is doubled, then twice as many molecules are in the light path. The absorption doubles, but the concentration remains the same. Usually, in spectrophotometry in the clinical laboratory, path length and absorptivity are constants, and the only variable is the concentration of the standards and unknowns.

Beer's law allows the determination of the concentration of unknown samples. To calculate the concentration of the unknowns, the absorbances of standards of known concentration are measured, then plotted on graph paper. As absorbance versus concentration has a linear relationship, a straight line will be obtained when plotted on linear graph paper (Fig. 6-4b). The concentration of the unknowns can then be read off of this graph.

Since $\% \, T$ versus concentration is a nonlinear relationship, a curved line will be produced when plotted on linear graph paper. To obtain a straight line, the concentration and $\% \, T$ values must be plotted on semilogarithmic graph paper.

The linear relationship between absorbance and concentration allows for an easier method to calculate unknown concentrations. If the substance being measured follows Beer's law, we can calculate unknown concentrations using a single standard and the following proportion:

$$A_{Standard}/A_{Unknown} = c_{Standard}/c_{Unknown} \qquad \text{(Eq. 6-11)}$$

Remember, this relationship is valid only if Beer's law is being followed.

Conditions of Beer's Law

The following conditions must be met for Beer's law to be valid: (1) Absorbances must be in the linear range. In general, absorbance readings between 0.05 and 2.0 are best. If high concentrations are being measured (outside the linearity of the test), the solution must be diluted to obtain accurate measurements. If the concentration is too

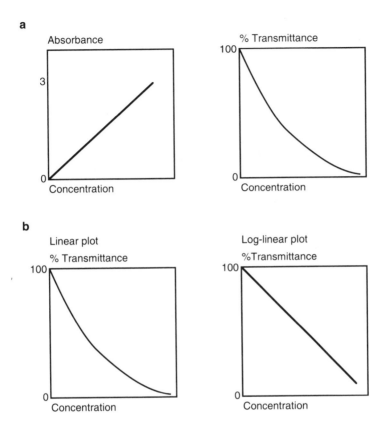

Figure 6-4. (a) The relationships between concentration and absorbance is linear for a substance obeying Beer's law. The relationship between transmittance (or percentage of transmittance) in nonlinear. (b) The percentage of transmittance plot from Figure 6-4a is shown alongside a log-linear plot made on semilogarithmic graphing paper. The result is a straight line for substances obeying Beer's law.

dilute, imprecision of measurements make the results less reliable. (2) The light passing through the solution must be monochromatic. Light can be nonmonochromatic when the spectral bandwidth of the instrument is too broad or when stray light is being detected. Stray light is radiant energy that reaches the detector without passing through the sample. Stray light can arise from scatter and diffraction inside the monochromator or from outside light reaching the detector. The intensity of the stray light is added to that of the transmitted light. The stray light falsely reduces the absorbance readings, thereby decreasing the calculated sample concentration in a nonlinear fashion.

Absorbance of light by other substances will cause errors. Some light is lost because of absorption by the sample holder or the solvent. Light transmitted through the sample can also be reflected from the inner surface of the sample holder.

Reflection or absorption by the sample holder are minimized by the use of cuvettes with parallel sides. Solvent absorption is minimized by the use of a blank consisting of the reagents in the procedure instead of just water or air.

Measurement of absorbance is most reliable at the optimum wavelength for the sample. This optimum wavelength is usually the absorption maximum of the sample. This wavelength is determined by performing an absorption spectrum on the compound to be measured. This absorption spectrum is characteristic of the absorbing compound. The wavelength that gives the highest absorbance reading (the peak absorption) is the absorption maximum for a given solution.

To determine the optimal wavelength several factors must be taken into consideration. These include the absorption maximum of the compound to be measured, the shape of the absorption peak, and the absorption spectra of any interfering substances (Fig. 6-5). Small deviations in wavelength or a widened bandpass produce little measurement error if the compound has a broad absorption peak. However, when the absorption peak is sharp, a small deviation in wavelength may produce a large measurement error because the reading will be taken on the slope rather than on the peak. Spectrophotometer measurements are usually made at the peak of the broadest absorption curve.

If another chemical compound (an interfering substance) absorbs at the same wavelength as the compound of interest, then an alternate wavelength must be chosen. This wavelength could be a different absorbance peak, if the compound of interest has more than one peak, or any other absorbing wavelength where the slope of the absorbance spectrum is low. Another method for measuring concentration in the presence of an interfering substance is to use a dual-wavelength instrument. Dual-wavelength photometry is discussed below under Categories of Photometric Instruments.

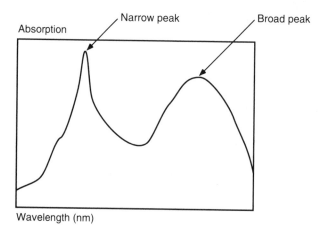

Figure 6-5. An absorption spectrum demonstrating a sharp or narrow peak at one wavelength and a broad peak at another. Wavelength selection accuracy must be high to use the sharp peak for determining concentration.

MEASUREMENT OF CONCENTRATION

Once the absorption spectrum of a compound has been obtained and the optimum wavelength to be used has been determined, a photometric method may be devised to measure concentrations.

The initial measurement of concentration requires a blank and a series of standards. Ideally, the blank consists of all of the constituents used in the analysis except the substance to be measured. It can then be assumed that the differences in light transmittance between the blank and the sample specimens are due only to that substance. The standards are known concentrations of the substance to be measured. The monochromator is adjusted to select the chosen wavelength for the analysis. The blank is inserted, and the absorbance readout of the spectrophotometer is adjusted to 0.000 (100% T). The absorbance or % T readings for each standard and then each unknown are recorded. A linear curve is made by plotting absorbance versus each standard's concentration (or transmittance versus concentration on semilog graph paper). The concentrations of the unknowns are determined from their absorbances by reading their corresponding concentrations from the plot. (Alternatively, an equation of the form $y = mx + b$ can be used. The unknown concentration $[x]$ is equal to its absorbance reading $[y]$, minus the intercept $[b]$, divided by the slope of the line $[m]$.)

Reflectance Spectroscopy

The concentration of a substance can also be determined by measuring light reflectance. Light striking a substance can be absorbed, transmitted, scattered, or reflected. The sum of all reflected light is the total reflectance (R_T). Reflectance (R) is the ratio of reflected light to incident light: $R = R_T/I_0$.

In reflectance spectroscopy, only a portion of the reflected light is measured. This depends on instrument design. Since R_T is not measured, the reflectance of an unknown substance is related to that of a known standard. The relationship is given in Equation 6-12.

$$R = R'/R'_{std} \qquad\qquad\qquad \text{(Eq. 6-12)}$$

where

R = reflectance
R' = measured reflectance of sample
R_{std} = measured reflectance of standard

Instruments that measure reflected light are known as *reflectometers* or *reflectance densitometers*. The concentration of a substance is inversely and logarithmically related to the reflectance. The negative logarithm of reflectance is known as the reflectance density (D_r). This is similar to the relationship between absorbance and transmittance. A typical plot of concentration versus reflectance density is shown in Figure 6-6. Standard curves are used to determine the concentration of an unknown from measurement of its reflectance density. This will be discussed in more detail in Chapter 18, under EKTACHEM analyzers.

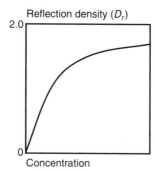

Figure 6-6. The relationship between reflection density and concentration is always nonlinear. In many cases it is not log-linear either.

Photometric Instruments

COMPONENT PARTS

The component parts of a spectrophotometer are a light source, monochromator, sample holder, detector, and readout device.

Light Source

The light source provides radiant energy over the wavelengths of interest. For work in the visible range, a tungsten-filament lamp has adequate output from 360 to 800 nm. This lamp may also be used for near infrared (IR) and ultraviolet (UV) ranges. Halogen lamps made with quartz iodide (which doesn't absorb in the UV range) can be used for a wider spectrum (290-800 nm). For work in lower UV ranges (200-375 nm), a hydrogen or deuterium lamp is needed. Deuterium lamps have absorption peaks at 486 nm and 656 nm that are used for wavelength calibration.

Monochromator

A *monochromator* isolates the desired wavelength and excludes all others. It does this by limiting which wavelengths from the light source will pass through or by dispersing the light and selecting the desired wavelength with slits.

The simplest monochromator is a filter that allows only discrete wavelengths to pass. An instrument that uses filters is called a *photometer.* There are two types of filters. Selective transmittance filters, such as Wratten-colored gelatin and colored glass filters, have a wide bandwidth (30-60 nm). They absorb all radiation except that of the specified wavelengths. Glass filters use two pieces of colored glass to absorb wavelengths on either side of the selected wavelength. Interference filters are made of multiple layers of reflective and transparent materials with selective refractive indices (Fig. 6-7). Light reaching the filter bounces off the reflective surfaces and is

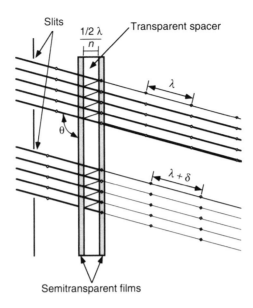

Figure 6-7. Interference filter designed to pass light of wavelength λ. Partial reflectance within the filter allows wavelengths that are multiples of λ to pass without interference. Light of longer or shorter wavelengths will be subjected to destructive interference.

refracted by the transparent material many times before exiting.[3] The peak wavelength of the exit beam can be calculated from Equation 6-13:

$$m\lambda = 2\,dN\,(\sin\theta) \tag{Eq. 6-13}$$

where

    m = order of diffraction pattern $(1, 2, 3, \ldots)$
    d = thickness of transparent layer
    N = refractive index of transparent layer
    θ = angle of incidence (usually $90°$)

Interference filters have a narrower bandwidth (5-15 nm) than glass or gelatin filters. Sharp cutoff filters are used to restrict incident light.

In contrast to filters, which block out unwanted wavelengths, prisms and gratings provide a continuous range of wavelengths. They disperse the polychromatic source light by refraction or diffraction. Instruments that use prisms or gratings are called *spectrophotometers.*

Prisms disperse white light into a series of wavelengths by refraction (Fig. 6-8). The angle of deviation depends on the wavelength. Red light deviates the least, violet the most. If projected on a plane surface, the light is spread with the shorter wavelengths at one end and the longer wavelengths at the other. The distribution of

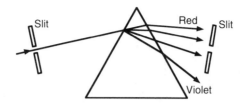

Figure 6-8. Light dispersion by a prism. The exit slit is selecting blue light. Note that the amount of bending increases from red through violet.

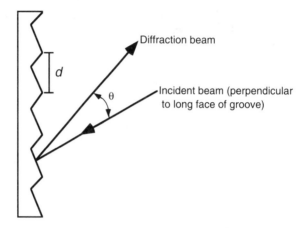

Figure 6-9. Portion of a diffraction grating. This grating is set up with the incident beam perpendicular to the diffracting face of the groove.

the wavelengths from a prism is more condensed at the red end than at the violet end. This property is known as a *nonlinear dispersion*. Prisms in a spectrophotometer are rotated to allow the wavelength of choice to pass through the exit slit.

    Diffraction gratings consist of many equally spaced parallel grooves etched on a glass or aluminum plate (Fig. 6-9). The gratings act as scattering centers for the rays of light. Each groove produces diffracted waves of light. The waves produced must travel different distances before reaching a specified point. The spacing and angle of the gratings determine the spectral bandwidth and the wavelength of the beam of light produced. The general equation for the wavelength of light diffracted by a grating is:

$$m\lambda = d\,(\sin\theta) \tag{Eq. 6-14}$$

where

        m = order of diffraction pattern (usually $1, 2, 3, \ldots$)
        λ = wavelength (nm)
        d = distance between gratings (nm)
        θ = angle of diffraction beam (deviation)

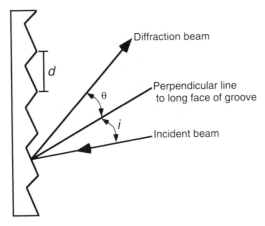

Figure 6-10. Portion of a diffraction grating. This grating is set up with the incident beam at any angle to the diffracting face of the groove.

Diffraction gratings produce integer multiples (m) of each wavelength. The distance between the gratings (d) is not usually given. Instead, the number of gratings per centimeter is recorded. Distance between gratings is calculated by taking the inverse of the gratings/cm and multiplying it by 10^7 (to convert the distance to nanometers).

The above equation assumes that the incident light is perpendicular to the surface of the diffraction grating. If the light strikes at any other angle (Fig. 6-10), the equation becomes:

$$m\lambda = d\,(\sin i + \sin \theta) \tag{Eq. 6-15}$$

where i = angle of incidence beam to perpendicular line of grating.

By passing the incident beam of light through a narrow slit, diffraction gratings achieve a much higher resolution (narrower bandpass) than other monochromators. Unlike with prisms and interference filters, all wavelengths are equally dispersed (linear dispersion). As with prisms, the grating is rotated so that the exit slot will pick up the desired wavelength. However, first-order, second-order, and third-order multiples of each wavelength are produced by diffraction gratings. Cutoff filters are used to isolate the desired multiple of the wavelength.

Prism and grating monochromators have entrance and exit slits. The entrance slit focuses light from the source lamp onto the monochromator. The entrance slit also collimates the light (makes it parallel) and reduces stray light. The exit slit determines the bandwidth of light that will be selected from the dispersed spectrum. Widening the slit allows more light to reach the specimen, but it also increases the bandpass, which may produce a condition in which Beer's law no longer holds.

The spectral bandwidths of monochromators have been referred to a number of times. What exactly is a spectral bandwidth? In spectrophotometry, the light that is transmitted and measured is monochromatic. In actual practice, monochromators

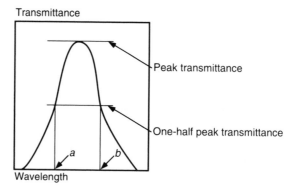

Figure 6-11.   Spectrum of light admitted by the exit slit of a monochromator. The wavelength scale is in nanometers. The width of the peak at half its height is the spectral bandwidth $(b - a)$.

allow a narrow range of wavelengths to reach the specimen. This range of wavelengths is referred to as the spectral bandwidth of the instrument or slit width, because the size of the slit affects the bandwidth. Spectral bandwidth is the difference, in nanometers, of the high and low wavelengths corresponding to half the peak height of the spectral transmittance curve (Fig. 6-11).[4]

A spectrophotometer with a narrow spectral bandwidth will produce high-resolution absorbance spectra and excellent linearity (due to a reduction in non-monochromatic light passing through the specimen). A narrow spectral bandwidth also allows analyses of compounds with sharp absorption peaks. In general, if the spectral bandwidth is less than one-tenth the width of the compound's absorption peak, then the spectrophotometer is sensitive enough for measurement of the compound.[5]

Sample Holder

Most specimens for photometric instruments are solutions. Therefore, most sample holders are built to hold cuvettes or flow cells. Some instruments have two holders, one for the sample and one for the blank. The cuvettes must be transparent across the wavelength region being measured. Glass cuvettes are transparent from 320 to 950 nm. However, because glass absorbs UV light, quartz cuvettes are used below 320 nm. The best cuvettes have flat surfaces. Rounded surfaces, such as those on test tubes, produce more stray light. Cuvettes must be clean and clear of fingerprints and scratches.

Flow cells also hold solutions. They are enclosed devices that allow liquid to flow into and out of the optical portion of the cell. Flow cells are used in semiautomated and automated photometers.

Plastic or metal racks hold solid samples such as glass filters or plastic electrophoresis plates. The racks may have one or more openings to admit light from the monochromator.

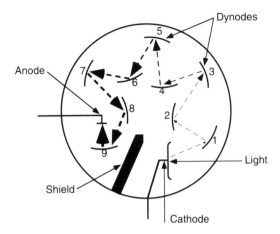

Figure 6-12. Partial schematic of a photomultiplier tube. Photons strike the cathode and transfer energy to free some electrons. These electrons are emitted and are passed on to a series of successively more positively charged dynodes (nine in this example). The number of emitted electrons increases by about a factor of 5 at each dynode (a total multiplication of about 2 million in this example).

Detector and Readout Device

The most commonly used types of radiant energy detectors are barrier layer cells and photomultiplier tubes. Detectors react to the light passing through the sample. The energy of the photons is converted to electrical energy by the detector. The electrical energy is sent to the readout device, which converts it to absorbance, transmittance, or concentration.

Barrier layer cells (photo cells) are composed of a crystal layer of cadmium or selenium on an iron backing. Photons strike the crystal layer, excite the selenium or cadmium, and release electrons. If the light intensity is great enough, a flow of electrons is produced. This electron flow (current) is proportional to the number of photons striking the detector. One drawback to the use of barrier layer cells is their slow response time.

Photomultiplier tubes (see Chapter 1) are electron tubes that amplify current (Fig. 6-12). Photons strike the cathode, which then emits electrons in an amount proportional to the energy of the photons. The emitted electrons jump to a positively charged dynode. The dynode then emits 4 to 6 electrons for every electron striking it. These emitted electrons are passed to the next dynode, which is more positively charged than the first. The number of emitted electrons is multiplied by each dynode. Finally, the electrons are collected at the anode. Photomultiplier tubes are very sensitive to low light intensities, and they have a fast response time.

A readout device picks up the electrical signal generated by either type of detector. The readout device may be analog (a scale) or digital (a light-emitting diode or a number sent to a screen or computer).

Figure 6-13 shows an analog photometer readout. The scale shows both absorbance

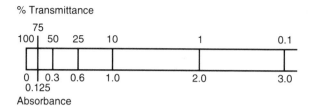

Figure 6-13.   Spectrophotometer readout scale that is linear for absorbance and logarithmic for transmittance.

and percent transmittance. Many instruments with digital readouts allow the operator to select absorbance, transmittance, or concentration units.

Categories of Photometric Instruments

Two basic types of instruments are available for measuring transmitted light: photometers and spectrophotometers. The difference is in the type of monochromator. Photometers have filters for wavelength selection. Spectrophotometers have prism or diffraction grating monochromators with entrance and exit slits. Both types of instrument are available in single-beam, double-beam, and dual-wavelength configurations.

SINGLE-BEAM SPECTROPHOTOMETERS

A *single-beam spectrophotometer* has one light path that passes from the light source through the monochromator system and sample cuvette and then to the detector (Fig. 6-14). A blank is used to set the instrument to 100% T (0 A), then the samples are read. Interferences from sample turbidity and light intensity changes from the radiant source and other instrument fluctuations are not compensated.

DOUBLE-BEAM SPECTROPHOTOMETER

A *double-beam spectrophotometer* has two light paths, both originating from the same light source (Fig. 6-15). One path is for the sample and the other for the blank or reference. The beam from the source strikes a vibrating or rotating mirror that alternately directs light through the reference cell and the sample cell. Light passing through each cell is sent to the detector. Two arrangements are available. In the double-beam-in-time spectrophotometer, the light source is alternated between sample and reference cells. This is usually achieved by placing a rotating mirror/chopper just past the exit slit of the monochromator. Light from each beam alternately strikes the detector. The detector output is an alternating signal with an amplitude proportional to the ratio of the intensities of the sample and reference beams. In the double-beam-in-space spectrophotometer, two detectors are present, one for light transmitted through the sample cell, the other for light transmitted through the reference cell. The readout device converts the electrical signals from each detector

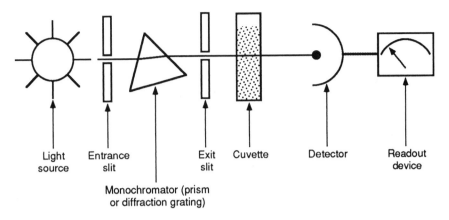

Figure 6-14. Single-beam spectrophotometer.

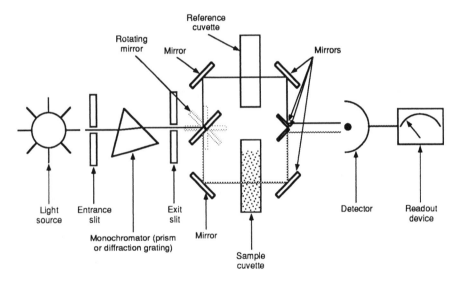

Figure 6-15. Double-beam spectrophotometer. A rotating mirror alternately sends monochromatic light to the sample or reference chambers.

to absorbance units. The ratio of the absorbances of the two beams is commonly displayed. However, most instruments allow the two signals to be added, subtracted, or presented in other fashions.

Double-beam systems automatically correct for changes in light intensity from the radiant source, fluctuations in instrument electronics, and absorption by the blank.[6] Scanning, double-beam spectrophotometers allow easy determination of a spectral transmittance curve.

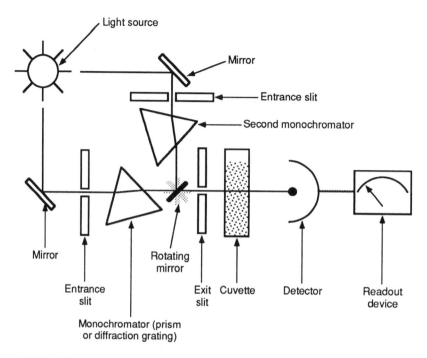

Figure 6-16. Dual-wavelength spectrophotometer. Two monochromators are present. A rotating mirror allows alternating signals from each monochromator to pass through the sample.

DUAL-WAVELENGTH SPECTROPHOTOMETER

A *dual-wavelength spectrophotometer* allows simultaneous measurement of a sample at two different wavelengths (Fig. 6-16). Two monochromators are present. A vibrating mirror or a rotating chopper is used to select either (or both) light beam(s). Other components in a dual-wavelength spectrophotometer are the same as in a single- or double-beam system. A reference and a measurement wavelength are used. In the most commonly used type, the reference wavelength is used to compensate for an interfering substance. The reference wavelength (λ_r) is chosen such that the absorbance of the interfering substance is the same as it is at the sample wavelength (λ_s). As long as the sample absorbs significantly more at λ_s than at λ_r, this method will completely compensate for the interference. The reference absorbance is subtracted from the sample absorbance to obtain the corrected value. This type of dual-wavelength procedure is used to measure neonatal bilirubin in the presence of hemoglobin. The sample wavelength is 453 nm; the reference wavelength is 540 nm. Hemoglobin's molar absorptivity is the same at both wavelengths; bilirubin absorbance at 540 nm is only about one-eighth its absorbance at 453 nm. Therefore, the reference absorbance can be subtracted from the sample absorbance, and the concentration of bilirubin can be calculated.

Maintenance and Quality Assurance

Quality assurance procedures are used to ensure consistent and reliable instrument performance, so that current results may confidently be compared with past or future results. Photometers and spectrophotometers must be regularly checked for wavelength accuracy, linearity, stray light, and photometric accuracy. These checks will ensure the accuracy and precision of spectrophotometric measurements. These instrument checks are performed in addition to standard methodological quality control and calibration procedures.

WAVELENGTH ACCURACY

Wavelength accuracy is important, especially when using a narrow bandpass instrument to measure a substance with a relatively sharp absorbance peak. Small errors in wavelength selection can then result in large errors in measured absorbance.[7] The best method for checking the accuracy of wavelength selection involves temporary replacement of the source lamp with a radiant energy source with strong emission lines (such as a mercury vapor lamp). Alternate methods use rare earth glass filters (holmium oxide or didymium) or solutions such as nickel sulfate ($NiSO_4$). ($NiSO_4$ is more commonly used as a secondary wavelength calibration standard after the wavelength accuracy has been checked with a primary calibration standard.) Accuracy should be checked at multiple wavelengths. At least three wavelengths should be used to calibrate instruments with prism monochromators. At least two points should be used for instruments with diffraction gratings.

Wavelength checks using a didymium filter are performed at 610 nm. The reading at this wavelength should be approximately 45% *T*. Other transmittance peaks should occur at 573, 586, and 685 nm.[8]

Wavelength calibration checks using $NiSO_4$ are made at 400, 460, 510, 550, and 700 nm against an HCl blank. The 510-nm wavelength is the maximum transmittance peak of $NiSO_4$. The 460- and 550-nm wavelengths on either side of the transmittance peak ensure wavelength accuracy and instrument linearity. The transmittances of the two wavelengths should have a 2:1 ratio. Inaccurate wavelength selection will result in a change in the transmittance: increased transmittance indicates that the actual wavelength is lower than the selected wavelength (and vice versa). A nonlinear instrument response will result in a change from the expected transmittance. The 400- and 700-nm wavelengths are outside the spectral transmittance curve of nickel sulfate; they are used to measure stray light (see Stray Light section).

If the wavelength calibration is off, realigning the source lamp will sometimes solve the problem. Another cause of wavelength selection inaccuracies is misalignment of the monochromator or its optics. If wavelength error is constant across the spectrum, the operator can correct for it manually.

LINEARITY OF INSTRUMENT

The determination of the linearity of detector response may be checked with solid glass filters or a solution that follows Beer's law. The purpose is to check for the accuracy of the absorbance versus concentration.

Linearity checks using cobalt ammonium sulfate ($CoSO_4 \cdot (NH_4)_2SO_4 \cdot 6H_2O$) are performed by using concentrations of 2, 4, 6, 8 and 10 g/100 ml of 1% sulfuric acid. (Note: These solutions must be made using scrupulously clean volumetric glassware and pipets. Otherwise what is being checked is the accuracy and precision of the person making the standards, not the linearity of the spectrophotometer.) The absorbances at 512 nm should be approximately 0.25, 0.50, 0.75, 1.00, and 1.25. Linearity is evaluated by plotting absorbance versus concentration.

A nonlinear response for a plot of absorbance versus concentration indicates either an error in preparation of the standards or an instrument problem. Nonlinear instrument response can be due to a faulty detector, stray light, or an excessively wide slit width.

STRAY LIGHT

Methods for detecting stray light involve the use of either filters or solutions. The substance chosen should have almost no absorption over a portion of the spectrum and extremely high absorption (opacity) below an abrupt cutoff wavelength. Possible substances are acetone (opaque below 320 nm), sodium bromide (opaque below 240 nm), and $NiSO_4$ (opaque below 400 nm and above 700 nm). For $NiSO_4$, readings greater than 4% T at 400 nm or greater than 2% T at 700 nm indicate a possible problem with stray light.[9] Stray light causes the greatest problems at the extremes of the spectral response of the radiant energy source. At these extremes, the intensity of source radiation is low, and stray light will have a greater effect. Stray light intensity greater than 1% of I_0 is unacceptable.

Corrective actions for excessive stray light include use of filters to eliminate most of the stray radiation, use of a different light source (such as a deuterium lamp instead of a tungsten lamp at 340 nm), or use of a better instrument.

BASELINE STABILITY

It is known that the output of many source lamps changes over time. This is due to the effects of lamp temperature on spectral output. That is why many instruments require a warm-up period. After the warm-up period, the rate of change of light intensity (drift) from the source should be low. Baseline stability testing detects excessive drift. Absorbance readings of a substance are made one minute apart. A change of more than 2% is unacceptable. This is usually caused by a failing source lamp.

PHOTOMETRIC ACCURACY

The purpose of checking photometric accuracy is to determine changes in spectral bandwidth and the amount of light energy falling on the detector. Photometric accuracy is determined using NIST filters,[10] neutral density glass filters for the visible range and metal-on-quartz filters for the ultraviolet range.

Instead of standard filters, solutions such as cobalt ammonium sulfate, copper sulfate, or potassium chromate can be prepared. For example, the absorbances of 0.0735 and 0.0367 M cobalt ammonium sulfate solutions in 1% sulfuric acid are

Table 6-2
Expected Absorbances for Spectrophotometry Standard Solution

Cobalt Ammonium Sulfate Concentration (M)	Wavelength (nm)	Absorbance
0.0735	512	0.346
0.0367	512	0.174
0.0367	400	0.012
0.0367	450	0.077
0.0367	500	0.163
0.0367	510	0.174
0.0367	550	0.077
0.0367	600	0.014

Table 6-3
Recommended Schedule of Spectrophotometer Maintenance Checks

Schedule	Maintenance Check	Method
Daily	Check for baseline stability (drift).	Read absorbance of a blank solution at 1-min. intervals, determine % change.
	Check for short circuits.	Gently tap instrument with hand and make certain instrument continues to function.
Monthly	Check wavelength calibration and accuracy.	Use emission lines of radiant energy source or holmium oxide or didymium filter.
	Confirm spectrum bandwidth.	Scan a standard filter or solution and determine spectrum bandwidth.
	Check 0% T.	Block light and measure % T.
	Check for stray light.	Use NIST filters or appropriate solutions.
	Check photometric accuracy and linearity.	Use NIST filters or cobalt ammonium sulfate solutions.

measured at 512 nm. In addition, the 0.0367 M solution is measured at six other wavelengths. Expected absorbances are shown in Table 6-2.[11] Problems with photometric accuracy may be due to improper alignment of the source lamp or to dirt on the lamp, mirrors, optical surfaces, or detector window.

ROUTINE MAINTENANCE

Periodic spectrophotometer maintenance is an important part of quality assurance in the laboratory. Consistent routine maintenance will prevent or detect subtle or gradual degradations in the instrument. Checks of photometric accuracy, wavelength calibration, linearity of detector response, and stray light should be performed at regular intervals. Table 6-3 gives a recommended schedule of maintenance checks.

Summary

Photometry is based on the linear relationship between absorbance of electromagnetic radiation and the concentration of the substance to be measured. Most photometric procedures are performed by using the visible portion of the electromagnetic spectrum that we call light (380–700 nm).

Beer's law is the mathematical relationship between absorbance or transmittance and concentration: $A = 2 - \log(\% \ T) = abc$.

Specific conditions must be met for Beer's law to be valid. These include the use of monochromatic light, a linear procedure, minimal light absorbance by other substances, and measurement at the optimum wavelength for the compound, usually the peak absorbance.

Photometric instruments are composed of a radiant light source, a monochromator system, a sample holder, a detector, and a readout device.

Photometers use filter monochromators; spectrophotometers use prism or diffraction grating monochromators with entrance and exit slits.

Photometric instruments must be regularly checked to ensure accurate and precise measurements. Check should include photometric accuracy, wavelength accuracy, linearity of detector response, and presence of stray light.

Questions and Problems

1. The $NiSO_4$ solution used in the wavelength calibration check is a 40% w/v solution in 1% HCl. Describe how this should be made.
2. What color is being absorbed when the $NiSO_4$ is being read at 512 nm? What color is being transmitted?
3. What are some possible causes of nonlinearity in a spectrophotometer?
4. What type of graph paper is used for plotting absorbance versus concentration? Percentage T versus concentration? Why?
5. What is the relationship between absorbance and % T?
6. Describe the components of a spectrophotometer and the function of each.
7. Why should methods be designed so readings fall between 20 and 80% T?
8. Indicate the complementary color for each spectral color below.

Violet	_____
Blue	_____
Green	_____
Yellow	_____
Orange	_____
Red	_____

9. Convert the following % T values to Absorbance values: A. 56.8; b. 81.1; c. 37; d. 95.6
10. Convert the following Absorbance values to % T: a. 0.98; b. 0.13; c. 0.66; d. 1.50.

11. A total protein biuret procedure is performed. Calculate the total protein concentrations of the controls and the patient sample.

	% *Transmittance*	*Concentration*
Standard 1	77.5	2.5 gm/dL
Standard 2	60	5.0 gm/dL
Standard 3	54.5	6.05 gm/dL
Standard 4	48	7.1 gm/dL
Control 1	47	?
Control 2	56.7	?
Patient sample	64.7	?

12. An albumin procedure is performed. The following data are gathered.

Specimen	*Absorbance*	*Concentration*
Blank	0.000	0.0 gm/dL
Standard	0.544	5.1 gm/dL
Control	0.456	?
Patient sample	0.307	?

What is the albumin concentration of the control and the patient sample?

13. An albumin procedure using BCG is performed. The molar absorptivity of the procedure is 10.6. The resulting absorbance reading is 0.656. What is the concentration? (Assume the cuvette is 1 cm.)

14. A wavelength of 340 nm is needed to perform an enzyme measurement using NADH. The diffraction grating has 600 grooves/mm. What angle of diffraction is needed in order for the 340-nm wavelength to be produced. (Assume an angle of incidence of 90°.)

15. Assume that in Problem 14 the angle of incidence is 15° for the perpendicular of the grating. What angle of diffraction is now needed?

16. An interference filter is made from magnesium fluoride (MgF_2) and silver (Ag). The refractive index of MgF_2 is 1.38, the angle of incidence is 90°, and the thickness of the MgF_2 is 250 nm. What wavelengths will be generated from this filter?

References

1. Hughes HK, Barnes RB, Bedell HM, et al. Suggested nomenclature in applied spectroscopy. Anal Chem 1952, 25:1349-54.
2. Serway RA, Faughn JS. College physics, 2nd ed. Philadelphia: Saunders College Publishing, 1989:781-28.
3. Treharne RW. Light intensity measurement; characteristics of light sources; filters and monochromators. Methods Enzymol 1972, 24:268-93.
4. Skoog DA, Leary JJ. Principles of instrumental analysis, 4th ed. Fort Worth: Saunders College Publishing, 1992:96.
5. James GP, DJang MH. Evaluation of clinical laboratory instruments, part III: Spectral bandwidth and wavelength accuracy. Am J Med Technol 1981, 47:477-83.
6. Willard HH, Merritt LL Jr, Dean JA, Settle FA Jr. Instrumental methods of analysis, 7th ed. Belmont, CA: Wadsworth Publishing, 1988:151-55.

7. Frings CS. Use of deuterium and hydrogen lamps in checking wavelength accuracy [Letter]. Clin Chem 1971, 17:568.
8. Rand RN. Practical spectrophotometric standards. Clin Chem 1969, 15:839-63.
9. Frings CS, Broussard LA. Calibration and monitoring of spectrometers and spectrophotometers. Clin Chem 1979, 25:1013-17.
10. American Society for Testing and Materials, Standard practice for describing and measuring performance of ultraviolet, visible, and near infrared spectrophotometers. Annual book of ASTM standards. Philadelphia, PA: 1989, 14.01:106-15.
11. Standards for checking the calibration of spectrophotometers (200-1000 μ). Villanova, PA. National Bureau of Standards, Letter Circular #1017, 1955.

Suggested Readings

Bender GT. Principles of chemical instrumentation. Philadelphia: WB Saunders, 1987.

Frings CS, Gauldie J. Spectral techniques. In: Kaplan LA, Pesce AJ, eds. Clinical chemistry: Theory, analysis and correlation. St. Louis: CV Mosby, 1990:49-72.

Caraway WT. Photometry. In: Tietz NW, ed. Textbook of clinical chemistry. Philadelpha: WB Saunders, 1986:55-77.

7

FLAME EMISSION AND ATOMIC ABSORPTION SPECTROSCOPY

Mary C. Haven
Martin R. Lohff

Objectives

After completing this chapter, the reader will be able to:

1. Outline the principles behind flame photometry.
2. Explain how atomic absorption differs from flame photometry.
3. Give at least two advantages of determining calcium by atomic absorption rather than flame photometry.
4. Give at least two advantages of determining sodium by flame photometry rather than atomic absorption.
5. Discuss important characteristics necessary for an internal standard for flame photometry.
6. Name at least three variables on which the intensity of light emitted by excited atoms depends.
7. Diagram the component parts of (a) a flame photometer, and (b) an atomic absorption instrument.
8. Discuss the types of interferences encountered in flame emission and atomic absorbtion spectrometry.
9. Establish and follow a maintenance program for both types of spectrometers.

Definitions

Emission Spectra: The characteristic spectra or color given off by atoms, ions, or molecules when excited by heat or other means.

Excitation Potential: The relative ease with which atoms entering a flame of constant temperature can be excited.

Excited State: An atom with an orbiting electron in an unstable higher energy state.

Flame Background Interference: The formation of continuous emission spectra by unknown substances in the solution to be analyzed, adding to the overall intensity of emission of light spectra.

Ground State: The lowest possible energy form of an atom or molecule in which orbital electrons have their normal unexcited energy potential and orbital planes.

I_i: Intensity of light transmitted after sample absorption.

I_o: Intensity of the incident light.

Interference: Changes in emission intensity from the expected of a standard or unknown due to the presence of certain anions, cations, overlapping emission spectra, or suppression of ionization through mass action.

Ionization Potential: The relative ease with which atoms in a gaseous state undergo ionization.

Resonance Line: The wavelength absorbed in exciting an atom from the ground state to the next highest energy state. This wavelength is the same as the wavelength emitted by an atom excited to the next highest energy level.

Self-Absorption: The absorption by a ground state atom of the emitted radiation from an excited atom of the same element.

Introduction

The fundamental principles of light emission and absorption by molecules discussed in the Chapter 6 also apply to atoms. The actual instrumentation differs for various types of spectroscopy; but the fundamental principles underlying excitation, emission, and absorption are similar. In this chapter we discuss atomic spectroscopy: *flame photometry,* which is atomic emission, and *atomic absorption.* Both techniques can be used for determining the concentration of some elements in biological samples. Flame emission is usually used for the alkali metals: sodium (Na), potassium (K), and lithium (Li). Atomic absorption is the method of choice for metals of lesser concentration in biological samples, often termed *trace metals.* These metals include, but are not limited to, calcium (Ca), magnesium (Mg), zinc (Zn), copper (Cu), lead (Pb), cadmium (Cd), and aluminum (Al).

Principles

All elements have the capability of absorbing electromagnetic radiation at the same wavelength that the element emits radiation. This elemental property is the basis of atomic absorption and emission spectrophotometry.

An atom is composed of a nucleus with electrons revolving around it in discrete orbits. If energy (thermal, electrical, or electromagnetic) is supplied to this atom, the electrons can move to an orbit of higher energy (Fig. 7-1). This occurs in atomic absorption. The atom in the ground state, the lowest possible energy form of the atom, absorbs a unit of radiant energy. The amount of light absorbed is directly related to the number of atoms in the ground state and is the principle of atomic absorption. Absorption of this energy moves an electron to a higher energy orbit. An excited atom is the result. The excited atom, in returning to the ground state, releases

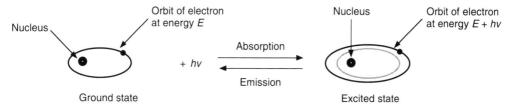

Figure 7-1. Atomic absorption or atomic emission.

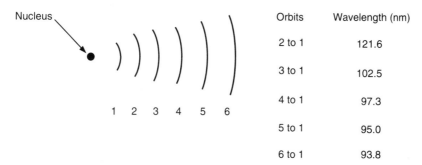

Orbits	Wavelength (nm)
2 to 1	121.6
3 to 1	102.5
4 to 1	97.3
5 to 1	95.0
6 to 1	93.8

Figure 7-2. Emission from excited hydrogen electron.

a photon. This is the principle of atomic emission or flame photometry. The intensity of the emitted light is proportional to the number of excited atoms.

Before going further in discussing atomic absorption and emission, it would be wise to digress a few moments into line spectra in order to understand some definitions.

The hydrogen atom is usually used for the example: As it absorbs energy, the electron can move to higher orbits; as the electron falls back to its original orbit, it emits radiation in specific lines (Fig. 7-2). Unlike molecules that may absorb and emit light over a broad band, atoms absorb and emit light in discrete, very defined, narrow lines (Fig. 7-2). The movement of an electron from the ground state of the next higher orbit requires the least amount of energy. Remember from Chapter 6 that energy is related to wavelength by the following equation.[1]

$$E = h\nu, \text{ but } \nu = c/\lambda, \quad \text{(Eq. 7-1)}$$

$$E = hc/\lambda \quad \text{(Eq. 7-2)}$$

where

h = Planck's constant
ν = frequency
c = velocity of light
λ = wavelength

That transition, which requires the least energy, has the longest wavelength. Therefore, the wavelength absorbed in exciting the atom from the ground state to the next higher orbit is the longest wavelength of the spectra. It is called the *resonance line.* This is the wavelength measured in atomic absorption or atomic emission. It is the strongest line of the atomic spectra of a particular element.

Although the principles of atomic absorption and emission theoretically hold true for all the elements, present application of the techniques has been limited to those elements with resonance lines in the ultraviolet and visible regions of the spectrum.

FLAME PHOTOMETRY

Flame photometry consists of four steps:

1. The sample is converted to an atomic vapor by a flame.
2. The thermal energy of the flame excites electrons in ground state atoms to higher energy orbits, which forms excited atoms.
3. As excited atoms fall back to the ground state, they emit light at wavelengths characteristic of the element being determined.
4. The intensity of the light emission at a specific wavelength is directly proportional to the concentration of the element being measured.

The intensity of the emitted light is related to concentration by the following equation:[2]

$$S = (N_1 E/\tau)(g^1/g^2)(e^{-E/kT}) \qquad \text{(Eq. 7-3)}$$

$$N_2 E/\tau \qquad \text{(Eq. 7-4)}$$

where

$$S = \text{intensity of emitted light}$$
$$N_1 = \text{number of unexcited atoms}$$
$$N_2 = \text{number of excited atoms}$$
$$\tau = \text{lifetime of an excited atom}$$
$$E = \text{energy difference } (h\nu) \text{ between excited state and ground state}$$
$$g^1/g^2 = \text{the ratio of atoms in the ground state and the excited state}$$
$$T = \text{temperature}$$
$$k = \text{Boltzmann distribution}$$

This equation shows that flame photometry depends on the temperature of the flame because temperature affects the number of excited atoms. The number of excited atoms increases 4% with only a 10°K increase in atomization temperature.[2] The number of excited atoms also depends on the energy difference between the excited state and the ground state. To correct for these variations, an internal standard (described later in this chapter) is usually added to samples and standards in flame photometric analysis.

ATOMIC ABSORPTION

Atomic absorption consists of three steps:

1. The sample is converted to an atomic vapor, usually by a flame.
2. The atomic vapor is irradiated at a wavelength characteristic of the element being sought.
3. Absorption of the light by the vaporized sample is related to the concentration of the desired element in it.

The degree of absorption (dv) follows the following relationship:[3]

$$\int K_v dv = (\pi e^2 / mc)\, Nf \qquad \text{(Eq. 7-5)}$$

where

K = absorption coefficient at frequency v
e = charge on the electron
m = mass of an electron
c = speed of light
N = number of atoms in the ground state
f = oscillator strength of the absorbing line

K, e, m, c, and f are all constants for a given element. The only variable is N, the number of atoms in the ground state.

The Beer-Lambert law ($I = I_0 e^{-abc}$) does not really apply to atomic absorption spectroscopy because the atoms are not in a steady state of homogeneous distribution. The sample is going from molecules to ions, to atoms in the ground state, to oxides. Valid values for a and b cannot be obtained. However, in actual spectrophotometric work, these values are rarely calculated either. Standards and samples are run at the same time under the same conditions, canceling out all values except c (concentration).

If we compare these two methods of measurement, we see some inherent advantages of absorption over emission. The intensity of the emission line in flame photometry is proportional to the number of excited atoms, but the number of excited atoms is also a function of the wavelength of emission and of the temperature of the system. An advantage of atomic absorption is that there are many more atoms in the ground state than the excited state. Even though sodium is easily excited, most of the sodium atoms in a flame remain in the ground state.

Na	1 excited	100 ground
Ca	1 excited	1000 ground
Zn	1 excited	1×10^9 ground

Interferences from temperature and wavelength variation are slight in absorption whereas emission is quite dependent on these parameters. A ratio of transmitted light to incident light can be used as the measurement of absorption; in emission, the absolute intensity of emitted light must be determined. Sensitivity between the two methods differs with the metals analyzed. For alkali metals (Na, K, Li), flame photometry is more sensitive; for other metals sensitivity is improved with atomic absorption methods.

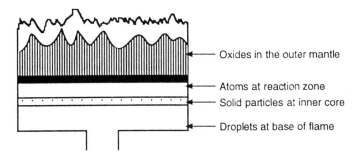

Figure 7-3. Composition of a flame.

Instrumentation

The individual components of atomic absorption and emission instruments are similar to other spectroscopic instrumentation. They include a radiation source, a sample cell, a monochromator, and a detector.

In *atomic emission* or *flame photometry,* the radiation source is the excited atoms themselves, excited by the thermal energy of the flame. The sample cell or sample cuvette is also the flame. The sample is aspirated into the flame by an atomizer. As the excited atoms fall back to the ground state, they emit light of a characteristic wavelength. That characteristic wavelength is isolated by a monochromator and detected by a photomultiplier tube or a photocell.

In *atomic absorption* the radiation source is a hollow cathode lamp. The sample cell is the flame itself. How can this be? How can the flame be both a source of excited atoms for flame photometry and a source of ground state atoms for atomic absorption? The flame provides the energy to break molecular bonds, to create atoms in the ground state, and to excite ground state atoms to excited atoms. The flame is a dynamic mixture: a mixture of droplets at the base of the flame, solid particles at the inner core, atoms in the reaction zone (compounds are dissociated to ions, ions are reduced to atoms, ground state atoms are excited) a little above the base, and oxides in the outer mantle (Fig. 7-3). The desired wavelength is isolated by a monochromator, and the amount of light absorbed is measured by a photomultiplier tube.

COMPONENT PARTS OF A FLAME PHOTOMETER

The basic components of flame photometer include a burner with gas supply and regulators combined with an atomizer, a monochromator, and a detector with a readout device.

Gas Supply

A steady flame with constant thermal output is required. A steady flame depends on a steady air or oxygen supply and gas pressure. Generally, piped-in gas supplies

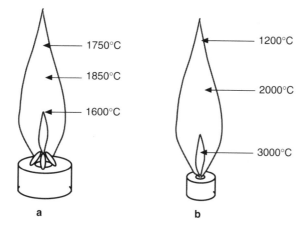

Figure 7-4.   Temperature distribution in flame zones: (a) natural gas-air flame; (b) acetylene-oxygen flame.

vary in pressure and must be carefully monitored and/or regulated. If bottled gas and oxygen sources are used as the supply for the flame, proper pressure reduction is necessary. Most air or oxygen tanks work best with two-stage automatic reduction valves for pressure regulation.

The composition of the various gas-oxidant combinations used for the flame varies considerably. In Figure 7-4, the two commonly used fuels and the temperatures generated are shown. These temperatures range generally from 1200 to 3000°C. Cyanogen and oxygen can generate flames up to 5000°C, but this heat can cause toxic products of combustion to be formed.

The external form of the flame depends on the quantitative ratio of combustible substance to oxidant. With a decreased oxidant (air or oxygen) ratio, a luminous yellow flame is obtained. With an increase in the oxidant ratio, the brightness of the flame decreases, and finally disappears to become a clear, blue, nonluminous flame. This results in a hotter flame with three cones: an inner, bright blue-green cone, an intermediate, almost invisible inner cone, and an outer blue-violet cone. The typical structure of a flame resulting from acetylene-oxygen is shown in Figure 7-4. The merging gases enter the inner cone and are heated to the ignition temperature. Primary combustion proceeds with a deficiency of oxidant and occurs over a period of approximately 10^{-4} seconds. The intermediate zone is the area usually used in flame photometry because it is often rich in free atoms. The outer zone (secondary combustion zone) is characterized by complete combustion and the formation of oxides.

It must be emphasized that the greater the thermal energy of a flame, the greater the number of atoms that will be excited. This increased emission intensity should result in increased sensitivity. However, increased background noise is often an unwanted by-product.

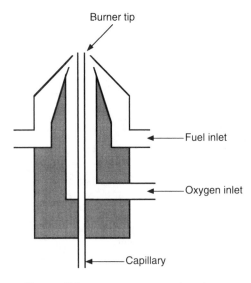

Figure 7-5. Combined atomizer-burner.

Atomizer-Burners

In the combined *atomizer-burner,* a stream of high-velocity gas passes over a capillary, causing reduced pressure. In this way the aqueous sample is pulled into the capillary tube where it is broken into droplets and vapor by the stream of gas (Fig. 7-5). This mist is introduced directly into the flame. All of the liquid sample aspirated is injected into the flame. This burner has several advantages, which include relative ease of cleaning, a rapid response; good sensitivity, and delivery of a completely representative aliquot of the entire sample into the flame. Its chief disadvantages include a wide variation in droplet size, problems with partial blockage of the burner tip, aspiration rate dependence on sample viscosity, density and surface tension, and turbulence, which makes the burners noisy, both physically and electronically.

Some atomizers use a spray chamber in which the larger particles settle out and only a fine aerosol mist is drawn into the burner (Fig. 7-6). The mist is mixed with fuel and oxidant before reaching the flame. The excess larger droplets of the sample are drained off. Advantages of this laminar flow burner include less blockage of the burner because the larger droplets are drained off, resulting in quieter burning with less turbulence and noise. However, this burner is more difficult to clean, and unburned mixtures of fuel and oxidant are explosive.

In either type of atomizer, the sample must be introduced at a rapid, stable, and reproducible rate. Atomization is the most critical step in flame spectroscopy. If compressed air is used, a pressure of approximately 10 lb/in^2 is needed for optimum atomization. Optimum pressure can be determined experimentally by finding the highest pressure attainable before an appreciable increase in background noise

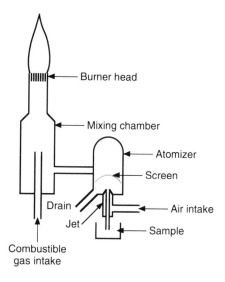

Figure 7-6.   Indirect atomizer with mixing chamber and burner (laminar flow).

results. Because viscosity, density, and surface tension of a solution affect the rate of atomization and droplet size, high dilutions of samples and standards in the same matrix are used to minimize these effects.

Burners may be made of glass, quartz, or metal. Glass is used only in work with relatively low-temperature flames, such as mixtures of natural gas or acetylene with air. Quartz is somewhat more widely used, but is difficult to manufacture. The most common types are made of metal; however, these corrode and plug up more often, particularly with heavy salt concentrations.

A portion of the emitted light from the sample in the flame is focused by lenses and mirrors through a process called *collimation*. This results in increased sensitivity.

Monochromators

A *monochromator* isolates the desired wavelength. Monochromation for spectral isolation in flame photometers is accomplished by prisms, diffraction gratings, or (more commonly) filters. Filters are relatively inexpensive, durable, reliable, and easy to use. Their major disadvantage is decreased resolution, which is a function of the half-bandpass (see Chapter 6). The advantages of a prism or grating for isolating wavelength are versatility, ease of operation, and the ability to analyze the spectral lines from many different elements. Major disadvantages include higher cost, loss of light, the use of front surface reflectors that cannot be cleaned, and the danger of destruction of the optical alignment by either heat or mechanical damage. For these reasons, the use of prisms or diffraction gratings is generally reserved for more complex emission spectrophotometry.

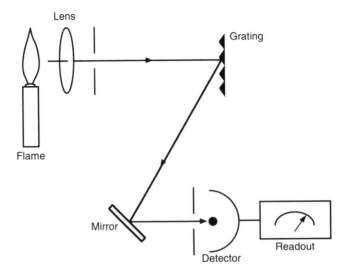

Figure 7-7. Flame photometer with a diffraction grating for monochromation.

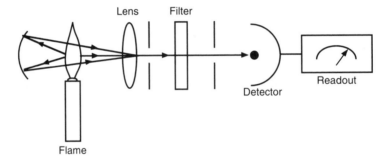

Figure 7-8. Flame photometer with a filter for monochromation.

Detectors

Detection of the emission intensity is similar to absorption spectrophotometry. It is generally accomplished by a photomultiplier tube, which converts the light emitted by excited atoms into electrical energy via multiple dynodes as a cascade effect. The current generated is indicated in a direct readout meter or is amplified and sent to a digital converter for readout or printout. For simple diagrams of flame photometers, see Figures 7-7 and 7-8.

Internal Standards

Because flame photometry is so dependent on temperature, degree of atomization, oxygen and fuel flow and pressure, and voltage fluctuations, an *internal standard* is commonly used.[4] This involves the addition of another element in known concentra-

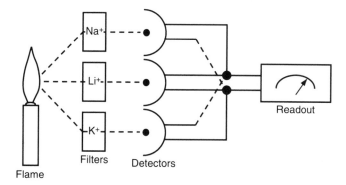

Figure 7-9. Plan of multichannel photometer: (1) flame; (2) light filters; (3) detectors; (4) readout.

tion to all standards, samples, and blanks, followed by simultaneous analysis for both the added reference element and the element of interest. The ratio of the intensity of the spectral emission line of the element of interest to the internal standard intensity is proportional to the concentration of the analyte. The use of an internal standard helps to eliminate many sources of instrumental error because both internal standard and the element being analyzed are affected in the same way.

In establishing a constant relationship between the internal standard and the element under measurement, it is important that several principles and procedures be followed.

1. The internal standard must be pure and of known concentration.
2. The internal standard should have physical and chemical properties similar to the element being analyzed.
3. The excitation potentials of the internal standard and the element to be analyzed should be matched as closely as possible.
4. The emission lines should be far apart to avoid spectral interference.
5. The concentration of the internal standard should be of the same order of magnitude as the element being analyzed.
6. The internal standard should not occur normally in significant concentrations in the samples under analysis.

The most common internal standard used for sodium and potassium analysis is a lithium salt, usually lithium nitrate or lithium sulfate. Its physical and chemical properties are similar to those of sodium and potassium. The excitation potentials of sodium, potassium, and lithium are similar. However the use of lithium would be less desirable for flame photometric determination of the alkaline earth metals such as calcium and magnesium.

The lithium internal standard is coupled with simultaneous potassium and sodium determination in many clinical instruments. A typical schematic diagram is shown in Figure 7-9. Some flame photometers also allow determination of lithium for therapeutic drug monitoring. In this case, potassium is added as the internal standard, and lithium concentration is determined from the ratio of lithium light emission to potassium.

Cesium has recently been introduced as an alternative internal standard. It shares many of the theoretical advantages of lithium, but unlike lithium, it is never used as a therapeutic drug. However, lithium therapy does not interfere in the clinical determination of sodium and potassium because the concentration of lithium as an internal standard (15 mEq/L in the diluent) far exceeds the maximum concentration in a patient's sample (<3 mEq/L), diluted 1 in 200. Of course, lithium cannot be determined in a sample with lithium as an internal standard. A cesium internal standard permits direct determination of sodium, potassium, and lithium in the same sample.

COMPONENT PARTS OF AN ATOMIC ABSORPTION SPECTROPHOTOMETER

Radiation Source

The most common radiation source is a *hollow cathode lamp* with the element of interest as the cathode filament. This lamp is filled with either argon or neon gas. When voltage is applied, the gas becomes charged and bombards the metal atoms of the filament. This bombardment causes excited metal atoms to be dislodged into the atmosphere of the lamp. Each excited atom, which can only exist for 10^{-6} to 10^{-8} seconds, returns to the ground state by emitting a photon. The photon's energy, $h\nu$, is the exact energy that the metal atom in the sample absorbs. The principle of the hollow cathode lamp is the same principle as for atomic emission.

High-intensity hollow cathode lamps are an improvement over conventional ones. They contain two extra electrodes that are coated with an easily excited material. A direct current flows between these auxiliary electrodes, causing more gas atoms to become ionized and bombard the sputtering metal atoms from the cathode. This causes an increase in the number of excited atoms, thereby increasing the intensity of the lamp. An additional power supply is required for these high-brightness lamps.

Another type of lamp, the *vapor discharge lamp,* is most often used for the determination of the alkali metals (sodium, potassium, cesium, and rubidium). This lamp is filled with a vapor at least partially composed of the element of interest. A current is passed through the vapor, and emission results. These lamps require special mounts and a special power supply.

Flame Atomizers

The function of the *atomizer,* whether combined with flame or furnace, is similar to what it is in flame photometry. The atomizer introduces the sample and reduces the metal being determined from an ion or molecule to the neutral atomic state (i.e., the ground state). This is the most difficult and least efficient step in the atomic absorption process. Calculations show that the flame atomization step may only reduce one atom per million in the sample.[5] Furnace atomization has vastly increased the efficiency of reducing elements to their ground state.

Flame atomizers can accommodate only liquid samples. The two most common burners are the total consumption burner and the Lundegardh burner. In the *total consumption burner,* all the sample that is aspirated is injected into the flame (Fig.

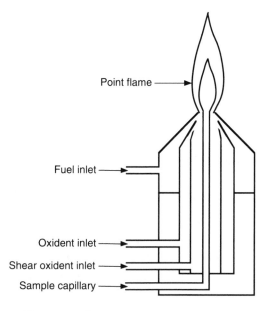

Point flame

Fuel inlet

Oxident inlet

Shear oxident inlet

Sample capillary

Figure 7-10. Total consumption burner.

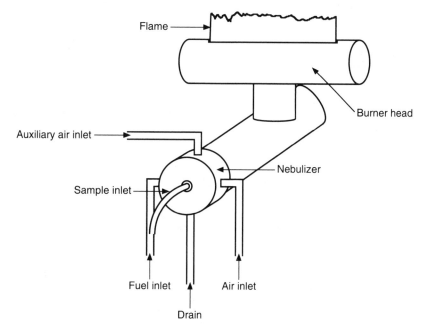

Flame

Burner head

Auxiliary air inlet

Nebulizer

Sample inlet

Fuel inlet

Drain

Air inlet

Figure 7-11. Lundegardh burner.

7-10). The advantages and disadvantages are the same as those for the direct burner in flame photometry, except that the burner does not give greater sensitivity in atomic absorption.

The *Lundegardh burner,* or premix burner, is shown in Figure 7-11. The oxidants and fuel are premixed in the barrel of the burner. The sample is aspirated into the same bowl, and an appreciable part of the sample evaporates in the fuel-oxidant mixture. The excess sample is drained off. This burner has improved sensitivity in atomic absorption because the elongated burner puts more atoms in the light path. Otherwise, the burner has the same advantages and disadvantages as the laminar flow in flame photometry.

The light absorbed, when passaging through different heights of the flame, is not constant. This is because the number of neutral atoms varies in different parts of the flame as previously described in this chapter.

Furnaces

The use of high-temperature furnaces significantly increases the number of ground-state atoms in the light path, which improves sensitivity and lowers the detection limit.[6] However, with increased sensitivity comes increased interference from the sample matrix (e.g., nonselective molecular absorption and light scattering), and some method of background correction is therefore necessary when using a furnace. These background corrections will be discussed later in the chapter. Commercially available furnaces are generally of two types: the L'vov graphite cuvette and the Massman furnace.

The *L'vov graphite cuvette* (Fig. 7-12) is a 30- to 50-mm long cylinder lined with pyrographite, which ensures uniform heating and is resistant to oxidation. The hollow cathode beam passes through the cylinder. The sample is placed on an auxiliary carbon rod electrode, 6 mm in diameter; the sample unit is then purged with nitrogen or argon gas, and the rod is heated to dry and ash the sample. The auxiliary electrode is then introduced into the center of the graphite cuvette. The sample is rapidly vaporized by running high current through the electrode, and a pulsed signal of maximum absorption is obtained and recorded. Analytical results can be calculated by peak height or peak integration.

Figure 7-13 shows a *Massman furnace,* a hollow graphite cylinder about 8 mm in diameter and about 28 mm long. The hollow cathode beam passes through this cylinder, and the sample (1 to 100 μl) is introduced through a hole in the center of the cylinder. Solid samples can also be introduced through the end of the cylinder. The system is purged with argon or nitrogen, and the cylinder is heated in three stages: The first stage dries the sample, the second chars and ashes the sample, and the third vaporizes the sample. Again, the absorption signal is monitored by a recorder.

Furnaces have several advantages over flame atomizers: high sensitivity due to increased concentrations of ground-state atoms within a well-defined volume,[7] smaller sample sizes, and no pretreatment of biological samples. The disadvantages of furnaces include less precision than flame burners, matrix interferences that demand background correction, and decreased sample throughput because furnaces must cool down between samples.

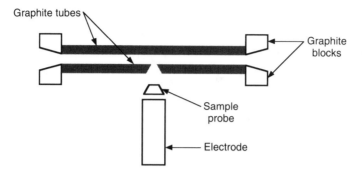

Figure 7-12. L'vov graphite cuvette.

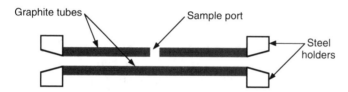

Figure 7-13. Massman furnace.

Monochromators

The *monochromator,* most commonly a diffraction grating, is used to separate the resonance line from other spectral lines in the immediate vicinity. These spectral lines originate from other metals in the hollow cathode and the filler gas. The wavelength range of this monochromator is the same as that of flame emission or ultraviolet-visible spectrophotometry, approximately 190 to 860 nm. The bandpass should be small enough to transmit only the resonance lines. For those elements whose resonance lines are closely surrounded by other lines, a bandpass of 0.2 nm is required. Yet, it is also desirable when working with other elements to increase the available light. This can be done by increasing the slit width, thereby widening the bandpass to as high as 4 nm. A good monochromator for atomic absorption should accommodate wide variations in slit widths. The wavelength accuracy for atomic absorption need not be greater than 1 nm, because the exact wavelength desired is "tuned-in" with the hollow cathode as the source.

Detectors

The *detector* is usually a photomultiplier tube, generally either a Bi-O-Ag or a Cs-Sb type of cathode. The most widely used is the Cs-Sb, but the more expensive Bi-O-Ag material has advantages in the far ultraviolet and red regions of the spectrum.

The commercial instruments differ in their *readout devices.* All readout devices are based on the fact that, in atomic absorption, the concentration is proportional to the negative logarithm of transmittance. The formula for converting the percentage of absorption to absorbance is the same as for percent transmittance to absorbance.

$$A = 2 - \log \% \, T \tag{Eq. 7-6}$$

$$= 2 - \log (100 - \% \text{ absorption}), \text{ where } A = \text{absorbance} \tag{Eq. 7-7}$$

Instruments with graphite furnaces usually record absorbance versus time and compute the area under the absorption peak. A standard curve of absorbance (or area under the absorbance peak) versus concentration is obtained with a set of known standards. The absorbance of the unknown sample is then read against the standard curve to determine its concentration.

Most instruments are now microprocessor controlled, with multistandard calibration programs that allow direct readout of concentration. The microprocessors may also control an automated sampling system and the programming for the furnace.

Modulated Equipment

The first atomic absorption spectrophotometers were made with direct current components; lamp source, flame, monochromator, and detector. However, certain problems arose and modifications were made. The first modification was modulated equipment.[8] If the source of radiation is considered I_0, then I_0 is reduced to I after passing through the flame. However, the element of interest emits radiation at exactly the wavelength it absorbs. As the atom that has absorbed radiation returns to the ground state, it emits the same energy it had just absorbed. Therefore, the detector would see $(I_0 - I) + S$, where S is the fraction of the emission signal that reaches the detector. The drop in the absorption signal, which should be $I_0 - I$, would now be reduced and equal to $(I_0 - I) + S$. This would cause a reduction in sensitivity. Also, S is the same signal used in flame photometry, and the process would then be subject to errors of both atomic absorption and flame spectroscopy. Modulation of the instrument is brought about by electrical or mechanical means. In the mechanical method, the output of the lamp, which is a dc signal, is modified to an ac signal with a chopper (Fig. 7-14). The detector is then synchronized to the same frequency. In this manner,

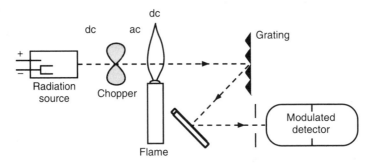

Figure 7-14.   Single-beam modulated atomic absorption spectrophotometer.

the detector sees only the ac signal from the radiation source and the absorption thereof. The emission signal from the flame is dc; the detector is unable to register it, and only $I_0 - I$ is detected.

Double-Beam Instruments

After a stable and instrumentally quiet burner was manufactured, it was noted that the weakest link in the system was the hollow cathode lamp. Lamps need a considerable warmup period before they'll give a constant emission. For this reason, the *double-beam instruments* (Fig. 7-15) were made. With a double-beam system, the light from a single lamp is split into two paths: a sample path and a reference path. The reference path goes directly to the detector. The sample path goes through the sample to the detector. In this system, the ratio between the reference and the sample beams is determined; thus, the absorbed light is monitored. A double-beam instrument usually produces a steadier baseline, but this does not compensate for variations in the flame, because the reference does not go through the flame.

Monitoring Channels

A further modification found in some atomic absorption instruments attempts to eliminate signal changes caused by flame variations. For this purpose, a second hollow cathode lamp, monochromator, and detector are used as a *monitoring channel*. The light paths of both lamps go through the flame, and the ratio of the monitoring channel signal to the measuring channel signal is computed (Fig. 7-16). This is similar to using an internal standard in flame emission photometry. Instead of using the second channel for monitoring, it can also be used for determining a second element.

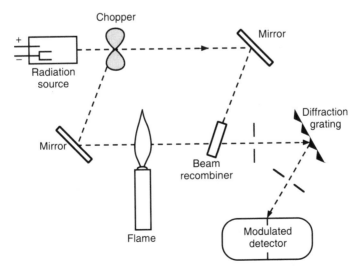

Figure 7-15. Double-beam atomic absorption spectrophotometer.

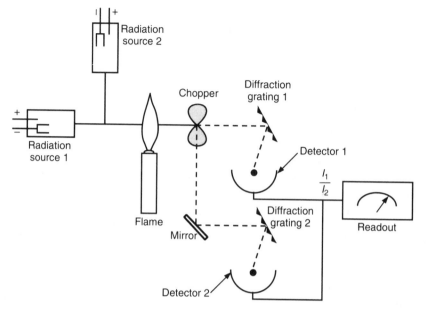

Figure 7-16.   Atomic absorption spectrophotometer with monitoring channel.

Background Correctors

When using graphite furnaces, correction for background absorption in the sample cuvette is necessary.[9] This background absorption can be caused by molecules, salt particles, or smoke. If no correction is made, erroneously high results will be computed. Background correction can be accomplished by means of a monitoring channel as explained in the previous paragraph, a deuterium arc, or the Zeeman effect. With the *deuterium background corrector*, light from the hollow cathode lamp and light from the deuterium arc alternately pass through the graphite tube or the flame. Absorption of radiation from the deuterium source by ground-state atoms being determined will be negligible, but background absorption should be the same for both beams, hollow cathode and deuterium. The ratio of the two beams is determined in the double-beam instrument electronics, and background absorption is automatically compensated. With the deuterium arc, compensation for background levels of 0.5 to 0.7 absorbance units can be achieved.

Correction by taking advantage of the splitting of spectral lines under the influence of a magnetic field *(Zeeman effect)* can compensate for background levels up to 2 absorbance units. When a magnetic field is applied to an atomic spectral line, the line is split into a π component at the original wavelength and into two σ components equidistant from the original line, one of slightly longer wavelength, the other of slightly shorter wavelength (Fig. 7-17). The magnetic field also causes polarization of these lines; the π component is polarized in the plane parallel to the magnetic field, the σ components are polarized perpendicular to the magnetic field.

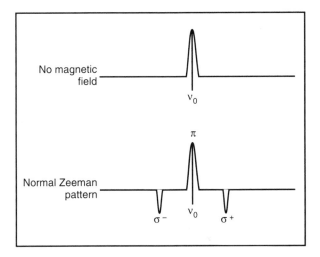

Figure 7-17. Zeeman effect; normal pattern.

More complicated splitting of the spectral line occurs with some elements, but the simple form is the easiest to use when explaining the background correction.

Because background absorption is largely broad-base molecular scattering or absorption and, usually, only atoms are affected by the Zeeman effect, instrument manufacturers have used this type of background correction in two ways: by placing the magnetic field around the source (source-shifted Zeeman correction) or around the furnace (analyte-shifted Zeeman correction).

When the hollow cathode is placed in the magnetic field, polarized light is passed through the atomized sample. Background correction is made with a rotating polarizer added to the system before the detector (Fig. 7-18). When polarized parallel to the magnetic field, only the π component is absorbed; thus, absorption of analyte and background occurs. When polarized perpendicular to the magnetic field, only the $\pm\sigma$ component is absorbed (i.e., background only). Subtraction of the perpendicular component from the parallel component yields absorption due to the analyte.

By placing the magnetic field around the furnace, the signal from the analyte is shifted. If the polarizer is fixed for the vertical component after the furnace (Fig. 7-19), application of the magnetic field measures the $\pm\sigma$ component or background only. When the magnetic field is off, both background and sample are measured. Subtraction yields a background correction a slight distance (≈ 0.01 nm) from the absorbing line. If the polarizer is fixed before the furnace (Fig. 7-20), allowing only the vertical component to pass, the application of the magnetic field does not allow the horizontal π component of the analyte to absorb any of the vertical incident light. Therefore, any absorption when the magnetic field is on is due to background. Without the magnetic field, both analyte and background can absorb the horizontally polarized incident light. Background is corrected at the exact wavelength of the absorbing line.

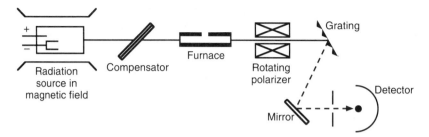

Figure 7-18.   Source-shifted Zeeman background correction.

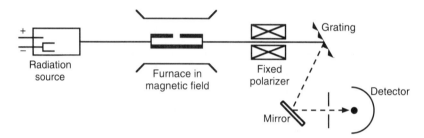

Figure 7-19.   Analyte-shifted Zeeman background correction; fixed polarizer after magnetic field.

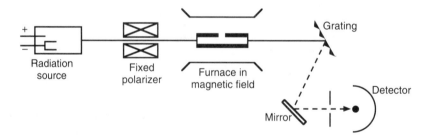

Figure 7-20.   Analyte-shifted Zeeman background correction; fixed polarizer before magnetic field.

Interferences

FLAME PHOTOMETRY

Although flame photometry is rapid, relatively inexpensive, and requires a small volume of sample, it has several major disadvantages. These include spectral interference between two or more substances in the solution to be analyzed, background interference, anionic and cationic interference, ionization, and self-absorption.

Spectral interference results when two or more elements in the sample under analysis have emission spectra in adjacent or overlapping wavelengths. A monochromator with precise spectral isolation characteristics (narrow bandpass) can usually solve this problem. Another wavelength, preferably toward the ultraviolet region, and one not associated with spectral line emissions from the interferent atoms can also be used.

Flame background interference occurs when continuous emission spectra formed by the flame itself add to the overall emission intensity. The maximum intensity of the line spectra generated by the elements under analysis, however, remains unchanged. Flame background interference can be eliminated by shifting the wavelength first to one side of the analyte wavelength, aspirating the sample solutions, noting the background, then to the other side of the wavelength, aspirating sample and finding the background. This is sometimes done electronically. Correction for this background noise can be accomplished, provided it does not exceed the emission signal from the analyte.

Other sources of interference include *chemical interference* caused by either anions or cations. When the element to be measured combines with an anion to form a thermally stable compound, this element will no longer be available as ground-state atoms. An example of this problem involves the marked decrease in emission intensity of calcium in the presence of sulfates and phosphates. Increasing flame temperature might improve this problem. The more common method for eliminating this type of chemical interference is to add another ion that will preferentially bind the sulfate or phosphate ion. (See chemical interference in atomic absorption below). Other anions can also interfere, usually with a negative effect. An example is the presence of hydrochloric acid, 0.01 M HCl results in a 15% decrease of sodium and 40% decrease in potassium emission intensity. Phosphoric acid shows an even greater effect. The degree of reduction in emission depends not only on the particular acid and its concentration but also on the alkali metal measured. The degree of interference from acids increases as the atomic number of the metal being determined increases.

Ionization is another cause of interference.[10] Those elements with low ionization potentials are more readily ionized in the flame, especially at low concentration. With few atoms in solution, all the energy available can go to these atoms, and ionization results. As the concentration increases, the energy is spread over more atoms, less ionization occurs, and greater spectral emission occurs. Ionization interference occurs mostly with the metals potassium, rubidium, and cesium. Lithium, which has a higher ionization potential, actually does not show such a phenomenon at the concentrations usually used in flame photometry. Ionization interference can be eliminated by adding an excess amount of a noninterfering, easily ionized element.

Self-absorption is another form of interference. Emitted radiation from one atom may be absorbed by a second atom. As the second atom absorbs the radiation, it becomes excited and emits radiation. In this case, although two atoms emitted light, the detector will see only one. Low results are obtained. However, self-absorption is a problem only with high sample concentrations and can be easily decreased or eliminated by further diluting the solution.

ATOMIC ABSORPTION

There are three major types of interference in atomic absorption spectroscopy: chemical, ionization, and matrix.

Chemical interference is quite common but can generally be overcome. The number of atoms in the ground state depends on the stability of the metal compounds in the flame atomizer. If the compound is readily dissociated, many neutral atoms are formed; however, if the compound remains partially undissociated, fewer neutral atoms are the result. Then, the predominant anion can have an effect on the number of neutral atoms if this anion binds strongly to the element of interest. This interference can be overcome by the addition of another metal that binds preferentially with the interfering anion. For example, in calcium and magnesium procedures, lanthanum is added in excess to complex the phosphate anion.[11]

Ionization interference results when a substantial number of atoms in the sample become ionized and no longer absorb at the atom resonance line. These ionized atoms are lost to the determination. A decrease in flame temperature may solve the problem, as may the addition of a large excess of a more easily ionized element. For example, in determination of lithium, excess sodium ions are added to decrease the ionization of lithium.[12]

A *matrix interference* is noted in solutions of high-salt concentration, resulting in a decrease in signal. This interference is caused by a decrease in atomizing efficiency of the flame, because much of the available flame energy will be used decomposing the other salts present. This effect can be overcome by simple dilution or by extraction. A viscosity effect can also be called a matrix effect. If the viscosity of samples and standards varies greatly, the amount of sample reaching the burner will not be the same as that of the standard. An apparent decrease in absorption will occur in the more viscous samples. This can be overcome by matching the viscosity of the standards to that of the samples[13] or by forcing the samples and standards into the burner at the same rate by using a peristaltic pump.[14] Matrix interferences are more prevalent and varied when furnaces are used instead of burners. Background correction as previously described in this chapter compensates for some matrix interference. Slavin[15] gives a more detailed discussion of minimizing matrix interferences.

Maintenance and Quality Assurance

FLAME PHOTOMETRY

Routine maintenance and function checks are required on flame photometers as for any other piece of laboratory equipment. The burner assembly, chimney, and appropriate optical surfaces should be checked for dirt and film accumulation and cleaned at periodic intervals. To prevent protein buildup in the aspirator tube, the atomizer should be periodically cleaned with the mechanical cleaning wires supplied with the instrument. The flow rate should be optimized at regular intervals. The burner head and aspirator should be flushed thoroughly with water each day of use. The operator should refer to specific maintenance manuals pertinent to the instrument being used. Whether lithium or cesium is used as the internal standard, the concentration of the internal standard should be maintained precisely. It is important that the same concentration of internal standard be used for establishing baseline or zero calibration, calibration of standards, and dilution of patient samples.

Whenever dilutions of calibrators and patient samples are performed, adequate precision of the diluters must be verified initially and routinely thereafter, at least weekly. If automatic diluters are used, it is important to check for possible viscosity effects. Calibrators are frequently aqueous and are readily aspirated, whereas patient samples, containing varying concentrations of proteins, may be less readily aspirated. Samples with high concentrations of lipids or proteins may have an apparent decrease in analyte concentration caused by decreased sample water for the analyte of interest to be found in (e.g., a greater proportion of plasma volume is due to solids).

ATOMIC ABSORPTION SPECTROPHOTOMETRY

Maintenance of an atomic absorption instrument centers around the hollow cathode lamp and the burner or furnace. As with all instruments, the maintenance instructions provided by the manufacturer should be followed. The lamp should be warmed up before use. Warmup ensures a steady emission of light at the metal's characteristic wavelength. After warmup the correct wavelength is optimized by decreasing the slit width and rotating the grating to maximum signal output.

Maintenance of the burner assembly is the same as for the burner maintenance described in flame photometry. Aspirator tubes and the aspirator itself should be cleaned periodically with the cleaning wire supplied by the manufacturer. The aspiration rate should be determined at least monthly. The burner and aspirator assembly should be washed thoroughly after each day of use. Before use the burner should be aligned so that the entire burner length is in the light beam. The burner height is adjusted for maximum absorbance while aspirating a standard of the analyte.

Quality assurance of a graphite-furnace spectrophotometer includes analyzing a standard reference material (e.g., SRM 1643c Standard Reference Material, Trace Elements in Water; National Institute of Standards and Technology, Gaithersburg, MD 20899) for three elements: silver, copper, and chromium. Slavin[16] explains that several different analyses are done and the average absorbance for each element determined, as well as the average Zeeman ratio (R):

$$R = Z/(Z + B) \tag{Eq. 7-8}$$

where

Z = Zeeman signal
B = background signal

Furnace misalignment results in a change in the Zeeman ratio for chromium; incorrect line voltage results in changes in the Zeeman ratio for copper.

The absorbance profile, absorbance on the y axis with time (sec) on the x axis, can detect problems in drying conditions when early background peaks are detected. Any other tests recommended by the manufacturer should also be done.

Summary

Flame photometry and atomic absorption are analytical techniques for determining the concentration of metals. Both techniques are based on the principle that all elements can absorb a unit of energy at the same wavelength at which the excited form of the element emits radiation. Flame photometry measures the intensity of the light emitted after excitation of atoms in a flame. Atomic absorption measures the amount of light absorbed by atoms in the ground state. The two techniques complement each other. For the easily excitable alkali metals (sodium, potassium, lithium), flame photometry usually gives better sensitivity. The alkaline metals, calcium and magnesium, can be determined by either method, although the reference method for calcium is atomic absorption. For trace metals such as zinc, copper, lead, cobalt, and aluminum, atomic absorption is used, because flame photometry has insufficient sensitivity.

Instrumentation for both methods includes a light source, a flame or furnace, a monochromator, and a detector. The flame is the sample cuvette for both flame photometry and atomic absorption. The light source in flame photometry is the excited atoms themselves (which are also in the flame). The usual light source for atomic absorption is the hollow cathode lamp. Both types of instruments can be constructed with diffraction gratings (flame photometers often use filters) for monochromators and photomultiplier tubes for detectors. Microprocessor control allows calibration from multiple standards and direct readout of sample concentration.

Interferences in both methods include chemical interference from anions that may bind with ionic forms of the element of interest, difference in the degree of ionization of the element of interest caused by other elements in the sample solution, variations in flame background noise, variation in atomization of the solution because of viscosity, density, or surface tension, and other matrix variations.

Questions and Problems

1. Discuss three similarities between atomic absorption and flame photometry.
2. Discuss the principle of flame photometry and how it relates to the hollow cathode lamp.
3. Known amounts of sodium (in mEq/L shown in the following list as theoretical) were added to a series of solutions. The following data were obtained on a flame photometer.

Theoretical	Manual Dilution	Automatic Dilution	Protein g/dL
145.9	143.8	142.5	6.5
142.8	142.8	139.9	7.9
141.3	141.5	135.5	10.4
133.6	135.2	126.3	15.4
121.3	121.4	85.9	26.4

Why do the results obtained by automatic dilution differ from results obtained by manual dilution as well as from the theoretical results?

4. The following data were found when determining zinc by atomic absorption. The wavelength was set at 214 nm, the standards were prepared in 6% albumin. Samples, standards, and controls were all diluted 1 in 3 with demineralized water.

Sample	*Absorbance*
0 μg/mL standard	0.026
0.5 μg/mL standard	0.071
1.0 μg/mL standard	0.115
1.5 μg/mL standard	0.160
2.0 μg/mL standard	0.207
Control I	0.077
Patient 1	0.182
Patient 2	0.154
Control II	0.190

Calculate the concentration of zinc in the unknown patient samples and in the controls.

5. Give at least three reasons why lithium is used as an internal standard in the flame photometric analysis of sodium and potassium in the clinical laboratory.

6. A grossly lipemic sample (triglyceride concentration = 5350 mg/dL) gave the following results for sodium concentration.

Sodium by specific ion electrode	139 mEq/L
Sodium by flame photometry	116 mEq/L

What do you think caused the discrepancy between the results?

References

1. Parsons ML. Atomic absorption and flame emission spectrometry. In: Ewing GW, ed. Analytical instrumentation handbook. New York: Marcel Dekker, 1990:141.
2. Skoog DA, Leary JJ. Principles of instrumental analysis, 4th ed. Fort Worth: Saunders College Publishing, 1992:203-04.
3. Robinson JW. Atomic spectroscopy. New York: Marcel Dekker, 1990:23-24.
4. Bender GT. Principles of chemical instrumentation. Philadelphia: WB Saunders, 1987:100-102.
5. Robinson JW. Atomic spectroscopy. New York: Marcel Dekker, 1990:78.
6. Sturgeon RE. Factors affecting atomization and measurement in graphite furnace atomic absorption spectrometry. Anal Chem 1977, 49:1255-67A.
7. Willard HH, Merritt LL Jr, Dena JA, Settle FA Jr. Instrumental methods of analysis, 7th ed. Belmont, CA; Wadsworth Publishing, 1988:234-49.
8. Walsh A. Application of atomic absorption spectra to chemical analysis. Spectrochim Acta 1955, 7:108-17.
9. Slavin W. Atomic absorption spectrometry. Methods Enzymol 1988, 158:117-45.
10. Risby TH. Flame atomic emission spectrometry. Methods Enzymol 1988, 158:180-90.
11. Trudeau DL, Freier EF. Determination of calcium in urine and serum by atomic absorption spectrophotometry. Clin Chem 1967, 13:101-14.
12. Ingle JD Jr, Crouch SR. Spectrochemical analysis. Englewood Cliffs, NJ: Prentice-Hall, 1988:201.
13. Parker MM, Humoller FL, Mahler DJ. Determination of copper and zinc in biological material. Clin Chem 1967, 13:40-48.
14. Hicks R, Haven M. Use of positive pressure sampling to minimize viscosity errors in atomic absorption spectrophotometry. Am J Clin Pathol 1970, 54:235-38.

15. Slavin W. Graphite furnace source book. Ridgefield, CT: Perkin-Elmer Corp, 1984.
16. Slavin W. Manning DC, Carnrick GR. Quality-assurance procedures for graphite-furnace atomic absorption spectrometry. Talanta 1989, 36:171-78.

Suggested Readings

Caraway WT. Photometry. In: Tietz NW, ed. Textbook of clinical chemistry. Philadelphia, WB Saunders, 1986:55-78.
Skoog DA, Leary JJ. Principles of instrumental analysis, 4th ed. Fort Worth: Saunders College Publishing, 1992:186-232.

8

NEPHELOMETRY AND TURBIDIMETRY

Gregory A. Tetrault

Objectives

After completing this chapter, the reader will be able to:

1. Define nephelometry and turbidimetry.
2. Explain the relationship between particle size, wavelength, and light scatter.
3. Calculate the concentration of particles in solution from a standard curve of intensity of scattered light versus concentration.
4. Describe end-point and kinetic methods of determining analyte concentration from intensity of scattered light.
5. Explain why sensitivity is increased when nephelometers measure forward light scatter.
6. Draw and label diagrams of a nephelometer and a turbidimeter.
7. Explain the advantages and disadvantages of laser light sources for nephelometers.
8. List the periodic checks needed to ensure quality results from turbidimeters and nephelometers.

Definitions

Backward Light Scatter: Light scatter in a direction opposite that of the incident light beam.

Dipole: A pair of separated electric charges, one positive and one negative. The magnitude of the dipole is the product of the charge and the separation distance between the charges (Fig. 8-1).

Electric Field (of light): A current that varies periodically (in magnitude and direction) perpendicular to the direction of propagation of the light ray (Fig. 8-1).

Forward Light Scatter: Light scatter in the same direction as that of the incident light beam.

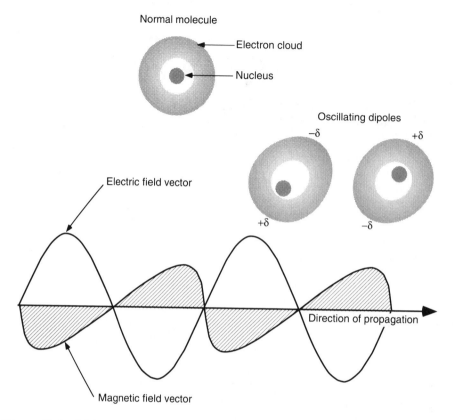

Figure 8-1.   Light ray with its electric field and magnetic field vectors (perpendicular to the direction of travel of the ray). Upper left: molecule with a symmetric electron cloud surrounding a nucleus. Above the electric field vector are two "snapshots" of the same molecule being converted to an oscillating dipole by the light ray. The charges of the dipole are represented by the symbol δ. The electron cloud is alternately pushed away from or pulled toward the light ray, resulting in shifts of the dipole in phase with the electric field wave.

Lambert-Beer Law: Another name for Beer's law, the relationship between concentration of a substance and absorption of light.

LASER: Acronym for light amplification by stimulated emission of radiation. A device that produces a coherent, nonspreading, high-intensity beam of monochromatic light.

Light-Emitting Diode: An electronic device that usually consists of a sealed, evacuated tube with a cylindrical anode surrounding a cathode. The cathode is heated (directly or indirectly) by current and emits electrons that are captured by the anode. The impact of electrons on the anode produces light.

Light Scatter: The phenomenon that occurs when a light beam's electric field induces an oscillating dipole in a particle. The oscillating dipole reemits light in all directions.

Logit: The natural logarithm of a number divided by 1 minus the number ($\ln [x/(1-x)]$).

Nephelometry: The quantitation of suspended particles by measurement of scattered light.

Polarizability: The ease with which a molecule becomes a dipole when exposed to an electric field.

Polarized Light: Light in which all vibrations are in a single plane perpendicular to the ray, instead of in all planes.

Reflectance: The ability of an object to throw light back from its surface.

Signal-to-Noise Ratio: The ratio of the lowest usable electrical signal (S) to noise (N)—undesirable, spurious signal components. S/N must be greater than 1 for reliable measurements.

Turbidimetry: The quantitation of suspended particles by measurement of the change in light intensity due to light scatter, reflection, and absorption.

Turbidity (t):   The loss of transparency due to particles. Units are cm^{-1}.

Introduction

Nephelometry and *turbidimetry* are related techniques that are commonly employed in clinical laboratories. Both are based on the measurement of light scatter. Quantitative relationships exist between the size and number of suspended particles and the amount of scattering that occurs. The instrumentation is similar to or identical to other photometric devices such as spectrophotometers and fluorometers. This chapter will discuss principles of light scatter by large particles, measurement of light scatter, component parts of nephelometers, and maintenance and quality assurance of instruments.

Principles

In Chapter 6 the relationship between concentration of a substance and the amount of light absorbed was discussed. For many circumstances, this relationship is defined mathematically by Beer's law. Similarly, for large particles in solution, there is a relationship between the total surface area of the particles and the amount of light scattered. Unfortunately, this relationship is far more complex than the linear one defined by Beer's law.

THE PHENOMENON OF LIGHT SCATTER

Light scatter is not the same as reflectance. Light scatter involves a direct interaction between a light beam and the particle it strikes.[1] When a light beam strikes a particle, its electric field (remember that a light beam consists of photons moving in a wavelike pattern that produces an alternating current [electric field] perpendicular to the direction of travel) moves the particle's electrons in one direction and its nucleus in the opposite direction. The maximum amount of movement is proportional to the electric field strength of the light beam. However, the movement is only at a maximum when the electric field of the light beam is closest to the particle. This occurs with each cycle of the photons. Thus, the electrons and nucleus move back and forth in phase with the light beam and produce an oscillating dipole (Fig. 8-1). The size of the dipole depends on the electric field strength of the light (which is determined by its frequency) and the polarizability of the particle's electrons.

The oscillating dipole is now a source of electromagnetic radiation. It radiates light in all directions. This light is the same frequency and wavelength as the original light beam. Hence, the appearance that light is simply scattered by the particle.

The basic mechanism of light scattering described holds for all conditions. However, the amount and distribution of scattered light depends on numerous factors besides light beam wavelength and polarizability of the particle's electrons. These factors include particle size, particle concentration, polarization of the light beam, and the ratio of particle size to wavelength. The simplest relationship is when polarized, monochromatic light interacts with immobile particles of uniform size and shape whose largest dimension is less than one-tenth of the wavelength of the incident light. This relationship (Equation 8-1) was derived by Lord Rayleigh in 1871.[1,2]

$$i_s = I_0 \frac{16\,\pi^2 a^2 \sin^2(90^\circ - \theta)}{\lambda^4 r^2} \tag{Eq. 8-1}$$

where

i_s = intensity of scattered light (erg/cm^2/s)
I_0 = intensity of incident light (erg/cm^2/s)
a = polarizability of particle (m^4 − cm^2)
θ = angle of observation from the incident light beam (degrees)
λ = wavelength of light (m)
r = distance from the particle to the detector (cm)

Figure 8-2 shows the intensity of scattered light for different observation angles (under the conditions just noted). Note that no scattering occurs perpendicular to the direction of the incident light beam.

Equation 8-1 does not allow calculation of particle concentration by measurement of light scatter intensity. However, for many small particles, Equation 8-2 can be used.[1,2]

$$i_s = I_0 \frac{16\,\pi^2 \left[\left(\dfrac{dn}{dc} \right)^2 \dfrac{Mc}{4N_a} \right] \sin^2(90^\circ - \theta)}{\lambda^4 r^2} \tag{Eq. 8-2}$$

where

dn/dc = rate of change of solution refractive index with concentration
M = molecular weight of the particle (g/mol)
c = concentration of the particle (g/mL)
N_a = Avogadro's number (6.023×10^{23})

Because the rate of change of refractive index with concentration is often constant, Equation 8-2 can be used to calculate the concentration of a particle by measuring scattered-light intensity.

The use of nonpolarized light alters the relationships shown in Equations 8-1 and 8-2. The relationship between intensity of scattered light and angle of observation from the nonpolarized light source is shown in Figure 8-3. Particles struck by

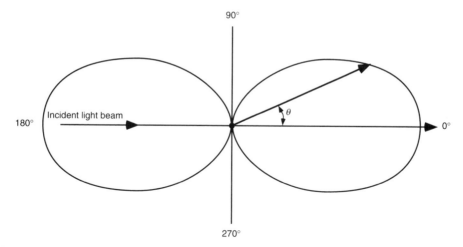

Figure 8-2. Two-dimensional plot of Rayleigh light scatter from an extremely small particle struck by polarized, monochromatic light. The intensity of light scatter at each angle is shown by the curve. Light scattering is symmetrical around all axes, and maximum scattering occurs at 0 and 180° to the incident light beam (forward and backward scatter). No light scatter occurs perpendicular to the light beam. In reality, light scatter occurs in three dimensions. This can be visualized by rotating the scatter intensity curve around the 0 to 180° axis.

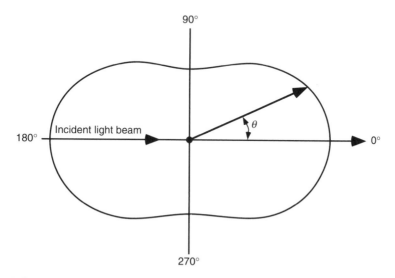

Figure 8-3. Two-dimensional plot of Rayleigh light scatter from a nonpolarized light source. Scatter is still symmetrical around all axes and maximal at 0 and 180°. However, now there is significant light scattering perpendicular to the light beam.

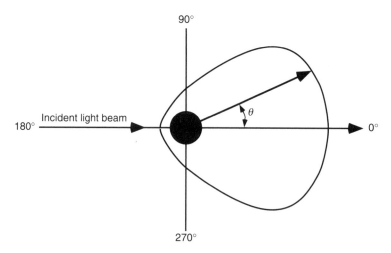

Figure 8-4. Two-dimensional plot of light scatter from a large particle. The intensity of light scatter at each angle is shown by the curve. Scatter occurs in all directions, but forward light scatter intensity is much greater than backward.

nonpolarized light will scatter light in all directions, although forward ($\theta = 0°$) and backward ($\theta = 180°$) scatter intensities are still greater than with other directions.

So far the discussion of light scattering has been restricted to particles less than one-tenth the diameter of the light beam's wavelength. This means that the particles must be smaller than 70 nm if visible light is used. However, many of the particles quantitated by nephelometry and turbidimetry (such as large proteins, immune complexes, latex particles, and oil droplets) are much larger than that. As particle size increases, backward light scatter decreases. Figure 8-4 shows the relationship between intensity of scattered light and angle of observation from the nonpolarized light source when particle size is the same order of magnitude as the wavelength of light. There is progressively less backward light scatter as particle size increases. Very large particles, such as erythrocytes, have almost no backward light scatter.

MODIFIED LAMBERT-BEER LAW FOR LIGHT SCATTER

Particles in solution scatter some light away from the forward direction of the incident light beam. The loss of light intensity in the forward direction is related to the scattering power of the solution. The relationship is described in Equation 8-3.[2]

$$I = I_0 \, e^{-tl} \qquad\qquad\qquad \text{(Eq. 8-3)}$$

where

      I = intensity of light passing through solution
      I_0 = initial intensity of light beam
      t = turbidity of the solution
      l = length of light beam travel through solution

The turbidity increases with the scattering power of the solution and is directly proportional to the concentration of particles in the solution (g/L). Therefore, for a solution with a single type of particle, its molar concentration can be determined from Equation 8-4.

$$C_p = \frac{-K \log \frac{I}{I_0}}{MW_p} = \frac{-K \log T}{MW_p} \qquad \text{(Eq. 8-4)}$$

where

C_p = concentration of particles (mol/L)
K = a constant incorporating turbidity, path length, and base e to base 10 conversion
MW_p = molecular weight of the particle (g/mol)
T = transmittance

It is evident from Equation 8-4 that particle concentration is directly proportional to transmittance. Even if the molecular weight of the particle is unknown, a standard curve can be used to determine the relationship between particle concentration and transmittance. This is the basis of turbidimetry. Note that the intensity of light passing through the solution is affected by light scatter, reflectance, and absorbance (if the particle absorbs at the wavelength of the incident light beam). However, because all three factors are directly proportional to the concentration of particles, Equation 8-4 still holds.

DIRECT MEASUREMENT OF SCATTERED LIGHT

Nephelometry measures a portion of the light scattered by particles in solution. The relationship between the intensities of the initial light beam and the scattered light reaching the detector depends on many factors: turbidity, particle size and shape, particle concentration, wavelength of incident light, reflectance, light absorption, size and shape of the slit between the sample holder and the detector, and the angle of observation. The last two factors depend on the design of the nephelometer. Therefore, no universal equation can be derived to calculate particle concentration from measured light scatter. Instead, nephelometry readings are treated in a manner similar to fluorometry readings. Light scatter units are measured and are plotted against known concentrations of analyte. The relationship between measured intensity of scattered light and concentration is nonlinear. Equation 8-5 shows a logit-log transformation that is often used to linearize nephelometric data.

$$\ln\left(\frac{I_s}{1 - I_s}\right) = a \ln(C_p) + b \qquad \text{(Eq. 8-5)}$$

where

ln = natural logarithm
I_s = intensity of scattered light reaching detector
C_p = concentration of particles (mol/L)
a = slope of line
b = intercept of line

TYPES OF TURBIDIMETRIC AND NEPHELOMETRIC REACTIONS

If the analyte of interest is a stable particle of uniform size and composition, then measurement of light scatter is straightforward. However, many clinical laboratory assays involve antibody-antigen interactions in which there is a mixture of particles of varying sizes and in which the concentrations of each type of particle change over time (Fig. 8-5). Also, some enzyme assays use large particulate substrates that are broken down and produce *less* light scatter. The turbidimetric lipase assay is one such method. The substrate is an aqueous emulsion of olive oil droplets. Lipase converts the triglycerides to soluble products, thereby reducing the size of the oil droplets and

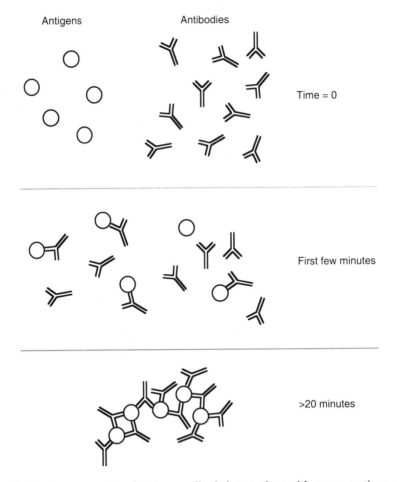

Figure 8-5. Representation of antigen-antibody interactions with concentrations at the equivalence zone. Mixing occurs at time 0. After a brief lag phase, antibody-antigen binding begins. Finally, a complex lattice of antigens and antibodies is formed. These very large particles require from 20 minutes to many hours to form.

decreasing light scatter. In these types of assays with changing particle size or composition, one may employ end-point or kinetic methods.

A stable equilibrium must be reached before making an end-point measurement of light scatter intensity. This can take hours when the solution contains only antigen and antibodies in buffer. Fortunately, the use of linear polymers such as polyethylene glycol (2-4%) increases the rate of reaction about tenfold.[3] The stable endpoint is reached after about 20 to 40 minutes.

Kinetic methods relate the rate of change in light scatter (dI_s/dt) to concentration of analyte. Reaction kinetics for antibody-antigen reactions are similar to the kinetics of enzyme-substrate interactions. Determination of (dI_s/dt) is usually made in the first few minutes after sample and reagents are mixed because the rate of increase in light scatter is highest during this period.[4] (Note that a brief lag phase exists, again similar to enzyme-substrate kinetics.) The main advantage of kinetic light scatter assays is the brief time required for analysis. Additional advantages include no requirement for a sample blank measurement and lower levels of interference from background light scatter or absorbance.[3] Disadvantages of kinetic light scattering assays include lower intensities of scattered light and the need for thorough and rapid mixing of sample and reagents.[3,4]

Turbidimetric Instruments

Turbidimetry can be performed on any standard spectrophotometer. See Chapter 6 for descriptions and diagrams of spectrophotometers. Photometers may also be used for turbidimetry. Photometers usually have wider bandpasses and greater background noise than spectrophotometers, so their lower limit of detection is much higher.

Nephelometric Instruments

Nephelometry can be performed on most fluorometers or spectrofluorometers. Instruments that use an "end-on" design (detector aligned with incident light beam) cannot be used for nephelometry. For nephelometry, the monochromators for incident light and emitted light are set to the same wavelength. Fluorometers that use nonremovable interference filters cannot be adapted to nephelometry.

There are a number of dedicated nephelometers available. Many of them are automated and computerized. These nephelometers all have the same basic design (Fig. 8-6). The major differences are in the light source, the types of monochromators, and the angle of detection. Most instruments used for nephelometry measure scattered light perpendicular to the incident light beam. This optical setup is simple and minimizes problems due to reflectance off the cuvette. However, since 90° light scatter is weak (compared to forward light scatter), the sensitivity is decreased. Stray light causes the greatest problems when a 90° system is employed. The best sensitivity is attained by placing the detector angle as close to 0° as possible. This requires a tightly focused incident light beam and excellent optics.

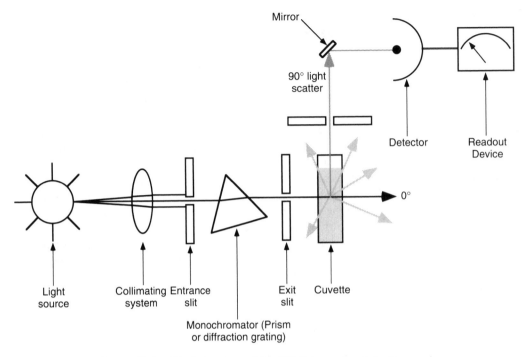

Figure 8-6. Nephelometer with a 90° light scatter detection angle.

COMPONENT PARTS

Nephelometers are composed of a light source, incident light monochromator, sample holder, scattered light monochromator, detector, and readout device (Fig. 8-6). The following descriptions apply to dedicated nephelometers and to fluorometers and spectrofluorometers adapted to measure light scatter.

Light Source

The common tungsten filament lamp can be used as a light source for nephelometry. However, its relatively low intensity makes it less useful for samples with low light scattering. Alternate light sources include quartz halogen lamps, xenon lamps, mercury-arc lamps, light-emitting diodes, and lasers.[2,5,6] All of these have higher intensities than tungsten lamps. Lasers are especially useful for nephelometry because they have extremely high intensity, narrow beams that do not require focusing or collimating optics. Laser nephelometers also have fewer problems with stray light. Disadvantages of laser light sources include high costs, operating hazards, and limited choices of wavelengths.

Monochromators

Any of the monochromators described in Chapter 6 and Chapter 7 may be used in nephelometers. Fluorometers or spectrofluorometers adapted for use as nephelometers must set the wavelength selector for the scattered (emitted) light to be the same as that of the incident light. Dedicated nephelometers do not require a second monochromator.

Detector

Photomultiplier tubes (Chapter 6 and Fig. 6-12) are the most commonly employed detectors in nephelometers. The photomultiplier tube must be well shielded to minimize interference from stray light. A high signal-to-noise ratio is necessary when analyzing samples with low intensities of scattered light.

Some nephelometers have movable detectors that allow the operator to vary the angle of detection.[2] This is useful for determining properties of particles such as mean molecular weight and radius of gyration.[1] Most nephelometers in clinical laboratories employ fixed-angle detectors.

Readout Device

Nephelometers measure the intensity of a small fraction of scattered light. Light intensity is converted to an electrical signal by the detector. This signal can be reported as arbitrary light scatter intensity units (similar to fluorescence intensity units). The scale is usually unimportant. Many nephelometers in clinical laboratories contain microcomputers that store standard curve data and report results in concentrations. Types of readout devices include analog meters, light-emitting diodes, and digital displays.

Maintenance and Quality Assurance

Turbidimeters and nephelometers are photometric instruments that require the same quality assurance checks and routine maintenance procedures as spectrophotometers (Chapter 6) or fluorometers (Chapter 9). Checks of photometric accuracy, wavelength calibration, linearity of detector response, and stray light should be performed at regular intervals. Stray light checks are extremely important in nephelometry.

Summary

Nephelometry and turbidimetry are measurement techniques based on light scattering by suspended particles. Nephelometers measure the intensity of a portion of scattered light. Turbidimeters measure change in light intensity due to scatter.

Light scatter occurs when a light beam impinges on a particle and produces an oscillating dipole (in phase with the light wave). The oscillating dipole reradiates light in all directions. The magnitude of light scatter by a particle depends on particle size, shape, and polarizability; the wavelength and polarization of light; and the ratio of particle size to wavelength.

A variation of the Lambert–Beer law describes the relationship between concentration of particles and transmitted light. Linear standard curves are used in turbidimetry to convert transmittance to concentration. Nonlinear standard curves are found with nephelometry.

When particle size varies over time, either end-point or kinetic methods may be used to convert change in the amount of light scatter to concentration of particles.

Turbidimetry is performed on spectrophotometers or photometers. Nephelometry is performed on spectrofluorometers, fluorometers, or dedicated nephelometers. The component parts of a nephelometer are high-intensity light source, monochromator, sample holder, shielded detector, and readout device. Sensitivity is maximized by measuring scattered light at a low angle (forward light scatter).

Maintenance and quality assurance procedures for nephelometers and turbidimeters are nearly identical to those of fluorometers and spectrophotometers.

Questions and Problems

1. For a very small particle, calculate the relative intensities of scattered light when monitored at 30° versus 60° from the incident light beam.
2. Given the following turbidimetric data, calculate the concentration of compound x in the patient sample.

Concentration of $\times$ (mol/L)	Transmittance
0.0	0.985
0.2	0.824
0.4	0.701
0.8	0.472
Sample	0.735

3. Give the advantages of kinetic or rate nephelometric methods over end-point methods.
4. Draw a diagram of a nephelometer.
5. List the quality assurance checks that should be performed regularly on a turbidimeter.

References

1. Tiffany TO. Fluorometry, nephelometry, and turbidimetry. In: Tietz NW, ed. Textbook of clinical chemistry. Philadelphia: WB Saunders, 1986:91-97.
2. Atkins PW. Physical chemistry, 2nd ed. San Francisco: WH Freeman, 1982:827-33.
3. Hurtubise PE, Bassion S, Gauldie J, Horsewood P. Immunochemical techniques. In: Kaplan LA, Pesce AJ, eds. Clinical chemistry: Theory, analysis, and correlation, 2nd ed. St. Louis: CV Mosby, 1989:178-89.
4. Buffone GJ. Principles of immunochemical techniques. In: Tietz NW, ed. Textbook of clinical chemistry. Philadelphia: WB Saunders, 1986:223-24.
5. Frings CS, Gauldie J. Spectral techniques. In: Kaplan LA, Pesce AJ, eds. Clinical chemistry: Theory, analysis, and correlation, 2nd ed. St. Louis: CV Mosby, 1989:66-70.
6. Behring nephelometer instruction manual. Marburg, Germany: Behringwerke AG, 1987:4.

Suggested Reading

Ritchie RF, ed. Automated immunoanalysis, Part 1. New York: Marcel Dekker, 1978.

9

FLUOROMETRY AND FLUORESCENCE POLARIZATION

Patricia K. Studts
David J. Studts
Jeffrey A. Huth

Objectives

After completing this chapter, the reader will be able to:

1. Explain the theory underlying molecular fluorescence.
2. Describe the basic principles of fluorescence and fluorescence polarization measurements.
3. Construct a simple diagram of a filter fluorometer, a fluorescence polarization analyzer, and a spectrofluorometer, and name the component parts of each.
4. Describe the similarities and differences between filter fluorometers, fluorescence polarization analyzers, and spectrofluorometers.
5. Name at least two advantages of fluorescence measurements over absorption measurements.
6. Name at least two disadvantages of, or problems associated with, fluorescence measurements.
7. Describe examples of fluorescence and fluorescence polarization applications used in the clinical laboratory.
8. Design a maintenance program for a spectrofluorometer.

Definitions

Emission Spectrum: The wavelengths at which a fluorescent compound will emit energy in the form of light.

Excitation Spectrum: The wavelengths at which a fluorescent compound will absorb energy in the form of light.

Excited State: A condition in which a molecule's electrons have undergone a transition from stable lower-energy orbitals to unstable higher-energy orbitals.

Filter: A device that will pass only light from a particular portion of the spectrum while absorbing other wavelengths.

Fluorescence: The emission of light energy from an excited molecule as it returns to the ground state.

Fluorescence Polarization: The emission of polarized light from a fluorophore that has been excited with polarized light.

Fluorometer: An instrument that is used to measure the intensity of fluorescence produced from a fluorophore. A fluorometer uses filters for wavelength selection.

Fluorometry: The quantitative measurement of the intensity of light produced by an excited fluorescent substance and the relationship between the measured intensity and the concentration of that substance.

Fluorophore: A molecule or portion of a molecule that is capable of being excited with high-energy radiation and that will subsequently emit lower-energy radiation.

Ground State: A condition in which a molecule's electrons are in stable lower-energy orbitals.

Inner Filter Effect: A phenomenon occurring at high fluorophore concentrations in which the molecules at the front of the cuvette absorb most of the incident radiation. This causes the molecules at the back of the cuvette to be exposed to less radiation, resulting in decreased fluorescence.

Monochromator: A device used to selectively pass light only at specific wavelengths.

Photomultiplier Tube: A vacuum tube containing a light-sensitive screen that generates an electrical signal proportional to the intensity of light striking the screen. Through the use of several electron emitter or collector cells, the tube amplifies the signal.

Polarizer: A device that filters the electronic component of electromagnetic radiation so that the radiation that passes through it lies in a single plane.

Quantum Yield: The efficiency with which a fluorophore emits light.

Raman Scatter: Optical emissions other than fluorescence, caused by solvent molecules, that appear at slightly longer wavelengths than the incident radiation.

Rayleigh Scatter: Optical emissions other than fluorescence, inherent to many solvents, solutes, and cells, that appear at the same wavelength as the incident radiation.

Scattered Light: Light that is of the same wavelength as that of the excitation beam and that emerges from the fluorescence cuvette in all directions.

Self-Absorption: A phenomenon occurring in fluorescence when the excitation band and emission band overlap. Some of the emitted fluorescence is reabsorbed, resulting in decreased fluorescence.

Self-Quenching: A phenomenon occurring at high fluorophore concentrations in which radiationless energy is given off as heat energy to the solvent molecules, resulting in decreased fluorescence.

Spectrofluorometer: An instrument that is used to measure the intensity of fluorescence produced from a fluorophore. A spectrofluorometer can select wavelengths continuously because it uses dispersion monochromators for wavelength selection.

Stokes Shift: The difference between the wavelength at which a fluorescent molecule is excited and the longer wavelength at which the molecule emits fluorescent radiation.

Stray Light: Light of unwanted wavelengths emerging from a monochromator.

Introduction

In the natural environment of a chemical substance, that substance will exist in what is called the *ground state.* As electromagnetic radiation or light energy impinges on that substance, enough energy may be absorbed to cause the substance to alter its electron configuration and place it in an *excited state.* The excited state is only short-lived, however, and the substance quickly returns to the ground state. If the substance is of unique chemical nature, the transition may be a multi-step process with the major step resulting in release of emitted light of lower energy than the excitation light. The other steps in the transition to the ground state are mostly vibrational energy loss due to electron collisions. This emitted light that is produced as the substance passes from an excited state to the ground state is called *fluorescence.*

Fluorometry is the quantitative measurement of the intensity of light produced by an excited fluorescent substance, and the relationship between the measured intensity and the concentration of that substance. *Fluorescence polarization* is defined as the emission of polarized light from a fluorophore that has been excited with polarized light. Fluorometry and fluorescence polarization are two of a group of techniques coined *multiparameter techniques,* or *multidimensional luminescence measurements.*[1] Because of the widespread use of fluorometry and fluorescence polarization in the clinical area, in this chapter we will focus only on these two multiparameter techniques.

Principles

As previously mentioned, for fluorescence to occur, a molecule must first be placed in an excited state through the absorption of light energy. Although the excitation process is not as complex or competitive as the process involved in returning to the ground state, the proper energy requirements must be met for the electronic transition to occur. Most often, for organic molecules the excitation process involves π electrons in a π-to-π^* transition. Although other electron transitions may occur, it is this difference in energy levels that favors fluorescence. These transitions are common for aromatic or highly conjugated double bonds in an organic molecule.

During the excitation process, both electronic energy and vibrational energy are absorbed from the photons of light striking the molecule. However, during the emission process, only electronic energy is given off in the form of light. Because the emission energy is less than the total excitation energy, the *emission spectrum* is shifted to longer wavelengths (lower energy) as compared to the *excitation spectrum* of shorter wavelengths (higher energy). This phenomenon is known as the *Stokes shift.*

The excitation of an organic molecule to a higher energy level is a rather simple process involving the absorption of electromagnetic radiation. The return to the ground state, or deactivation, however, is not quite so simple and involves a competition between several different pathways.[2] The emission process found in fluorescence is only one mechanism through which the excited molecule may return. The following is a list of deactivation processes, and a complete description of these processes can be found in the book by Skoog and Leary.[2]

Deactivation Processes for Excited Molecules[2]

Fluorescence (photon emission)	Dissociation
Vibrational relaxation	External conversion
Internal conversion	Intersystem crossing
Predissociation	Phosphorescence (photon emission)

Of important concern in the evaluation of all these deactivation processes is the concept of *quantum efficiency,* or *quantum yield, ϕ.* The quantum yield may be defined as the number of molecules that fluoresce divided by the total number of excited molecules.

$$\phi = \frac{\text{number of fluorescent molecules}}{\text{total number of excited molecules}} \qquad \text{(Eq. 9-1)}$$

Accordingly, the total number of molecules that are excited includes molecules that fluoresce plus all those excited molecules that deactivate by other processes. Therefore, a molecule whose quantum yield approaches 1 would have a high degree of fluorescence because of less competing deactivating processes, whereas a quantum yield that approaches zero indicates that a competing process would be more favored and less fluorescence would be produced.

From the discussion so far, it is evident that a number of molecular events may occur, reducing the probability that fluorescence will be produced. Many of these events may be the result of the chemical nature of the molecule itself, or they may be produced because of an incompatible environment. The importance of π-to-π^* transitions has already been discussed. Those molecules that fluoresce are most likely highly conjugated organic molecules, aromatic hydrocarbons, and heterocyclics with fused benzene rings. Other important parameters that affect fluorescence are chemical substitution, structural rigidity, and polarity. Environmental parameters that may affect fluorescence are solvent viscosity, temperature, pH, heavy atoms, and dissolved oxygen. Table 9-1 lists the parameters and whether they tend to enhance ($\uparrow$) or decrease ($\downarrow$) fluorescence.

In fluorometry, it is common practice to develop a standard curve for measured fluorescence intensity versus solute concentration. A linear curve is obtained with an equation of

$$F = kc \qquad \text{(Eq. 9-2)}$$

where F is fluorescence, k is a constant, and c is the concentration of the species being measured. Mathematically, this equation is derived from the Beer–Lambert law.

Table 9-1
Factors That May Affect Fluorescence

Factor	Fluorescence
Chemical substitution	$\uparrow$ or $\downarrow$
Structural rigidity	$\uparrow$
Polarity	$\uparrow$
Solvent viscosity (increase)	$\uparrow$
Temperature (decrease)	$\uparrow$
pH	$\uparrow$ or $\downarrow$
Heavy atoms (Cl, Br, I)	$\downarrow$
Dissolved oxygen	$\downarrow$

Similar to absorption methods, the fluorescence concentration curve deviates from linearity at high concentrations. In fluorometry, the deviation may occur for several reasons. First, at high concentrations in which the absorbance approaches 0.02, the mathematical equation derived from Beer's law for fluorometry cannot be simplified to $F = kc$. Therefore, a linear equation for the curve is not obtained. High absorption of the solution also promotes a phenomenon called the *inner filter effect.* As light impinges on the front of the cuvette containing the fluorescent sample, those molecules in the front will absorb the incident radiation. Because of this, the molecules at the back of the cuvette will be exposed to less radiation resulting in less fluorescence. Another problem encountered at high fluorophore concentrations is *self-quenching.* If an abundant quantity of excited molecules are in solution, collisions between the molecules occur more frequently. Radiationless energy is then given off as heat energy to the solvent molecules, which results in decreased fluorescence. In each of these cases, appropriate dilution of the concentrated solution would eliminate these problems and would result in a linear fluorescence concentration curve. One instrumental technique to eliminate absorption problems has been designed by Adamsons and associates.[3] Through the use of cell rotation methods, absorption-corrected fluorescence measurements have produced linear curves from solutions with absorbances as high as 2.5.

The excitation or emission phenomenon that occurs in molecular fluorescence also occurs when the excitation beam is polarized. The fluorescence that results from a polarized excitation beam is also polarized. The design feature added to fluorescence polarization analyzers to use this phenomenon is a set of *polarizers,* one positioned in the excitation path, and the other in the emission path. The excitation source is polarized so that the light energy that impinges on the molecules does so in a well-defined plane. The resultant polarized emission is then measured in the dimension of a well-defined plane relative to the excitation source.

Two different instrumental techniques are used in fluorescence polarization analyzers. In one design, the excitation source is polarized only in one direction. The resultant emission is measured in planes both parallel and perpendicular to the excitation source. An instrument that uses this approach for fluorescence polarization measurements is Roche Diagnostic Systems' (Branchburg, NJ 08876-1760) COBAS FARA™ II analyzer. The other design, examples of which are Abbott Laboratories' (Abbott Park, IL 60064) TDx® and TDxFLx® fluorescence polarization analyzers, uses the opposite approach. The excitation source is polarized alternatingly in horizontal and vertical planes. The emission is measured only in the vertical plane. In either of these designs, fluorescence intensities are measured both parallel to, and perpendicular to, the plane of the excitation beam.

The resultant degree of polarization (P) is calculated as follows:

$$P = \frac{I_{\parallel} - I_{\perp}}{I_{\parallel} + I_{\perp}} \qquad \text{(Eq. 9-3)}$$

where P is the degree of polarization, $I_{\parallel}$ is the fluorescence intensity measured parallel to the plane of the excitation beam, and $I_{\perp}$ is the fluorescence intensity measured perpendicular to the plane of the excitation beam.

On a molecular level, if polarized light is used to excite a fluorescent substance, only those molecules that are electronically aligned properly will be excited and have potential for fluorescence. Should these aligned molecules be in a fixed state (no molecular rotation), the fluorescence produced would be emitted in the same polarized plane as the excitation source. However, in solution, molecules are free to rotate and do so. Because fluorescence is not an instantaneous process, some time will elapse between the moment when the molecule becomes excited and the moment when the emission of light occurs. This time lapse is approximately 10^{-9} seconds, which is sufficiently long for molecular rotation to occur. Therefore, the plane of the emitted fluorescence will deviate from the plane of the excitation beam and some depolarized fluorescence will be emitted in all rotational planes.

From this discussion it is evident that depolarization depends on molecular rotation. Because of this dependency, small molecules with a greater freedom of rotation will produce less polarized fluorescence as compared to larger, slower rotating molecules. This principle is the key to fluorescence polarization assays. In these assays, a competitive binding immunoassay is performed in which a substrate and a covalently bonded fluorescent-labeled substrate compete for binding sites on an antibody. The binding of the fluorescent-labeled substrate to the antibody causes the fluorescent tag to be part of a large molecule that rotates slowly. Thus, the fluorescence produced by this bound fluorescent tag will remain highly polarized. Conversely, the fluorescent-labeled substrate that is unbound is free to rotate more rapidly and will produce depolarized fluorescence. In competitive binding fluorescence polarization immunoassays, the presence of large amounts of natural substrate causes less binding of labeled substrate and results in less fluorescence polarization. If the natural substrate concentration is low, more labeled substrate binds to the antibody, which results in a higher degree of fluorescence polarization.

Applying this to Equation 9-3, one can determine that $I_{\parallel}$ is a measure of the polarization from the bound fluorescent tags plus the few unbound fluorescent tags that by chance were oriented in the same plane as the bound fluorescent tags when fluorescence occurred. Because of the high rotational speed of the unbound fluorescent tags, their fluorescence intensity is the same in all rotational planes. Therefore, $I_{\perp}$ is a measure of the unbound fluorescent tags. The difference between the two signals ($I_{\parallel} - I_{\perp}$) is therefore a measure of the concentration of the bound fluorescent tags. These two quantities are customarily expressed as the ratio of Equation 9-3. The degree of polarization (P) will therefore vary between a value of zero when there are no bound fluorescent tags (very high analyte concentration) and a value of 1 when there are no unbound fluorescent tags (very low analyte concentration).

Basic Components

The basic components of a fluorometer are essentially identical to those of a photometer. These components include a light source, an excitation filter, a cell or cuvette, an emission filter, a detector, and a readout device. In addition to these components, a fluorescence polarization analyzer has both an excitation and an emission polarizer. A spectrofluorometer differs from a fluorometer in that it uses monochromators (prisms or gratings) instead of filters for the selection of monochromatic light. As a result, spectrofluorometers permit continuous wavelength selection, whereas fluorometers do not.

LIGHT SOURCES

The light source used for fluorescence measurements serves the purpose of supplying the radiant energy that is necessary to excite the fluorescent molecule, or *fluorophore*. The desired features for a source are intensity, stability, and wavelength variability.[4] The source must supply intense radiant energy, because fluorescence is a function of source intensity, that is, the more intense the source, the greater the fluorescence produced. Stability is the second desired characteristic of a source. If the source flickers, fluorescence measurements will not be reproducible. The third area to be considered is the spectral range of the source. Fluorescent molecules are generally excited at specific wavelengths. The source must supply energy for excitation at these wavelengths if any fluorescence is to occur.

Lasers are a source of very intense radiation and high stability. Although these light sources have great potential for molecular excitation, wavelength variability is a major drawback in that these sources are monochromatic. The fluorophore must be able to be excited at the specific wavelength to which the laser has been "tuned," or no fluorescence is observed. The high cost of these sources is another major drawback.

The more commonly used sources in fluorometry are the deuterium lamp, the mercury vapor lamp, and the xenon arc. The deuterium lamp provides for an intense source; however, its wavelength range is limited to the 200- to 350-nm range.

The mercury vapor lamp provides a very intense and stable source. Its major drawback is that this source does not provide a continuous spectrum. The mercury lamp emits radiation only at well-defined wavelengths; therefore, it is called a line source. The source will give off light at the following wavelengths: 257.7 nm, 313.0 nm, 365.0 nm, 404.7 nm, 407.8 nm, 435.8 nm, 546.1 nm, 577.0 nm, 579.1 nm.[4] The advantage of this source is its intensity and stability. In addition, mercury lines provide a monochromatic beam at each wavelength. If other lines are efficiently filtered, stray light is minimized. As a result, mercury lamps are quite often used in filter fluorometers. Although this source is discontinuous, most fluorescing molecules will absorb some radiation at one of the mercury lines. By setting the excitation source at the line nearest to the absorption maximum, fluorescence can be achieved.

The xenon arc is the other commonly used source in fluorescence. This source produces a continuous spectrum from 250 to 600 nm; however, the intensity varies with wavelength. Peak intensity is at 470 nm. The major advantage of the xenon source is its continuous spectrum. Through this, optimal fluorescence can be obtained by setting the source at the wavelength at which absorption is maximum. The disadvantages are that some lamps need a cooling apparatus for proper operation. The removal of ozone that may be produced by the xenon arc also poses instrumental limitations. Use of this source over the deuterium lamp extends the working excitation wavelength range and adds considerably more selectivity.[5]

As with fluorescence, the source in fluorescence polarization must supply the intensity and proper wavelength for excitation of the fluorophore. However, the use of intensity ratios for polarization calculations permits less sophistication in lamp design. Through the use of ratios, lamp instability as a source of error is significantly reduced. Generally, a tungsten halogen lamp is used as the source for fluorescence polarization. This source provides a continuous spectrum in the visible range. The use of highly efficient fluorophores (high quantum yield) facilitates the use of this less intense source while retaining accurate fluorescence measurements. One wavelength in the range is optimally chosen to match the excitation maximum of the fluorescent tag chosen. The major advantages of the tungsten halogen lamp in fluorescence polarization are the instrumental simplicity required for operation and its low cost.

FILTERS AND MONOCHROMATORS

Filters may be classified as either short-pass, long-pass, or bandpass filters. A *short-pass filter* will permit light at wavelengths below that given for the filter to pass. Similarly, *long-pass filters* permit light at wavelengths above that given for the filter to pass. A *bandpass filter* permits light between two given wavelengths to pass and performs similarly to a monochromator. Each of these types of filters is good for eliminating different sources of interfering light. The reader is referred to the article by Weinberger and Sapp[5] for a detailed description of filters.

As stated, the mercury vapor lamp is most often used in fluorometers. Because the lamp supplies narrow lines of radiation, a bandpass filter is often used to select the desired wavelength for excitation. Other undesired wavelengths are excluded. On the emission side of the fluorometer, a long-pass filter is commonly used. Of importance is that the excitation bandpass filter and the long-pass emission filter have no wavelengths in common. Through this, stray light is essentially eliminated.

Filters are often made of glass or are dye-containing Wratten filters. Through proper selection of the glass or dye, optical transmission can be regulated. The glass or dye acts by absorbing those wavelengths that are not desired. In other words, the undesired wavelengths are filtered out. Accordingly, those wavelengths that are desired are not absorbed and pass through the filters.

The monochromators used in spectrofluorometers are the same as those used in spectrophotometers. Although prisms were used in early instruments, gratings are more prominent today. Gratings may be classified as either ruled or holographic, with the ruled type being more common. Generally, the holographic gratings are better at reducing stray light, but the efficiency of these is less than that of the ruled gratings,[5] which permit greater intensity to pass for a given wavelength as compared to holographic gratings.

As explained in Chapter 6, monochromators operate by adjusting the angle at which the incident radiation strikes the surface of the grating. By rotating the gratings, the monochromator separates the incident light into its component wavelengths and focuses it on to the sample through the use of slits. In the case of emission, the fluorescent sample serves as the light source and the gratings are used in the same manner for selection of the emission wavelength.

CUVETTES

Generally, glass cuvettes can be used when the excitation wavelength is greater than 320 nm. At wavelengths below this, the glass cuvette itself will absorb significant amounts of radiation; therefore, glass cuvettes are used mainly in the visible range. For ultraviolet excitation or for very sensitive fluorescence measurements, quartz cuvettes should be used. In addition, matched quartz cuvettes are available so that both the reference and the sample are contained in identical cuvettes. Elimination of cuvette variability is obtained and enables sensitive measurements to be made.

In the clinical laboratory, matched quartz cuvettes are seldom required. In fact, for routine fluorescence measurements using a filter fluorometer, round glass test tubes are satisfactory. Stray light may cause significant problems with round tubes; however, the optical and electronic null of the instrument usually permits compensation for this. In addition, appropriate use of baffles blocks stray radiation and permits only the radiation emitted from the sample to be focused onto the detector.

DETECTORS

The *photomultiplier tube* is the detector commonly used in fluorometry. Generally, for emission that is measured in the visible range, a glass-encased tube is sufficient. In the ultraviolet range, glass absorbs the radiation; therefore, special ultraviolet-responsive tubes are required for ultraviolet fluorescence measurements.

The photomultiplier tube, explained in Chapter 1, operates on an amplification principle. As light strikes the surface of a light-sensitive screen in the detector, a potential proportional to the intensity of the light is generated. This potential is magnified through the use of several electron emitter or collector cells. As an electronic signal passes from one cell to the next, it is amplified until the end-stage collector is reached. At this point, the potential is measured and recorded on a meter, digital display, or other recording device.

Many instruments are now equipped with microprocessors that permit concentration calculations and direct printouts. The instrument is calibrated with a series of standards, and the fluorescence concentration curve is stored in instrument memory. Subsequent samples are analyzed, and the fluorescence is compared to the stored curve for the calculation of analyte concentration.

POLARIZERS

Electromagnetic radiation consists of both electronic and magnetic components. Only the electronic component of electromagnetic radiation interacts with electrons during the absorption process. This electronic component is composed of radiation vibrating in two planes perpendicular to each other. Thus, for any given radiation beam, the electronic component may be defined in terms of two planes perpendicular to each other.

Certain noncubic (anisotropic) crystals are used as polarizers because they have the capability of filtering one of the two perpendicular planes. Depending on the orientation of the crystal to the incident beam, one plane of light will pass directly through the crystal while the other plane of light is absorbed. The resultant light that passes through the crystal is plane-polarized.

Systems

Generally, fluorometers and fluorescence polarization analyzers are designed such that the emitted fluorescence is measured from a light path that is at a 90° angle from the excitation light path, as shown in Figure 9-1. Because fluorescence is emitted in all directions, the fluorescence signal could theoretically be measured at any angle. However, at 90°, stray light is at a minimum; thus, the fluorescence signal at this point has less background interference. One system has been described in which the optical path has a "straight-through" geometry.[6] Through the use of special filters and an attenuated light source, stray light and high background problems are eliminated.

FILTER FLUOROMETERS

As discussed, filter fluorometers employ a mercury vapor lamp with wavelength selection achieved through the use of filters. In the simplest form, the instrumentation design of a fluorometer would follow the schematic in Figure 9-1. This simple fluorometer uses a single-beam design. The advantage of such a system is its simplicity and low cost. In addition, the stability of the mercury lamp provides for accurate measurements. Extreme sensitivity can be achieved if the maximum excitation wavelength of the fluorophore coincides with one of the mercury lines. The major disadvantage of this system arises from its lack of versatility.

However, from these basic filter fluorometers a number of specialized systems have evolved. One example of such a system is Abbott Laboratories' IMx® immuno-

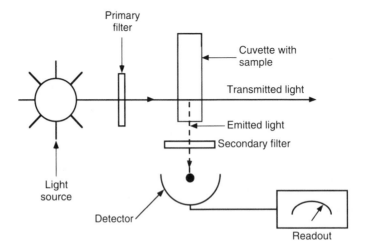

Figure 9-1.   Simple, right-angle fluorometric system.

chemistry analyzer (described in Chapter 19), which uses a front surface filter fluorometer design.[7] In this system, excitation energy is directed downward by means of a dichroic mirror on to the surface of a reaction cell matrix. The resulting fluorescence produced on the matrix surface passes upward through the dichroic mirror and a pair of bandpass filters to a photomultiplier tube where the intensity is measured. Another example is the Stratus® Immunoassay System[8] (Baxter Diagnostics Inc., Miami, FL 33152-0672), which measures reaction rates with a front-surface filter fluorometer (see Chapter 19 for an explanation of this system).

SPECTROFLUOROMETERS

Spectrofluorometers, like spectrophotometers, are available in either single-beam or double-beam configurations. Generally, these instruments use the xenon arc lamp for the source. The use of monochromators in these instruments adds versatility.

Single-Beam Spectrofluorometers

In a single-beam instrument, as illustrated in Figure 9-2, the light from the source passes through the entrance slit into the excitation monochromator. The monochromator grating disperses the light, and the resulting spectrum is focused on the monochromator exit slit. A selected portion (bandwidth) of the spectrum is allowed to pass to the sample. The fluorescence emitted at a right angle to the excitation

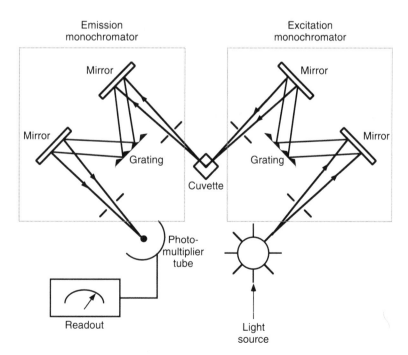

Figure 9-2. Single-beam spectrofluorometer.

beam then passes through the entrance slit of the emission monochromator. This monochromator passes only energy of the desired emission wavelength on to the photomultiplier tube. The output of the photomultiplier is amplified and sent to the readout device.

One area of concern in the single-beam spectrofluorometer is the error caused by xenon arc lamp flicker. To compensate for this instability, the single-beam instrument may be operated in the ratio mode, in which the source light is focused on a rotating chopper. This device alternates the direction of the beam between the sample and a reference photomultiplier tube. The signal from the sample photomultiplier tube is compared with the signal from the reference photomultiplier tube. Through the use of this ratio mode, any alteration of the fluorescence as a result of a change in source intensity is corrected. In other words, any change in the source would be detected by both photomultiplier tubes. Because a ratio is employed, error due to an unstable source would be minimized. Filter fluorometers may also be operated in a ratio mode.

Double-Beam Spectrofluorometers

As stated, spectrofluorometers are also available as double-beam instruments. Essentially, the design is very similar to that of double-beam spectrophotometers. The beam of light from the source is focused on a rotating chopper. The source light is then split between a sample cuvette and a reference cuvette, and the fluorescence produced by each cuvette is monitored by a single photomultiplier tube synchronized with the chopper. The synchronization permits distinction between sample and reference signals. Use of the double-beam design permits correction of background fluorescence that may be produced by the sample matrix. The double-beam design also compensates for source flicker in the same manner as the single-beam design in the ratio mode. For very sensitive measurements, matched quartz cuvettes are used to eliminate any difference that may result from cuvette variances.

FLUORESCENCE POLARIZATION ANALYZERS

Fluorescence polarization analyzers are basically filter fluorometers to which a set of excitation and emission polarizers has been added. Generally, the fluorescent tag used in fluorescence polarization immunoassays is fluorescein. As a result, narrow-width bandpass filters are used for both excitation and emission wavelength selection. The excitation filter permits light at 485 nm to pass for excitation, whereas the emission filter permits light at 525 nm to pass for subsequent measurements. Because fluorescein absorbs light in the visible range, a tungsten halogen lamp can be used as the source.

Figure 9-3 illustrates the schematic diagram for the optical system of a fluorescence polarization analyzer.[9] The beam of light from the tungsten halogen lamp is split and passes to both a sample and a reference detector. The reference detector is used to monitor and regulate the intensity of the source. The other portion of the beam strikes a polarizer or liquid crystal device. Here, the beam is polarized in the horizontal plane. The liquid crystal serves to rotate the polarized beam 90°. When a voltage is applied to the crystal, no rotation occurs. When no voltage is applied, the

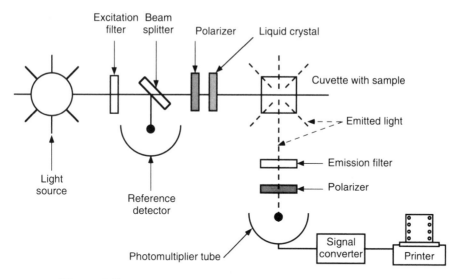

Figure 9-3. Components of a fluorescence polarization analyzer.

plane is rotated 90°. Therefore, by turning the voltage to the crystal on and off repeatedly, the excitation beam alternates between horizontal- and vertical-plane-polarized light.

The polarized light next strikes the sample. Baffles surround the sample to prevent excitation light from striking the detector. Upon excitation, the sample emits fluorescence. The fluorescent beam passes through the emission filter and on to an emission polarizer. This polarizer only passes light in the vertical plane. This design enables measurement of polarized fluorescence relative to the excitation polarization. Depending on the relative binding of the native analyte and the fluorescent-tagged analyte, different degrees of polarized fluorescence are obtained.

The photomultiplier senses the vertical fluorescence intensity produced by both the horizontal and vertical excitation beams. Through the use of a microprocessor and a counter-timer device, the fluorescence intensities for each excitation component are determined and used to calculate the degree of polarization obtained for a particular sample. For quantitative purposes, a calibration curve, as shown in Figure 9-4, is obtained. Through the use of the microprocessor, the curve is mathematically stored and can be used for subsequent sample analysis with direct concentration printout. An automated system of that design has been described and is commercially available.[10] This system, the TDx® analyzer, is commonly used for the measurement of a wide range of drugs in serum by fluorescence polarization immunoassay. In addition, a variety of other types of analytes are measured by this automated technique. Of importance in the shape of the calibration curve is the high degree of polarization at low analyte concentrations. This characteristic gives fluorescence polarization excellent sensitivity and precision at low analyte concentrations.[11]

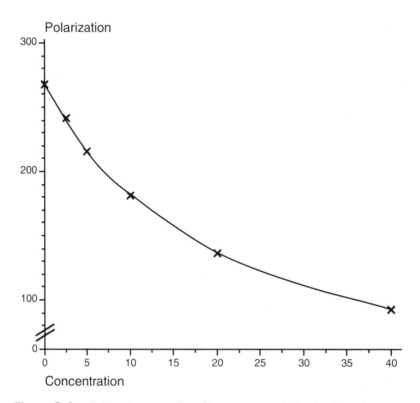

Figure 9-4.   Calibration curve for a fluorescence polarization immunoassay.

The instrument uses a fixed emission polarizer and a rotating excitation polarizer controlled by an electric signal. Another type of instrument is available that uses a different orientation of the polarizers.[12] The fluorometric components of the system operate similarly to the previously described system and produce similar data; however, operation of the polarizers is different.

The excitation polarizer is fixed so that polarized light in only one plane is allowed to strike the sample. The emission polarizer is variable and is used to pass alternatively horizontal-and vertical-plane-polarized light for subsequent detection by the photomultiplier tube. The emission polarizer is varied in direction through the use of a motor that mechanically turns the crystal. The motor is synchronously driven so that fluorescence measurements coincide with the horizontal and vertical orientation of the crystal. A microprocessor collects the fluorescence data and calculates polarization values.

Routine Operation

In the development of a fluorometric assay, optimization of fluorescence intensity is desired to achieve maximum sensitivity. To optimize the fluorescence for a given analyte, some understanding of the absorption spectrum is helpful. With an analyte standard placed in the instrument, the excitation wavelength is set at the absorption maximum for the analyte. The emission spectrum is scanned to find the wavelength at which fluorescence intensity is maximum. The emission monochromator is then set at this wavelength, and the excitation spectrum is scanned to check for maximum fluorescence. For subsequent analyses, the excitation and emission monochromators are at the wavelengths found for maximum fluorescence.

If little is known about the absorption spectrum before checking for fluorescence maximum, a good starting place for the excitation wavelength adjustment may be nonspecific wavelengths of 254, 280, or 340 nm. Subsequent increases of 25 or 50 nm may be needed until a fluorescence signal is obtained, after which the delineated procedure may be followed.

Another point of consideration in finding optimum wavelengths is specificity. Although maximum fluorescence intensity is found at one set of wavelengths for a standard, possible interferences in the sample matrix may prohibit using these. By choosing a secondary set of wavelengths, fluorescence for the desired analyte may still be obtained, but the new wavelengths exclude the interference through lack of excitation or through filtering of the interferant emission.

Once the desired wavelengths are obtained, a fluorescence assay may be performed. Because fluorescence measurements are relative numbers and are not absolute, a reference must be established. Generally, a calibration curve is generated using standards in an appropriate matrix. The background of the matrix is subtracted using a blank consisting of the matrix. Once the curve is established, samples may be read relative to the standards. Concentration of the sample is determined from the calibration curve.

In fluorescence polarization operation, the analyzer generally performs all functions through microprocessor control.[10] Because only one fluorescent compound (fluorescein) is analyzed, wavelengths need no adjustments. The analyzer also generates the calibration curves through the use of a standard set. Background fluorescence for each sample is measured and stored for subsequent subtraction. Calculations are performed by the analyzer, and a direct printout of concentration is obtained.

ADVANTAGES

The use of fluorometry over absorption has several advantages. The first is the increase in sensitivity. In fluorometry, measurements are not based on difference as in absorption. Generally, a signal is obtained on a very low background. If increased sensitivity is desired, increasing the lamp intensity will increase fluorescence. Similarly, an increase in the voltage to the photomultiplier tube will increase sensitivity. Both of these adjustments increase the fluorescence signal without significant alteration in the background intensity. Electronic noise and stray light may become a problem if the components are set near their respective limits. Adjustments to the source and detector tube in absorptivity measurements also increase the background, rendering the absorption measurement less sensitive. Fluorescence measurements are generally 10 to 1000 times more sensitive than absorption measurements.

Specificity is also an advantage of fluorometry. Through the use of two wavelengths, various interferences are eliminated. The emission of light in fluorescence adds inherent specificity. Many substances may absorb at a given wavelength, including the fluorophore; however, not as many substances will fluoresce. This limited degree of fluorescence coupled with the variance of the emission wavelengths greatly adds specificity to this technique.

In fluorescence polarization, excellent sensitivity and specificity are also achieved. Through the use of a highly efficient fluorophore, fluorescein, and of the polarization technique, sensitivity in the nanogram range is obtained. In addition, specificity is significantly increased by several factors. Sample background subtraction ensures that analytical measurements result only from the desired analyte. The use of narrow-bandwidth bandpass filters reduces stray light and potential fluorescent interferences. The use of specific antibodies directed only to the analyte of interest ensures that the polarization values obtained are from the competitive binding assay between the analyte of interest and its fluorescent-tagged analog.

DISADVANTAGES

Fluorometry has several disadvantages because of the unique nature of fluorescence. Interferences are a problem from both a positive- and negative-bias standpoint. Drugs that may be present in the sample matrix may fluoresce at the same wavelengths as the analyte of interest does, thereby giving an abnormally high measurement. Signal intensity may also be affected by interference from *Rayleigh scatter* and *Raman scatter,* two scattering phenomena that occur when light passes through a solution. From a negative-bias viewpoint, quenching of fluorescence for various reasons described in the Principles section may occur and reduce the measured intensity. In fluorescence polarization, interferences may result from the binding of substances that have a similar immunoreactivity as the analyte of interest. The interference would decrease binding of the fluorescent tag and would produce analyte concentrations that were falsely elevated.

A second disadvantage is the environmental sensitivity of fluorescence and fluorescence polarization. The solvent and *p*H are important and should be kept as constant as possible to minimize errors. Temperature is important, particularly in fluorescence polarization measurements. These analyzers typically have a thermoregulated sample chamber to minimize this variable.

Another potential problem in fluorometry is *self-absorption.* This phenomenon occurs when the excitation band and emission band overlap. As some molecules are excited and fluoresce, the emitted fluorescence is of a wavelength that may cause excitation of other fluorophores. As a result, emitted fluorescence is absorbed, causing an overall decrease in fluorescence intensity. Finally, as discussed in the Principles section, high fluorophore concentrations cause self-quenching and the inner-filter effect to occur, which result in decreased fluorescence and nonlinearity of the fluorescence concentration curve.

APPLICATIONS

Most fluorometric methods used in clinical chemistry laboratories either measure a fluorescent compound directly, chemically produce a fluorescent molecule that is then measured, or measure an analyte that has been chemically coupled to a fluorescent molecule.

In order to measure a substance directly, it must fluoresce naturally in a solvent. After appropriate isolation, the concentration of the substance is determined by means of its inherent fluorescence. Analysis of phenylalanine, porphyrins, LSD, imipramine, phenothiazines, and quinine are a few examples of this technique.

Methods that quantitate nonfluorescent compounds by a chemical reaction and production of a fluorescent molecule have also been used in the clinical laboratory. Catecholamines have historically been quantitated by measuring the fluorescent compound produced by oxidation in the presence of a strong alkali.

However, methods that quantitate analytes by immunochemical reactions and the ultimate production of a fluorescent-labeled molecule are the most widely used fluorescent applications in the clinical laboratory today. With the development of fluorescent labels for immunoassays, new technologies have evolved that combine the sensitivity of fluorescence measurements with the inherent specificity of antigen-antibody reactions.

Enzyme immunoassays designed to measure large molecular weight analytes have been developed for use in automated fluorometric systems.[7,8] available assays include tumor marker assays such as AFP, CEA, and PSA; antibody assays for CMV and rubella; hormone assays; hepatitis serology assays; reproductive hormone assays such as hCG, FSH, LH, and prolactin; and other assays such as vitamin B_{12}, CK-MB, and ferritin. The Stratus® automated fluorometric systems also include assays for therapeutic drugs.

The use of fluorescence polarization in the clinical laboratory has been increasing dramatically since the 1980s, and much of the therapeutic drug monitoring being performed uses fluorescence polarization immunoassay (FPIA) technology. Types of drugs assayed include antiarrhythmics, antiasthmatics, antibiotics, anticonvulsants, antineoplastics, and cardiac glycosides. In addition, drug-of-abuse detection, toxicology, endocrine function, and specific protein assays are available with this technology.

Maintenance and Quality Assurance

The manufacturers of most fluorometric instrumentation on the market today publish operating manuals that include a section containing information on maintenance required for their particular instrument as well as procedures for ensuring that the instrument is performing acceptably. These procedures should be performed at the intervals specified by the manufacturer. Because not all clinical laboratories have the latest fluorometric instrumentation with the most complete operating manuals, this section will help to identify important checks that should be performed periodically and will suggest general methods to accomplish these.

FILTER FLUOROMETERS

Because filters are used to select the optimum excitation and emission wavelengths for a given analyte, wavelength calibration checks are not required. The filters should, however, be carefully cleaned and checked for scratches or fingerprints to minimize light scattering.

Nondisposable cuvettes and cells should be handled with care and must be thoroughly cleaned before and after use. Because of the high sensitivity of fluorescence measurements, it is important to avoid even slight contamination of both the inside and the outside of the cuvette.

To check the day-to-day fluctuations of the instrument, a standard such as 0.01 μg/mL quinine sulfate in 0.1 N sulfuric acid solution should be read using suitable filters and the fluorescence recorded. Periodic checks of the instrument's sensitivity and linearity may also be performed with appropriate dilutions of the quinine sulfate solution.[13]

SPECTROFLUOROMETERS

The calibration of excitation and emission monochromator wavelengths should be checked periodically to ensure optimum instrument sensitivity. Although an instrument may appear to be functioning properly, errors in wavelength may render results unreliable. It is best to check the wavelength as close as possible to the emission characteristics of the compound under investigation. The use of a source that emits intense lines of known wavelength is needed for the wavelength calibration check. This source may be the instrument's own radiation source, such as xenon lines at 450.1, 462.4, 467.1, and 473.4 nm from the xenon lamp or any of the mercury lines found in the light of a mercury vapor lamp (257.7, 313.0, 365.0, 404.7, 407.8, 435.8, 546.1, 577.0, and 579.1 nm). The source may also be fluorescent lamp light if the instrument is equipped to allow for the introduction of room fluorescent lamp light into the emission monochromator.[14] The mercury line of 435.8 nm is contained in room fluorescent light.[14] The mercury line may also be provided by the use of a small lamp such as a mercury light pen, which fits into the cuvette well.[7] Solutions that produce sharp fluorescent peaks at known wavelengths have also been used to check the wavelength calibration. For each line being checked, the wavelength is adjusted to give maximum signal, and the wavelength reading is recorded. If the true and observed readings are different, the instrument operation manual should be consulted to adjust the monochromator. Once the emission monochromator is checked, the excitation monochromator can be checked against it.[15]

Instrument sensitivity is another important check to ensure optimum instrument function, especially at the minimum level of response or limit of detectability. Sensitivity properly relates to response at all levels, although an instrument with high sensitivity is likely to have low detectability. The signal-to-noise ratio is one of the parameters that affect the sensitivity of an instrument. One of the methods commonly used for checking instrument sensitivity is the measurement of the Raman spectrum of water and determination of the noise at the peak wavelength in the spectrum.[14] The excitation wavelength should be set at 350 nm and the emission wavelength at 398 nm. Sensitivity in this case is determined by dividing the peak height of the Raman spectrum of water by the noise value. This ratio should be reproducible and within the recommended specifications of the instrument manufacturer. Another method for checking the sensitivity of a spectrofluorometer has been described, in which dilutions of quinine sulfate in 0.1 N sulfuric acid are read at an excitation wavelength of 350 nm and an emission wavelength of 450 nm.[13] These readings should be recorded and observed for changes that may occur from day to day.

FLUORESCENCE POLARIZATION ANALYZERS

Fluorescence polarization analyzers are generally self-contained units that process a specimen completely from presentation of sample to printed result with little operator intervention. Function checks, used to verify proper analyzer operation, are generally provided by the instrument manufacturer and are performed as part of periodic maintenance. These checks test the function of the analyzer's major subsystems independent of the chemistries performed. The subsystems that should be checked periodically include the pipetting, optical, and temperature systems. The operation of all moving parts for proper positioning and motion should also be checked.

To ensure accurate, reproducible pipetting of sample and reagents, the analyzer's pipetting system should be inspected at least daily. This should include inspection of the sample probe or needle, syringes, tubing, and other pipetting components for signs of wear, leakage, or dried reagent residue. Periodic cleaning or replacement of these items should also be performed and documented. Another important check of the dispenser system is an evaluation of the system's ability to perform precise pipetting. This is usually accomplished by multiple samplings of a fluorescent solution. To evaluate the accuracy and reproducibility of the photometer and optical system, a set of fluorescent standards should be run and the readings compared to known values. Because assay standard curves are stored for several weeks at a time, and because fluorescence measurements are temperature dependent, monitoring the operation of the system's temperature circuitry is another important function check. Because of the computerization incorporated into many of these analyzers, many of these checks are performed automatically and the results flagged as acceptable or unacceptable. Experience and a complete understanding of the troubleshooting section of the instrument manual are very helpful in correcting problems revealed by an unacceptable function check.

Summary

When electromagnetic radiation impinges on a molecular substance, the electron configuration of the substance may be altered in such a way that the substance is placed in an excited state. If the substance is of unique chemical nature, radiant energy, at a wavelength longer than that absorbed, may be given off as the substance returns to the ground state. This radiant energy is called fluorescence. Fluorescence is favored in highly conjugated organic molecules, aromatic hydrocarbons, and heterocyclics with fused benzene rings. However, fluorescence is only one of several possible deactivation processes by which a substance may return to the ground state. These other deactivation processes reduce the probability that fluorescence will occur and reduce the quantum efficiency of the substance. In addition to these processes, a number of other factors, both intrinsic and environmental, may result in either increased or decreased fluorescence.

Fluorometry is the quantitative measurement of fluorescence and the relationship between the measured fluorescence and the concentration of the fluorescent substance. Instruments designed to perform such measurements are called fluorometers. The basic components of a fluorometer include a light source, an excitation filter, a cell or cuvette, an emission filter, a detector, and a readout device. A spectrofluorometer uses monochromators instead of filters for wavelength selection. Of these components, the light source is perhaps of the utmost importance, because intensity, stability, and spectral range of the source are all critical parameters in fluorescence measurements. The most commonly used sources in fluorometry are the deuterium lamp, the mercury vapor lamp, and the xenon arc.

Fluorescence polarization, a unique application of fluorometry, is the measurement of polarized light emitted from a fluorophore that has been excited with polarized light. To accomplish this measurement, fluorescence polarization analyzers contain polarizers located in the excitation and emission paths, and a device for rotating the plane of either the excitation or emission beam. In all designs, fluorescence intensities are measured both parallel and perpendicular to the plane of the excitation beam. The key to fluorescence polarization assays is the fact that the degree of polarization depends on molecular rotation, which depends on molecular size. In these assays, a competitive binding immunoassay is performed in which a substrate and a covalently bonded fluorescent-labeled substrate compete for binding sites on an antibody. The binding of the fluorescent-labeled substrate to the antibody causes the fluorescent tag to be part of a large molecule that rotates slowly. Thus, the fluorescence produced by this bound fluorescent tag will remain highly polarized. Conversely, the fluorescent-labeled substrate that is unbound is free to rotate more rapidly and will produce depolarized fluorescence.

Fluorometers, spectrofluorometers, and fluorescence polarization analyzers are often designed so that the emitted fluorescence is measured at a right angle to the excitation light path, because at 90°, stray light is at a minimum. However, designs employing measurements at angles other than 90°, as well as "straight-through" and front-surface designs are also used. Fluorometers typically use a mercury vapor lamp with wavelength selection accomplished by the use of filters. The advantage of these systems is simplicity and low cost, and the specialized designs are well suited for repetitive high-volume measurements. However, they lack versatility. Spectrofluorometers, which are available in single-beam and double-beam designs, generally use a xenon arc source and permit selection of both excitation and emission wavelengths. Single-beam instruments may be operated in the ratio mode to compensate for changes in source intensity, which can be a problem. In addition, double-beam designs permit correction of background fluorescence that may be produced by the sample matrix.

The major advantages of fluorometric and fluorescence polarization measurements over absorption measurements are the increase in sensitivity and specificity of these techniques. Disadvantages include interferences from other fluorescent compounds, scattering phenomena, quenching, and, potentially, self-absorption. Fluorescence is also sensitive to environmental factors such as temperature and *p*H.

Fluorometric methods used in clinical chemistry generally measure a fluorescent compound directly, measure a fluorescent molecule that has been produced chemically, or measure an analyte which has been coupled to a fluorescent tag. Methods that quantitate analytes by immunochemical reactions and the ultimate production of a fluorescent-tagged molecule are the most widely used fluorescent applications in the clinical laboratory today. Enzyme immunoassays designed to measure large molecular weight analytes have been developed and are being used on automated fluorometric systems. The use of fluorescence polarization in the clinical laboratory has also increased, and much of the therapeutic drug monitoring being performed uses FPIA technology.

Because quality assurance is so vital in today's laboratory, it is very important that routine maintenance and function checks for all instruments be performed and documented. The manufacturers of most fluorometric instruments publish operating manuals that describe maintenance and performance checks in detail. These procedures should be performed at the intervals specified by the manufacturer. When such documentation is not available, the general methods suggested here may be used as a guideline to accomplish these procedures.

Questions and Problems

1. Explain similarities and differences between (a) absorption spectroscopy and fluorometry; (b) reflectance measurements and fluorometric measurements.
2. What additional component parts are necessary in a fluorescence polarization analyzer compared to a filter fluorometer?
3. One screening test for phenylalanine in serum is a fluorometric assay. Phenylalanine in the serum (after precipitation of protein with trichloroacetic acid) and standards reacts with ninhydrin in the presence of L-leucyl-L-alanine and succinate buffer at pH 5.8 to form a fluorescent product. The fluorescent intensity after excitation at 365 nm and emission at 515 nm is determined. The following results were obtained.

Standard Concentration (mg/dL)	Fluorescent Intensity
0	2.5
2.5	65.4
5.0	127.5
10.0	250.9
Sample 1	57.1
Sample 2	85.5

Construct a calibration curve. Calculate the concentration of samples 1 and 2.

4. Why is the standard curve for theophylline on a TDx® analyzer a different shape from the standard curve for phenylalanine on a spectrofluorometer?
5. Explain why fluorometry can be more sensitive than photometry.
6. What are some disadvantages of fluorometric analysis?

References

1. Warner IM, Patonay G, Thomas MP. Multidimensional luminescence measurements. Anal Chem 1985, 57:463A-83A.
2. Skoog DA, Leary JJ. Principles of instrumental analysis, 4th ed. New York: Saunders College Publishing, 1992:174-83.
3. Adamsons K, Sell JE, Holland JF, Timnick A. Absorption corrected measurements in molecular fluorescence. Am Lab 11/1984, 16:16-29.
4. Willard HH, Merritt LL Jr, Dean JA, Settle FA Jr. Instrumental methods of analysis, 7th ed. Belmont, CA: Wadsworth, 1988:206-07.
5. Weinberger R, Sapp E. Fluorescence detection in liquid chromatography. Am Lab 5/1984, 16:121-29.
6. Khalil OS, Routh WS, Lingenfelter K, Can DB, Ladouceur P. Automated in-line ratio-correcting filter fluorometer. Clin Chem 1981, 27:1586-91.
7. Fiore M, Mitchell J, Doan T, et al. The Abbott IMx® automated benchtop immunochemistry analyzer system. Clin Chem 1988, 34:1726-32.
8. Heller ZH, D'Aquino M, Alvite A, et al. Design principles of the Stratus® fluorometric immunoassay instrument. Biomed Sci Instrum 1984, 20:63-72.
9. Popelka SR, Miller DM, Holen JT, Kelso DM. Fluorescence polarization immunoassay II. Analyzer for rapid, precise measurement of fluorescence polarization with use of disposable cuvettes. Clin Chem 1981, 27:1198-201.
10. Jolley ME, Stroupe SD, Schwenzer KS, et al. Fluorescence polarization immunoassay III. An automated system for therapeutic drug determination. Clin Chem 1981, 27:1575-79.
11. Jolley ME, Stroupe SD, Wang CJ, et al. Fluorescence polarization immunoassay I. Monitoring aminoglycoside antibiotics in serum and plasma. Clin Chem 1981, 27:1190-97.
12. Muira H. Application of fluorescence polarization to the determination of urinary lysozyme activity. Clin Biochem 1985, 18:40-47.
13. Udenfriend S. Fluorescence assay in biology and medicine, vol. II. New York: Academic Press, 1969:594-614.
14. Hitachi instruments instruction manual for model F-2000 fluorescence spectrophotometer. Tokyo, Japan: Hitachi, Ltd, 1988.
15. Udenfriend S. Fluorescence assay in biology and medicine, vol. I. New York: Academic Press, 1962:110-23.

Suggested Readings

Skoog DA, Leary JJ. Principles of instrumental analysis, 4th ed. New York: Saunders College Publishing, 1992:174-95.
Warner IM, Patonay G, Thomas MP. Multidimensional luminescence measurements. Anal Chem 1985, 57:463A-83A.

10

PHOTON COUNTERS: SCINTILLATION AND CHEMILUMINESCENCE

Mary C. Haven

Objectives

After completing this chapter, the reader will be able to:

1. Describe the differences between solid scintillation counting, liquid scintillation counting, and luminometers.
2. Describe the similarities between solid scintillation counting, liquid scintillation counting, and luminometers.
3. Name the three major unique ways that γ radiation interacts with material.
4. Construct a block diagram of a liquid scintillation counter, and explain the component parts.
5. Discuss a pulse-height analyzer.
6. Correct a sample for chemical quenching by at least two different methods.
7. Construct a block diagram of a luminometer.
8. Design a quality control program for a photon counter.

Definitions

Alpha (α) Particle: A helium nucleus ejected from a larger nucleus during radioactive decay. It contains two protons and two neutrons and is positively charged, $^4_2He^{2+}$.

Annihilation Radiation: The production of two 0.51-MeV γ rays resulting from the combination and subsequent annihilation of an electron-positron pair.

Beta (β) Particle: An electron ejected from the nucleus during radioactive decay.

Bioluminescence: A chemical reaction producing light that occurs in nature.

Chemiluminescence: A chemical reaction that results in the emission of light.

Cocktail: In this context, an undrinkable mixture of organic solvent and a fluor.

Compton Effect: The interaction of a γ ray with an atom, resulting in ejection of a weakly bound electron with incident energy being divided between the ejected electron and a photon (γ ray) of less energy.

Crossover: The detection of γ rays in crystals adjacent or near an isotopic source in another well in a multiwell system.

Excitation: The process wherein orbital electrons are raised to a higher energy state.

Flash point: The lowest temperature at which vapors above a volatile combustible compound reach an adequate concentration to ignite in air if exposed to a flame.

Fluor: A substance that emits light when exposed to energetic electrons.

Gamma (γ) Rays: In electromagnetic radiation, a unit of energy emitted by a radioactive atom.

Half-life: The time required for the disintegration of one-half of the radioactive atoms.

Ionization: The formation of an ion pair; an electron and a positively charged ion, from an atom.

Isotopes: Nuclides of the same atomic number (Z) but different atomic mass (A); number of protons = Z = atomic number, number of neutrons + protons = A = atomic mass.

keV: 10^3 eV (thousand [kilo] electron volts).

Luminometer: A photon counter that detects and measures the amount of light generated by chemical reactions.

MeV: 10^6 eV (million electron volts).

Normalization: The process by which the efficiencies of multiple crystals in a multiwell counter are matched.

Pair Production: γ ray interaction with the field surrounding the atomic nucleus, resulting in the formation of an electron-positron pair.

Photoelectric Effect: The interaction of a γ ray with an atom, resulting in the ejection of a tightly bound electron with all incident energy transferred to the electron.

Positron: A positively charged β particle with the same mass as an electron.

Pulse Height Analyzer: A device for selecting a range of amplitude pulses to be counted.

Radioactive Decay: A nuclear reaction that occurs spontaneously in unstable nuclei as the nuclide approaches stability.

Radioactivity: A spontaneous reaction of unstable nuclei as they approach stability.

Resolution: A measure of the energy width of the actual counted spectrum in a particular crystal.

Scaler: An electronic method of counting the number of output signals from a detector.

Spilldown: Counts from a higher energy isotope that overlap into the window of a lower-energy isotope when more than one isotope are being counted.

Introduction

In preceding chapters measuring light intensity or light absorbance was discussed. In this chapter we present another type of photometric instrumentation that counts the number of light photons emitted. When light pulses come from the interaction of radioactive materials with a sensing compound, the instrument is called a scintillation counter. When light pulses result from a chemical reaction, the instrument is called a luminometer, and the process of light emission is called luminescence. In this chapter we discuss several photon counters: solid scintillation counters for detecting and measuring γ radiation, liquid scintillation counters for detecting and measuring β radiation, and luminometers for detecting and measuring luminescence.

Applications for photon counters in the clinical laboratory include immunoassay technics where the labeled compound is detected with this type of instrumentation. Chemiluminescent, β, and γ tags are also used in DNA probes and Scatchard plots.

Luminometers simply measure the light emitted by a chemical reaction, but instruments measuring radiation require a sensing element that converts the energy of radiation to electrical energy. The electrical energy is then detected by its interaction with a fluor that produces light flashes (scintillation). Scintillation counters are used to detect both β and γ emissions. A brief discussion of radioactivity forms a basis for understanding how radiation is measured.

NUCLEAR DECAY

Radioactive isotopes undergo spontaneous radioactive decay, releasing both nuclear particles and energy. The rate of nuclear decay and the character of the emissions identify specific isotopes. The rate of nuclear decay is usually described in terms of half-life ($t_{1/2}$). In one half-life, the initial activity of an isotope will have decreased by one-half; in two half-lifes, another one-half of that activity decays, thus one-quarter of the original activity remains. The equation below, derived from the decay constant,[1] can be used to calculate the remaining activity:

$$A = A_0 e^{-\lambda t}$$

(Eq. 10-1)

where

A = activity at time t
A_0 = activity at time t_0
e = logarithm to the base e
$\lambda = 0.693/t_{1/2}$
$t_{1/2}$ = half-life of isotope
t = time elapsed

Each isotope has a characteristic half-life as well as characteristic energy emission. The radiation emitted from a radioisotope can be α, β, or γ rays.

Beta particles represent electrons derived from nuclear events, and their energy spectrum depends on the speed with which the electron leaves the nucleus. Beta particles are emitted from a given radioisotope over a continuous range of energy up to a maximum value (E_{max}), which is characteristic of each radioisotope. However, only a very small fraction of the emitted particles have energies near the maximum, and most of them have a much lower energy. In general, the average energy is about one-third the maximum ($\frac{1}{3} E_{max}$). Commonly used isotopes such as ^{3}H and ^{14}C emit β particles of relatively low energy (Figs. 10-1 and 10-2). Beta particles, because of both their mass and charge, readily interact with matter and travel only short

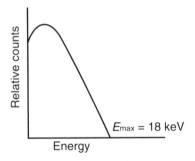

Figure 10-1.   Beta spectrum of ^{3}H.

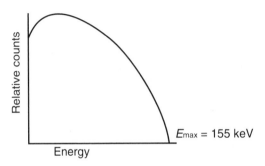

Figure 10-2.   Beta spectrum of ^{14}C.

distances. As the β particle traverses material, it causes ionization and excitation of orbital electrons.

Gamma rays represent pure energy emissions that are analogous to x rays, except for their origin. Gamma rays are emitted from specific radioisotopes at characteristic energies generally ranging from 10 keV to 6 MeV. The spectrum of each γ-emitting isotope is unique and can be used to identify the isotope (Figs. 10-3 and 10-4). Because γ rays have neither mass nor charge, they are capable of traveling great distances through matter (e.g., cosmic rays represent high-energy γ rays, and they travel through light-years).

INTERACTION OF GAMMA RAYS WITH MATTER

Gamma rays characteristically interact with matter in three unique ways, all producing energetic electrons: photoelectric effects, Compton effect, and pair production.

Photoelectric effect refers to the total transfer of the γ ray's energy to an orbital electron; the energy is therefore transformed to the kinetic energy of the electron. This process is especially prevalent with low-energy (<0.5 MeV) γ rays (Figs. 10-5 and 10-6).

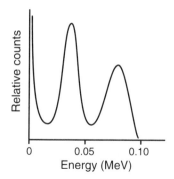

Figure 10-3.   Gamma spectrum of ^{125}I.

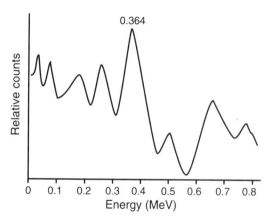

Figure 10-4.   Gamma spectrum of ^{131}I.

The *Compton effect* occurs most commonly with γ rays of medium energy (0.5–1.0 MeV). Here, only a portion of the γ ray's energy is imparted to the electron, the result of the Compton effect being the production from the incident γ ray of an energetic electron and a photon of lesser energy. These Compton electrons may possess any amount of energy up to a defined maximum. Compton recoil electrons thus have a wide energy spread even when they result from monoenergetic γ rays (Figs. 10-7 and 10-8).

Pair production is a unique process in which high-energy γ rays are transformed into matter. It occurs only with γ rays that have energy in excess of 1.02 MeV. The energy of the incident γ ray becomes mass in the formation of an electron-positron pair. The resulting positron reacts with surrounding matter by colliding with an electron. The mass of both positron and electron are annihilated to become two 0.51 MeV photons. This represents annihilation radiation, which always accompanies pair production (Figs. 10-9 and 10-10).

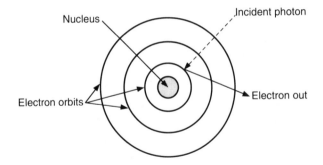

Figure 10-5.   Photoelectric effect.

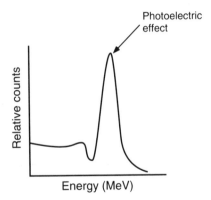

Figure 10-6.   Spectrum showing photoelectric effect.

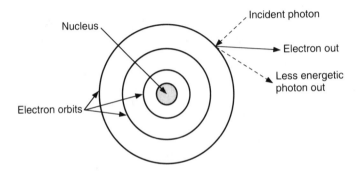

Figure 10-7.   Compton effect.

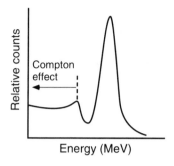

Figure 10-8. Spectrum showing Compton effect.

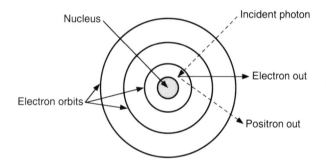

Figure 10-9. Pair production.

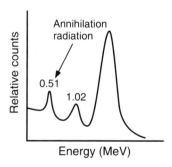

Figure 10-10. Spectrum showing pair production.

Both β and γ emissions are referred to as ionizing radiation, because during their interaction with matter they produce ions. Several devices for the detection of radioactivity are based on the measurement of this ionization in gas-filled chambers. Gas ionization detectors such as ion chambers, proportional counters, and Geiger-Mueller counters, however, are now only rarely used in clinical laboratories. These instruments are too imprecise for analytical work.

Solid Scintillation Counters

BASIC COMPONENTS

The three effects—photoelectric, Compton, and pair production—all ultimately yield energized electrons that, in solid scintillation systems, can interact with the fluor.[2] When these electrons pass near the orbital electron of the fluor, part of the energy is imparted to the orbital electron, raising the electron to a higher energy level. On return of this electron to the ground state, a characteristic photon is emitted. The number of photons released by the fluor depends on the kinetic energy of the electrons and therefore on the total energy of the incident γ ray.

The fluor generally used for solid scintillation counting is a single large crystal of sodium iodide containing thallium. This crystal, usually well-shaped (i.e., like a well), virtually surrounds the sample to increase counting efficiency. The thallium-activated sodium iodide (NaI [Tl]) crystal characteristically emits photons at a visible wavelength suitable for detection by photomultiplier tubes. The sodium iodide crystals are hygroscopic (absorb water) and are therefore completely enclosed. The crystal is sealed in light-reflecting aluminum, except where attached to the photocathode through a transparent window. Through this window, photons may pass from crystal to the photocathode. This arrangement both protects the crystal from moisture and maximizes the light reaching the photomultiplier tubes.

By using photomultiplier tubes, the photons arising from the interaction of a single γ ray with the crystal are transformed to an electrical pulse; the magnitude of this pulse is increased by more than a million times. If this multiplication is to be useful, it must be reproducible so that a γ ray of 1 MeV might always result in the production of 1×10^8 electrons at the photomultiplier anode, whereas a γ ray of 2 MeV would result in the production of 2×10^8 electrons. Reproducible multiplication within the photomultiplier tube requires great stability of the high-voltage power supply. Ideally, the output of these power supplies, which provide overall gradients of up to 3000 V, should vary 0.01 V or less with a line voltage change of 1 V. The line voltage should be monitored before installing scintillation counters, and auxiliary voltage-regulation devices should be installed if necessary.

Closely coupled to the photomultiplier tube is a preamplifier, which further amplifies or multiplies the photomultiplier output. Thus, the amplifier, upon receiving 1×10^8 electrons from the photomultiplier tube, might generate a pulse of 0.6 V, and upon receiving 2×10^8 electrons, a pulse of 1.2 V would result. The duration required from the impingement of a γ ray on the crystal to the generation of a measurement voltage pulse is measured in nanoseconds. This allows high counting rates to be achieved using scintillation counting.

The combination of crystal, photomultiplier tube, and preamplifier produces discrete voltage pulses proportional in magnitude to the energy of incident γ rays. The addition of a pulse-height analyzer to this system results in a spectrometer that will discriminate among energies of the incident γ rays. This analyzer classifies the pulses according to their height or amplitude.

A single-channel pulse-height analyzer consists of two variable discriminators that allow selection of lower and upper levels of detection. The lower discriminator setting is termed the *base*. The upper discriminator setting is selected by adding a voltage increment (a window) to the base. These two discriminators, in conjunction with an anticoincidence circuit, allow only those energies between the two discriminator levels to pass to the scaler.

Discriminator I, the base, establishes the lower limit of detection. Pulses with an amplitude less than the base are rejected and do not appear as analyzer output. Discriminator II rejects all pulses with an amplitude less than the base plus the window. The anticoincidence circuit is designed to block all pulses arriving simultaneously (i.e., all pulses with amplitudes greater than both discriminators). Only those pulses passed by discriminator I and rejected by discriminator II will reach the scaler.

Figure 10-11 represents an example of a single-channel pulse-height analyzer with the base set at 1 V and the window at 0.5 V. In this case, a pulse of 0.5 V will be rejected by both discriminators. A pulse of 1.2 V will be passed by discriminator I and rejected by discriminator II and will reach the scaler. A pulse of 2.0 V will be passed by both discriminators I and II, arrive simultaneously at the coincidence counter, and therefore be rejected. Only those pulses greater than 1 V and less than 1.5 V will reach the scaler.

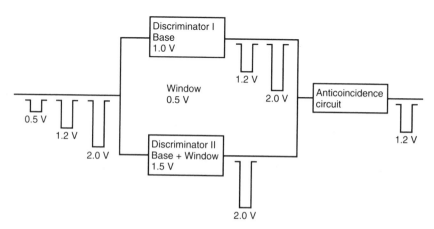

Figure 10-11. Single-channel pulse-height analyzer.

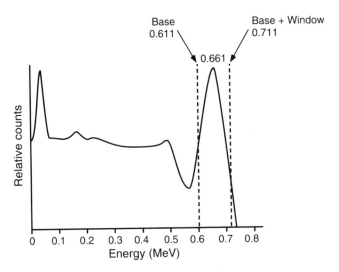

Figure 10-12.   Isolation of ^{137}Cs photopeak.

To illustrate how a pulse-height analyzer can isolate and count only the principal photopeak of a spectrum, the example of ^{137}Cs will be used. The principal photopeak has an energy of 0.661 MeV. The assumption will be made that the base setting can be varied between 0 and 1000 keV; that is, 0 and 1 MeV. The base sets the lower discriminator, and the window sets the increment increase above the base that will serve as the upper discriminator. If the base can vary between 0 and 1 MeV and a 10% window is employed, this window is 10% of 1 MeV, or 0.1 MeV. The Poisson distribution peaks at 0.661 MeV, but there are a significant number of counts on each side of 0.661 MeV. To center this peak in a 10% window, or, in this case, a 0.1-MeV window, one-half of this 0.1 MeV should be on either side of 0.661 MeV. Therefore, the base should be set 0.05 MeV lower than the 0.661-MeV peak, or at 0.611 MeV; the 10% window would set the upper discriminator 0.1 MeV higher than the base, or at 0.711 MeV. At these settings, most of the counts resulting from the photopeak of ^{137}Cs will reach the scaler (Fig. 10-12).

The counts derived from the scintillation process and isolated according to amplitude are recorded and shown on a scaler that displays the counts accumulated during the counting period selected. A device that counts pulses as well as controls the timing is called a scaler-timer. The pulses, after being discriminated by the pulse-height analyzer, pass through an electronic "gate" to a series of decimal counter assemblies (DCAs). Each DCA counts from 0 to 9 pulses; at 10 pulses the DCA resets at 0, but passes 1 count to the next DCA for a total of 10 counts. The process continues through the series of DCAs. If there are 6 DCAs, the count capacity is 999,999. At 1 million counts the scaler of 6 DCAs would reset to 0, usually with some sort of signal that maximum counts had been attained.

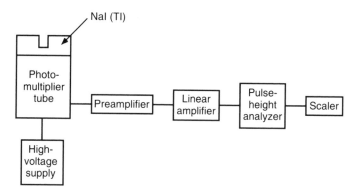

Figure 10-13. Gamma spectrometer.

A single-channel γ-ray spectrometer (Fig. 10-13) includes a NaI (Tl) crystal attached to a photomultiplier tube. A high-voltage supply is necessary for the photomultiplier tube. The signal is transmitted by a preamplifier to a linear amplifier, where further amplification occurs. A pulse-height analyzer then classifies the pulses according to their height or amplitude, and a scaler registers the number of pulses received.

MODES OF OPERATION

A scintillation counter can be used for two types of counting, integral and differential. In *integral counting,* a rejection of low pulses can be set, but no limit is set on higher-energy pulsing. In Figure 10-14, which shows a ^{131}I emission spectrum, pulses below 0.314 MeV are rejected (0.314 MeV is the base), but all higher pulses are counted. *Differential counting* employs the pulse-height analyzer. It not only rejects pulses lower than the base but also sets a limit on high-energy pulses. The same ^{131}I sample, set to count differentially with a 10% window, would count only the principal photopeak (Fig. 10-15).

Differential Counters

In the discussion of pulse-height analyzers, the assumption was made that the base could be varied between 0 and 1000 keV (0 and 1 MeV). In order for the pulse to be calibrated in γ-ray energy, the optimum high voltage to be applied to the photomultiplier tube must be determined experimentally. By adjusting the voltage to the photomultiplier tube and the amplification of the linear amplifier (called *attenuation* or *gain*), the pulse height can become a multiple of the incident γ-ray energy. To accomplish this calibration,[3] a monoenergetic source, usually ^{137}Cs, with a photopeak at 0.661 MeV is used. The attenuation to the linear amplifier is set to correspond to a maximum amplified pulse of 10 V. The 0.661 MeV peak can be perfectly centered between 0.611 and 0.711 MeV by a base setting at 0.611 and a window of 10% or 1 V

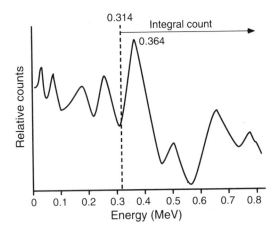

Figure 10-14.   Integral count of ^{131}I spectrum.

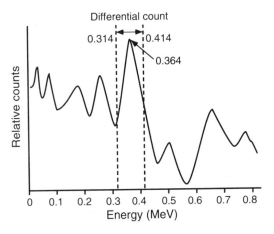

Figure 10-15.   Differential count of ^{131}I spectrum.

(Fig. 10-12). The voltage to the photomultiplier tube is then varied in small increments until a maximum count rate is obtained. As the voltage is increased, the pulse height produced by the γ-ray will be increased until the pulses fall within the area set by the base and window. When the applied voltage causes some of the pulses to exceed the upper discriminator level, the count rate begins to decrease. When the maximum count rate is achieved, the high voltage is fixed, placing the instrument in calibration. Now a 0.661 MeV γ-ray will give a pulse of 6.61 V at this attenuation and high-voltage setting. The high-voltage setting is not changed after this calibration regardless of the γ-emitting isotope counted. An amplified pulse of 10 V now

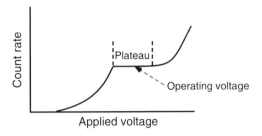

Figure 10-16.   Scintillation detector response curve for integral counting.

corresponds to a 1 MeV γ-ray. The high-voltage adjustment is usually done by the instrument manufacturer and checked by the manufacturer's service representative at routine intervals. Once the high voltage is calibrated, the response to the incident γ ray is linear over the 0- to 1-Mev range. Most instruments are factory adjusted for base and window selection for optimum counting of the commonly used isotopes, ^{125}I, ^{57}Co, and ^{51}Cr. In these instruments, the technologist relies on regular quality control procedures to detect changes in instrument performance.

Integral Counters

A simpler scintillation counter without a pulse-height analyzer, only a lower-level discriminator (base), is used for integral counting. If a detector is to be used for integral counting, adjustment of the voltage applied to the photomultiplier tube is needed, and the optimum voltage again is determined experimentally. While counting an isotope, the applied voltage is varied, and a graph of count rate versus voltage is prepared. A typical response curve is shown in Figure 10-16. An applied voltage midpoint of the resulting plateau will ensure a count rate relatively independent of small voltage changes, thereby increasing instrument stability. This operating voltage should be determined for each isotope to be counted in the instrument. Integral counting is rarely used in the clinical laboratory because it sets only a lower limit for the energy counted.

Multiwell Counters

Speed in reporting results was the impetus for the introduction of multiwell γ counters into the clinical laboratory. With these counters, multiple samples (usually 10 to 24) can be counted simultaneously in closely matched scintillation crystals. These crystals are usually smaller (1 to 1.5 inches) than the more standard crystals (2 to 3 inches) used in the single-well counters. They are not as efficient for counting high-energy γ rays but are suitable for the low-energy isotopes, ^{125}I and ^{57}Co, commonly used in clinical diagnostics. Most multiwell instruments have dual pulse-height analyzers so that these two isotopes can be counted simultaneously. High voltage to the photomultiplier is adjusted at the factory; the individual laboratory matches the various detectors through a normalization process. Each detector is surrounded by lead to decrease the amount of radiation detected in wells adjacent to the sample being counted; these unwanted counts are usually called *crosstalk* or *crossover*. The multiwell counters frequently include software for normalization, crosstalk correction, spilldown (counts from a higher-energy isotope that overlap into the window of the lower-energy isotope), as well as data reduction of standard curves and calculation of unknown samples.

Liquid Scintillation Counting

BASIC COMPONENTS

Low-energy β emission is detected in a unique way. The emission is too low to penetrate the thin aluminum film surrounding the NaI (Tl) crystal. Instead, the β emissions of the commonly used isotopes, ^{3}H, ^{14}C, ^{32}P, ^{35}S, are determined by liquid scintillation counting. An intimate admixture of solvent, sample, and fluor is necessary to detect the low-energy and slight penetration of these β particles. The entire solution is placed in a capped vial and counted in a light-tight chamber. The energy of the β particle is transferred via the solvent molecule to the solute, the fluor. The excited fluor molecule emits photons of light as it returns to its molecular ground state. The photons of light are then counted by a scaler, as in solid scintillation counting.

Other radioactive decay, including γ emission, can be detected by liquid scintillation counting, but the problems associated with the process (see Problems section) usually preclude its use for counting higher-energy radiation.

The *solvent* in liquid scintillation counting must dissolve the fluor as well as transfer the energy from the β emission to the fluor without significant loss. The original solvents (toluene, dioxane, and xylene) have largely been replaced by a newer generation of less hazardous organic solvents. Pseudocumene (1, 2, 4-trimethylbenzene) has the highest efficiency for transferring energy to the fluor and has a flash point of 50°C that classifies it (according to the U.S. Department of Transportation classification) as a combustible liquid rather than a flammable liquid.[4] Combustible liquids have fewer shipment and storage restrictions. Pseudocumene can be placed in plastic vials during counting, but it diffuses through plastic slowly and, therefore, is not suitable for storage in plastic. All of the mentioned solvents, after the addition of the β emitter, must be disposed of as mixed low-level radioactive and hazardous waste (since July 1986), which increases the cost and inconvenience of using them. The newer alkylbenzene and diisopropylnaphthalene solvents have higher flash points (>130°C), which classify them as nonhazardous by Environmental Protection Agency (EPA) regulations.[5] These solvents exceed all current (December 1992) environmental and safety requirements. In addition, some of these newer solvents have been termed "biodegradable" and can be disposed of through the sanitary sewerage system. In the next few years manufacturers will continue to search for solvents less hazardous to personnel and to the environment.

The addition of a *solubilizing agent*, a surfactant or emulsifier, provides a method for making a homogeneous solution from the sample (usually in an aqueous phase) and the organic solvent. Some surfactants used are Triton X100, Triton N57, dodecylbenzene sodium sulfonate, and Hyamine 166.

The fluor must accept energy from excited solvent molecules, form an excited molecule itself, then release photons of light as it returns to the ground state. Most fluors are complex, heterocyclic, organic compounds that emit light in the near ultraviolet and visible regions of the electromagnetic spectrum. Secondary fluors are sometimes added as a "wavelength shifter" to change the wavelength to the spectral response of the photomultiplier tube. In the clinical laboratory the most commonly used fluor is PPO (2, 5-diphenyl oxazole) in combination with the wavelength shifter POPOP (1, 4-bis-2-[5-phenyloxazolyl]-benzene), or dimethyl POPOP. Figure 10-17 shows how the wavelength shifter changes the spectrum to match the response of the photocathode. The mixture of fluors, solvent, and solubilizer is termed a *cocktail.* Kessler[6] gives a more detailed description of various cocktails.

As β emissions from the sample interact with the material (solvent) surrounding them, they cause excitation, that is, they excite solvent molecules. This excitation energy of the solvent is transferred to the solute, the fluor, causing excitation of fluor electrons. The excited electrons in the fluor emit photons of light as they fall back to the ground state. This energy transfer and emission of light photons takes about a nanosecond. The photons of light are detected by the photomultiplier tube and result in electrical pulses as in solid scintillation counters. The high-voltage supply to the photomultiplier tube is similar to that used in γ-ray spectrometry, except that liquid scintillation counters have paired photomultiplier tubes. Each tube requires its own

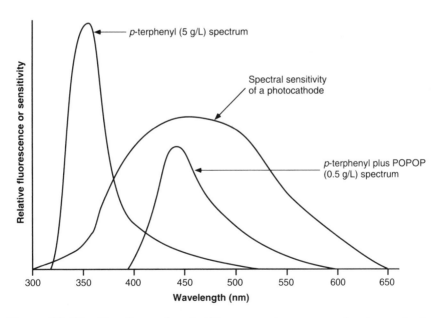

Figure 10-17.   Use of a wavelength shifter to match response to the photocathode.

power supply. Because the low-energy ranges of γ emission result in photomultiplier outputs of the same order of magnitude as thermionic emission (noise), coincidence circuitry has been employed. The use of paired photomultiplier tubes and coincidence circuitry ensures that only pulses seen simultaneously (usually within less than 20 nsec) are passed on to the spectrometer. Pulses simultaneously observed are most often due to β emission. By contrast, the thermionic emission arising in each photomultiplier tube is random, and this background noise is unlikely to be detected simultaneously. Thermionic emission is also often decreased by refrigeration of the entire detector unit. Refrigeration is of relatively less importance with solid-state electronics, and many current instruments can be operated at ambient temperature. Preamplifiers are often attached to the photomultiplier tubes to provide initial amplification. Pulses from the two detection circuits are passed through a coincidence circuit and are electronically summed. Pulses then pass to one or more channels, each consisting of a linear amplifier, pulse-height analyzer, and scaler, much like in γ scintillation counting (Fig. 10-18). Some manufacturers amplify the summation pulse proportionally to its logarithm, called logarithmic amplification. In this design, separate amplifiers for each channel are not used. Neither type of amplifier seems to be superior to the other.[7] Because of the multiplicity of instrument types available for liquid scintillation counting, it would be impractical to describe instrument setting for counting a specific γ-emitting isotope. The directions provided by each manufacturer should be carefully followed.

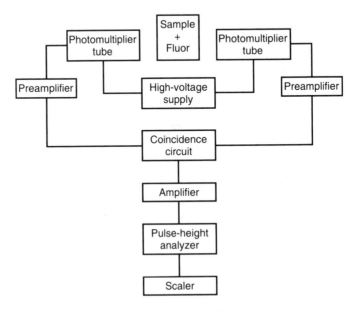

Figure 10-18.   Liquid scintillation counter.

PROBLEMS

Chemiluminescence

Chemiluminescence, described later in this chapter, can be an interferant in liquid scintillation counting. If a chemical reaction that releases light occurs within the vial, the photomultiplier tubes will detect this light. This problem occurs most frequently when quaternary amines, which are strong bases, are used as solubilizers. The presence of peroxides or dissolved oxygen in the sample can also increase the incidence of chemiluminescent interferences. If chemiluminescence is suspected (because of a high initial and unstable count rate), a basic solution can be neutralized with acid, peroxides can be destroyed with reducing agents, or the sample can be stored 12 to 24 hours before it is counted.

Photoluminescence

Some samples exposed to normal fluorescent light in the laboratory will phosphoresce, that is, emit light. This interference can be detected by a high, unstable, initial count rate. However, storage in the dark for ½ hour should eliminate the problem.

Quenching

The admixture of sample and fluor in liquid scintillation can lead to the problem of *quenching.* This is especially true of biologic samples that may contain a great variety of chemical compounds. Even the oxygen in air, as well as any number of chemicals in the sample, may result in quenching. As noted previously, β particles are emitted at a continuous spectrum of energies, the characteristic feature of each isotope being the maximum energy of β emission, the E_{max}. Quenching shifts this β emission curve to the left, lowers the energy of the E_{max}, increases the number of counts in the lower-energy range, and decreases the total detectable count (Fig. 10-19). Quenching may be of three types: chemical, chromatic (color), and optical.

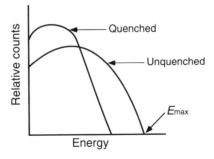

Figure 10-19. Beta spectrum showing effect of quenching.

Chemical quenching is caused by a variety of polar organic compounds that can absorb energy from the excited solvent molecules, preventing, in part, excitation of the fluor (Fig. 10-20). Color quenching occurs when color in the scintillation vial absorbs part of the light emitted by the fluor before it reaches the photomultiplier tube (Fig. 10-20). Color quenching can be expected whenever the scintillant solution does not have its usual light blue color because of colored impurities in the sample. Yellow and red solutions especially may absorb the blue light that is emitted by the fluors. Finally, optical quenching results when the mixture of scintillation cocktail and sample is not a true solution but a suspension that interferes with the passage of light through a heterogeneous solution. Because quenching decreases the detectable energy of β-emitting isotopes, it should be minimized whenever possible. Quenching is sometimes unavoidable, however, and the degree of quenching unpredictable; therefore, it must be recognized and corrected.

Compared to most γ emissions, the β emissions of ^{14}C and especially ^{3}H are of very low energy. Even in the absence of quenching, only approximately 90% of the ^{14}C emissions and 60% of the ^{3}H emissions will be detected. These percentages are referred to as counting efficiency, and they equal detected counts per minute divided by disintegrations per minute $\times$ 100 (% E = [cpm/dpm] $\times$ 100). Disintegrations per minute (dpm) is an absolute number proportional to the isotopic content of the sample, whereas counts per minute (cpm) refers only to the observed count. By correcting for quenching (i.e., determining efficiency), an estimation of the dpm of each sample and consequently of the isotopic content is obtained. Chemical and

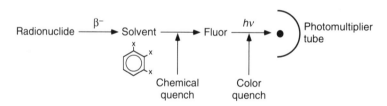

Figure 10-20. Quenching interferes with the basic scintillation process.

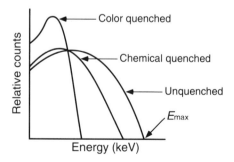

Figure 10-21. Beta spectrum shifts due to quenching.

color quenching both result in a decrease in cpm and a shift of the energy spectrum to a lower range, but the shapes of the resulting curves are different (Fig. 10-21).

Quench Correction

The *internal standard method* for determining counting efficiency and thus correcting for quenching is considered by some to be the most reliable method.[8] The sample is counted once, and then a sample aliquot of radioactive standard with known dpm is added, and the sample is again counted.

$$\% E = \frac{\text{cpm due to added standard}}{\text{dpm of added standard}} \times 100 \qquad \text{(Eq. 10-2)}$$

The drawbacks of this method include a small pipetting error, the inability to re-count unaltered sample because it has become contaminated with standard, and the necessity for counting the sample twice. However, the internal standard method corrects equally well for all types of quenching.

The *channels ratio method*[9] is based on the observation that the β spectrum is always displaced to the left when quenching occurs. The first channel of a two-channel instrument used to measure a single isotope is set to encompass all energies of a given isotope. The second channel is set to encompass approximately 50% of the counts in an unquenched sample, usually in the lower-energy range. As the degree of quenching increases, the count rate in the first channel decreases proportionately more than in the second channel because of the spectral shift. The channels ratio method is standardized by counting multiple samples containing a standard amount of radioisotope with known dpm in the presence of varying quantities of chemical quenching agents. A curve relating the percent efficiency ($\% E = [\text{cpm} \times 100]/\text{dpm}$) to the ratio of counts in the two channels is constructed. When unknown samples are counted, the ratio between the two channel counts is determined and the percentage of efficiency is determined graphically. Channels ratio corrections are most applicable to chemically quenched samples; small errors are produced when mild optical quenching is present. Large errors may be introduced when quenching is due to color or precipitation of the sample. A major weakness in this method occurs when samples of low activity are counted, necessitating very long counting periods to accumulate statistically significant counts in each channel. Despite these disadvantages, the channels ratio method is less time-consuming than the internal standard method, is not subject to pipetting errors, and does not result in contamination of the sample.

In the *external standard method,* the sample is irradiated by a γ source that produces Compton electrons. The assumption is made that the Compton electrons behave as β particles in solution and that quenching in the sample results in proportionate quenching of Compton electrons. After the sample is counted, the external standard is automatically positioned near the sample vial, and the sample is again counted for an additional minute. Depending on the γ-emitting isotope used as external standard, the energy range of the Compton electrons may or may not overlap with the energy range of the β-emitting isotope within the sample. Depending on the instrument used, either the gross counts of the external standard or the channels ratio of the external standard counts in two separate channels can be plotted against percentage of efficiency to generate a curve. This curve is produced experimentally and used in the same manner as channels ratio curves. The major advantage of the use of the external standard is that it allows one to rapidly determine counting efficiency regardless of the amount of radioactivity in the sample. The reproducibility of the technique depends on a constant geometric relationship between γ source and sample. Thus, the γ source must be positioned automatically in the identical position for each count, and sample volume and vial characteristics must be constant. Because the Compton electrons produced are all of relatively high energy compared to the β emissions of tritium, it is possible that minor quenching of low-energy β emissions from tritium may go undetected.

Electronic quench correction is currently available on several instruments. In general, the instrument monitors the external standard ratio of the sample and adjusts instrument performance to produce results proportional to dpm when subsequently counting the sample. Automatic instrumental adjustment consists of either varying amplifier gain or altering the efficiency of the photomultiplier tubes by varying a magnetic field surrounding the photomultiplier tubes. This technique is least efficient in correcting low-energy samples such as tritium or highly quenched samples from other β emitters. In another electronic method, a mathematical transformation of the Compton spectrum of ^{133}Ba (as the external standard) corrects for quenching independent of counting interferences from various tube sizes and plastic vials. However, van Cauter and Roessler[10] have concluded that such computer software techniques, although an improvement over previous automatic quench correction methods and more convenient, are no substitute for a quench curve when extreme accuracy is required.

Luminometers

A recent introduction to the clinical laboratory is another photon counter, the luminometer. This instrument is used to detect and measure luminescence, usually chemiluminescence, but in some applications bioluminescence. *Chemiluminescence* is light resulting from a chemical reaction. If the chemical reaction producing light occurs in nature, the phenomenon is called *bioluminescence.* The firefly we chased as children is an example of bioluminescence. Luminescence results in excited molecules, which emit light photons as they return to the ground state. In chemi- and bioluminescence the energy that causes the excitation of the molecules comes from a chemical reaction instead of heat, electricity, β, γ, or other electromagnetic radiation (the causes of excited state atoms and molecules described in this and earlier chapters).

CHEMILUMINESCENCE

Applications of chemiluminescence in the clinical laboratory have been described by several authors.[11-15] Much of the interest involves chemiluminescent labels in immunoassays as replacements for radioisotopic or enzymatic labels. Chemiluminescent methods of analysis promise extreme sensitivity, low cost, fast analysis for high-sample throughput, and a lack of the regulatory paperwork associated with radioisotopes. Other promising clinical applications are protein blotting and DNA probe assays.[16]

In some reactions the chemiluminescence is a burst of light lasting less than 1 s. Other reactions result in a longer glow lasting several minutes or even hours. The efficiency of the light production can be nearly 1 (for each molecule reacting, one molecule is emitting light), as in the bioluminescent firefly luciferase reaction, but is nearer 0.01 to 0.25 in chemiluminescent reactions. The chemical reaction is usually an oxidation, and several chemiluminescent compounds have been synthesized (see Table 10-1).

Table 10-1
Chemiluminescent Compounds

Compound	Oxidant	Catalyst	Product	Light $h\upsilon$	Reference
Luminol	H_2O_2	OH^-		425 nm	12, 14, 15
Isoluminol	H_2O_2	OH^-			12
Acridinium esters	H_2O_2	OH^-		470 nm	12, 14, 15
Dioxetanes	none	Alkaline phosphatase		477 nm	16, 17

Luminols need a catalyst such as peroxidase or hemin for the reaction to occur. Luminols are easily conjugated to other molecules, but the resultant compound has about one-half the quantum efficiency of the original luminol. For this reason, luminol is often used as the substrate for peroxidase-labeled immunoassays rather than the labeled analyte itself. Primary labels for some derivatives of isoluminol have been prepared as these compounds retain more of their light-producing abilities.

The aryl *acridinium esters* do not require a catalyst and undergo oxidation in the presence of dilute alkaline hydrogen peroxide. Stable conjugates can be prepared readily with little loss of quantum efficiency. The reaction generates an immediate signal, over a 5 s period. Acridinium esters are used in several commercial chemiluminescent immunoassay systems.

Dioxetanes have not been widely used because of their instability—they undergo spontaneous decomposition as they generate light. Recently a highly stable derivative, phenylphosphate-substituted dioxetane, has been discovered.[17] When cleaved by alkaline phosphatase, this stable form converts to the luminescent form that spontaneously decomposes and generates chemiluminescence. An enhancer of fluorescent micelles can be added that increases the chemiluminescence efficiency to 0.48%.[17] The reaction produces light intensity that increases with time, reaching a plateau in 60 minutes and lasting for several hours. This enhanced dioxetane is currently used as a chemiluminescent substrate in some alkaline-phosphatase-labeled immunoassay systems.

INSTRUMENTATION

For the weak sources of electromagnetic radiation emanating from chemiluminescent compounds, photon counting is appropriate. Counting the pulses provides greater sensitivity and more accurate intensity data than measuring average currents, which is done in emission spectroscopy (flame photometry). Photon counting of the chemiluminescent signal demands a rapid response time from the photomultiplier tube when one counts the bursts of light from luminols and acridinium esters. Rapid response is not as critical when measuring the dioxetanes because the signal lasts for hours.

A luminometer is a simple, inexpensive instrument. The signal pulses are a great deal stronger than the background noise of the photomultiplier tube, detector, and

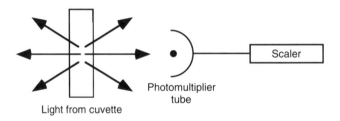

Figure 10-22. Luminometer.

associated electronics. The light source is the sample itself, the detector is a photomultiplier tube with rapid response, and a scaler counts the number of pulses. It is not necessary to discriminate energy; therefore, a pulse-height analyzer is not necessary. The final readout is in relative light units per unit time. For reactions yielding a burst of light, the sample must be placed in front of the photomultiplier tube (encased in a light-tight measuring chamber) with access to an injection port through which one can add reagents. Because chemiluminescence is temperature dependent, the measuring chamber is often temperature controlled, usually at 37°C. At the same time, photomultiplier tubes must be cooled to decrease thermionic noise. The measuring chamber can also be mirrored to collect all of the available light emissions. A simple optical filter filters out the low-energy thermionic noise. Figure 10-22 shows a simple diagram of a luminometer.

Quality Control of Photon Counters

GAMMA COUNTERS

Peak resolution should be checked in the instrument at the time of installation and occasionally thereafter, to ensure that the instrument meets specifications. The energy width of the actual counted photopeak depends on the quality of the crystal. A perfect crystal would have a peak width of 1 pulse height. The lower the percent resolution, the sharper the photopeak and the better the signal-to-noise ratio because narrower windows may be set. Peak resolution is determined from the spectrum of a standard isotope. To determine this spectrum, a narrow window is selected, 1%; the base of the pulse-height analyzer is varied in small increments, 5 keV, across the entire photopeak; and the standard isotopic source is counted at each setting for the same time unit. A graph of counts versus energy yields the isotope spectrum. The full width at half maximum (FWHM) of the photopeak expressed in energy divided by the energy of the γ ray times 100 equals the percent resolution (Fig. 10-23).

$$\frac{\Delta E}{E} \times 100 = \text{\% resolution} \tag{Eq. 10-3}$$

For ^{137}Cs, resolutions of 7% to 12% can be found with clinical laboratory instruments.[18]

Counting efficiencies of ^{137}Cs and/or ^{125}I should also be determined at installation, at regular intervals thereafter, and when troubleshooting the instrument. A source of known activity (corrected for decay since calibration) is counted, and percentage of efficiency is calculated from the following equation:

$$\frac{\text{cpm}}{\text{dpm}} \times 100 = \text{\% efficiency} \tag{Eq. 10-4}$$

The counting efficiencies found with clinical laboratory instruments are approximately 20% for ^{137}Cs and 80% for ^{125}I and ^{57}Co.

The counting reproducibility of each crystal should be checked at regular intervals. The standard method for checking the assumed normal distribution (the Poisson distribution of radioactive decay approaches a normal Gaussian distribution

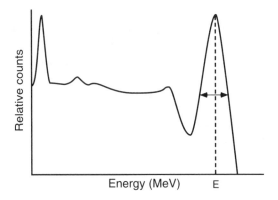

Figure 10-23.   Determination of photopeak resolution: FWHM of the photopeak divided by the energy of the γ ray.

as *N,* the number of observations, becomes larger[19]) is by using the chi-square test. An isotopic standard (count rate $\approx$ 100,000 cpm) is counted several times, usually between 15 and 30, but the same number of observations is checked each time. The mean of the multiple observations is considered the *expected count rate;* the individual count is considered the *observed count rate.* The chi-square is calculated from the following equation:[20]

$$x^2 = \Sigma \frac{(O - E)^2}{E}$$ (Eq. 10-5)

where

O = observed count or each individual count
E = expected count or mean of all observations
x^2 = chi-square

The calculated chi-square should fall between the two chi-square values found in standard chi-square tables[21] for $N - 1$ degrees of freedom (df)(N = number of observations) at the selected probability range (usually 99%, or $p = 0.01$). When the chi-square is within limits, the observed count rate does not differ significantly from what was expected. If the calculated chi-square falls outside the selected limits, the observed count rate differs significantly from that expected of a normal distribution, and the process should be repeated. The second time the criteria are not met, the instrument service representative should be notified.

Each day a particular isotope is counted, a standard isotopic source (about 100,000 cpm) of the isotope of interest or one of similar γ-ray energy should be counted at the exact instrument settings used for routine clinical work.[22] Records should be kept, and limits of count rate variability should be established by calculating the standard deviation (SD) as the square root of the mean counts. Because radioactive decay is a random event per time unit, the probability distribution of this random occurrence follows a Poisson distribution;[19] the SD of a Poisson distribution is the square root of the mean.[23] If the high-voltage supply were to drift, the count rate of the standard source would fall outside the established day-to-day limits (e.g., mean ±6 SD of the initial standardization corrected for isotope decay).

In multiwell γ counters, the standard source of the isotope of interest should be counted in each crystal; alternatively, a set of matched sources may be counted simultaneously. Any detector that differs more than 10% from the mean count rate of the others should be disabled and the service representative notified. After recording individual counts in each crystal, all crystals should be normalized within 1% to the crystal of lowest efficiency. Software for multiwell counters includes the normalization process.

A record of background counts in each crystal for each isotope used should be maintained. Background counts at the beginning and end of each batch of samples ensure that the crystal has not been contaminated. This is not as practical in multiwell instruments with separate trays of samples as it is in single-well instruments. The trays, themselves, should be cleaned at least weekly.

When both pulse-height analyzers are being used, the higher-energy isotopic standard should be counted, and the spilldown into the lower-energy window should be noted and documented. If the high-voltage supply has drifted and the two isotopes are no longer centered in the window, the spilldown into the lower window will have changed significantly and the voltage should be readjusted. When the spilldown is as expected, instruments with microprocessors correct samples and standards for the spilldown from the high-energy isotope.

BETA COUNTERS

Records of counts obtained from standard isotopes of interest should be maintained with the standard isotopic source counted each day the instrument is used for counting that particular isotope. The value of the external standard for quench correction should be obtained at the same time and recorded; background counts in all channels should be used as well. The quench curve, if quench correction is used, can be monitored at less frequent intervals.

LUMINOMETERS

Cold light sources sealed in glass ampules can be purchased for standardizing equipment. These decrease in intensity over time but can be used for a year or more. Some luminometers are equipped with a light-emitting diode (LED) or other standard light source. Either of these standards can be used to monitor day-to-day performance of the instrument. The relative light units of the standard and of the background should fall between defined acceptable limits. Absolute calibration of the instrument is not done because there are currently no absolute photon standards with which to calibrate.

If the instrument is capable of injecting reagent into the measuring cuvette, the accuracy of the injection device must be monitored periodically, at least quarterly. Because chemiluminescence is temperature dependent, it is important to monitor the temperature of the measuring chamber. This should also be done on a routine basis, at least quarterly.

Summary

In this chapter we described photon counters, those that count the photons produced by radioactivity reacting with the scintillator surrounding it, and those produced by a chemical reaction.

The scintillator used for detecting gamma energy (which is more energetic than beta radiation) is a NaI(Tl) crystal. The sample is placed adjacent to the well or in a hole drilled into the crystal. The scintillator used for detecting beta rays is a fluor dissolved in an organic solvent. The sample is then added and also dissolved in the solvent. As the radiation, either β or γ, reacts with the material surrounding it, energetic electrons are formed. These energetic electrons excite the fluor, and, as the excited fluor returns to the ground state, photons of light are emitted. Emitted photons are detected and changed to electrical energy by a photomultiplier tube. In a luminometer the photomultiplier tube detects the photons produced by a chemical reaction.

The photons of light are detected and changed to electrical pulses by a photomultiplier tube. The number of pulses is counted by a counter-scaler and is proportional to the number of photons emitted. When a standard curve is run with the assay, the end result (in cpm, dpm, or relative light units) is related to concentration.

All three instruments, then, have the basic components of sample, photomultiplier tube, and scaler-counter. In addition, scintillation counters, both beta and gamma, have a pulse-height analyzer to separate only those photons emitted by the isotope selected.

How the sample is presented to the photomultiplier tube differs in the three instruments. For γ counting, the sample is adjacent to the crystal or in a well drilled into the crystal; for β counting the sample is dissolved in a mixture of sample, solvent, fluor; for chemiluminescence the sample (in front of the photomultiplier tube) usually must have a reagent added immediately before the signal is detected.

Beta counting has the most interferences, with quenching causing most problems. There are several ways to correct for quenching, the internal standard method being the most accurate. However, it is also the most cumbersome. The usual method for routine clinical work is the external standard method; in newer instruments the correction is done electronically by transforming the Compton spectrum of the external standard and reporting the result in dpm.

Quality control for the instruments involves counting background and a standard each day of use to make certain there has not been a contamination of the sample chamber (if background counts are excessive) or a change in the gain to the photomultiplier tube (if the standard counts fall outside the defined range). If multiple counting wells are used, the wells or counting chambers must be balanced to one another so they are all giving the same response to a particular standard or sample. The volume of the reagent injected and the temperature of the measuring chamber also need to be monitored in some luminometers.

Questions and Problems

1. A 100-μL aliquot of ^{3}H standard was calibrated at 115,000 dpm on January 3, 1991. How much activity is left in a 100-μL aliquot on April 3, 1993? The half-life for ^{3}H is 12.43 years.
2. Construct a quench curve using 100 μL of the ^{3}H standard from Question 1. The external standard ratio as well as the cpm of the series of quenched standards was determined on April 3, 1991. The results follow:

μL Quenching Agent	cpm 100 μL ^{3}H Std.	External Std. Ratio
0	42,600	0.77
10	33,300	0.62
25	24,500	0.50
50	15,000	0.34
75	10,100	0.25
100	6,600	0.19

3. The following sample containing ^{3}H was counted on that same day under identical conditions. The sample was 30,000 cpm and the external standard ratio was 0.75. How many dpm of ^{3}H were in the sample? What was the efficiency with which it was counted?
4. Each day a multiwell gamma counter is used, identical ^{125}I standards are counted as part of routine quality control of the instrument. On a particular day the following counts were obtained for wells 1 through 10: 35,447; 35,777; 35,636; 35,359; 35,247; 35,227; 35,581; 39,552; 35,576; 35,704. Control limits were 35,528 $\pm$1130. Is the instrument performing satisfactorily? If not, what is a probable cause of the problem and what action should be taken?
5. The relative light units (RLUs) of a standard LED are determined each day the luminometer is operated. Control limits for this LED are 112,000 $\pm$3000. On a particular day the RLUs are 78,000. Is the luminometer acting satsifactorily? If not, what is a probable cause of the problem and what action should be taken?
6. Construct a block diagram of a scintillation counter.
7. Explain why a pulse-height analyzer is not used in a luminometer.

References

1. Powsner ER. Basic principles of radioactivity and its measurements. In: Tietz NW, ed. Textbook of clinical chemistry. Philadelphia: WB Saunders, 1986:182.
2. Knoche HW. Radioisotopic methods for biological and medical research. New York: Oxford University Press, 1991:89-92.
3. Haven MC, Haven GT. Scintillation Counters. In: Hicks MR, Haven MC, Schenken JR, McWhorter CA, eds. Laboratory instrumentation, 3rd ed. Philadelphia: JB Lippincott, 1987:202-03.
4. ter Wiel J, Hegge T. Advances in scintillation cocktails. In: Ross H, Noakes JE, Spaulding JD, eds. Liquid scintillation counting and organic scintillators. Chelsea, MI: Lewis Publishers, 1991:51-67.
5. Neumann KE, Roessler N, ter Wiel J. Safe scintillation chemicals for high efficiency, high throughput counting. In: Ross H, Noakes JE, Spaulding JD, eds. Liquid scintillation counting and organic scintillators. Chelsea, MI: Lewis Publishers, 1991:35-41.
6. Kessler MJ. Liquid scintillation analysis. Meriden, CT: Packard Instrument Co, 1989:Pub. #169-3052, 6-1 to 6-27.

7. Knoche HW. Radioisotopic methods for biological and medical research. New York: Oxford University Press, 1991:169.

8. Powsner ER. Basic principles of radioactivity and its measurement. In: Tietz NW, ed. Textbook of clinical chemistry. Philadelphia: WB Saunders, 1986:192.

9. Kobayashi Y, Maudsley DV. Biological applications of ligand scintillation counting. New York: Academic Press, 1974:28-29.

10. van Cauter S, Roessler N. Modern techniques for quench correction and dpm determination in widowless liquid scintillation counting: A critical review. In: Ross H, Noakes, JE, Spaulding JD, eds. Liquid scintillation counting and organic scintillators. Chelsea, MI: Lewis Publishers, 1991:219-37.

11. Boeckx RL. Chemiluminescense: Applications for the clinical laboratory. Hum Pathol 1984, 15:104-11.

12. Whitehead TP, Kricka LF, Carter TJN, Thorpe GHG. Analytical luminescence: Its potential in the clinical laboratory. Clin Chem 1979, 25:1531-46.

13. Seitz WR. Immunoassay labels based on chemiluminescence and bioluminescence. Clin Biochem 1984, 17:120-25.

14. Stabler TV. Chemiluminescence. Clin Chem News 1991, Oct:12,16.

15. Nieman TA. Detection based on solution-phase chemiluminescence systems. In: Birks JW, ed. Chemiluminescence and photochemical reaction detection in chromatography. New York: VCH Publishers, 1989:99-123.

16. Kricka LJ. Chemiluminescent and bioluminescent techniques. Clin Chem 1991, 37:1472-81.

17. Schaap AP, Akhavan H, Romano LJ. Chemiluminescent substrates for alkaline phosphatase: Application to ultrasensitive enzyme-linked immunoassays and DNA probes. Clin Chem 1989, 35:1863-64.

18. Howard PL, Trainer TD. Radionuclides in clinical chemistry. Boston: Little, Brown, & Co, 1980:27.

19. Harbert J, DaRocha AFG. Textbook of nuclear medicine, vol. 1: Basic science. Philadelphia: Lea & Febiger, 1984:71.

20. Shott S. Statistics for health professionals. Philadelphia: WB Saunders, 1990:207.

21. Tietz NW. Textbook of clinical chemistry. Philadelphia: WB Saunders, 1986:1807.

22. Johnson RF. Well-type scintillation counting systems and their care: A procedural approach. The Ligand Review 1980, 2:65-69.

23. Colton T. Statistics in medicine. Boston: Little, Brown, & Co, 1974:77-79.

Suggested Readings

Bernier DR, Christian PE, Langan JK, and Wells LD. Nuclear medicine technology and techniques, 2nd ed. St. Louis: CV Mosby, 1989.

Gollnick, DA. Basic radiation protection technology, 2nd ed. Altadena, CA: Pacific Radiation Corp, 1988.

11

ELECTROCHEMICAL METHODS OF ANALYSIS

Ellen R. Goshorn
Steven M. Faynor
Mary C. Haven

Objectives

After completing this chapter, the reader will be able to:

1. List various electrochemical methods that have been applied to clinical chemistry.
2. Describe the principles of potentiometry.
3. Draw an electrochemical cell for determining pH.
4. Compare and contrast the electrochemical measurements of $P\text{CO}_2$ and $P\text{O}_2$.
5. Discuss the electrochemical methods available for measuring electrolytes.
6. Discuss the electrochemical methods available for measuring glucose.
7. Explain the importance of sloping a pH meter.
8. Discuss the use of anodic stripping voltammetry for lead analysis.
9. Calculate pH from a given concentration of hydrogen ion.

Definitions

Acid: A hydrogen ion donor. An acid dissociates to a hydrogen ion plus a conjugate base. Example: hydrochloric acid.

$$\text{HCl} \rightleftharpoons \text{H}^+ + \text{Cl}^-$$
$$\text{acid} \quad \text{conjugate base}$$

(Eq. 11-1)

Activity: The thermodynamic expression for the effective concentration of a substance in solution. Activity (a) is equal to the concentration (C) times an activity coefficient (γ).

$$a = \gamma C$$

(Eq. 11-2)

The activity coefficient varies with the ionic strength of the solution. In dilute solutions (most biological systems), the activity coefficient approaches 1, so activity is roughly equivalent to concentration.

Ampere: The unit of current. One ampere (A) is one coulomb of charge per second.

Amperometry: An electrochemical technique that determines the concentration of a substance by measuring the amount of current produced by an oxidation or reduction of that substance at an electrode that is maintained at a single applied potential. In coulometry, amperometry is used to determine the endpoint of the titration by signaling the appearance of an excess of titrant.

Anode: The electrode where oxidation takes place.

Automatic Temperature Compensation: A device used to automatically change the gain of a pH meter to compensate for changes in sample temperature.[1]

Cathode: The electrode where reduction takes place.

CO_2 Content: The sum of the concentrations of all CO_2 species in solution. Although CO_2 is present in plasma in many forms, including that physically dissolved as well as attached to proteins and hemoglobin (carbamino groups), for practical purposes, CO_2 content is approximately equal to the sum in millimoles per liter of the bicarbonate plus carbonic acid.

Combination Electrode: An electrode where the indicator and reference electrodes are combined into a single unit.

Conductivity: Measure of the ability of a solution to carry an electrical charge.[2]

Coulomb: The unit of charge. One coulomb (Q) is equivalent to the charge on 6.24×10^{18} electrons.

Coulometry: A titration that uses an electrochemically generated titrant.

Direct-Reading Electrode: An electrode that is exposed to an undiluted specimen as the sample. It is usually applied to sodium and potassium electrodes.

Dissociation Constant: An acid present in dilute aqueous solution will dissociate predictably. The constant (K) is calculated by multiplying the hydrogen ion concentration by the conjugate base concentration and dividing this by the undissociated acid concentration.

$$K = \frac{[H^+][HCO_3^-]}{[H_2CO_3]}$$ (Eq. 11-3)

Electrode: The site of an oxidation or reduction reaction in solution.

Electrode Response: The change in potential of an ion-selective electrode in response to changes in the concentration of the ion the electrode is designed to measure. Predicted by the Nernst equation (q.v.).

Electrolyte: An ionizable substance in solution capable of conducting electricity.

Equivalence Point: That point in the titration at which stoichiometrically equivalent amounts of the main reactants have been brought together. It is the point at which there is no excess of either reactant.

Faraday: The charge carried by an equivalent weight of an ion. One faraday (F) equals 96,487 Q/equivalent weight.

Faraday's Law: The law according to which the passage of 1 F of electricity (96,487 Q) will oxidize or reduce one gram-equivalent of the substance under investigation.

Henderson-Hasselbalch Equation: In a weak aqueous solution such as blood, the pH can be predicted on the basis of the following equation using the observed pK$'$ (q.v.) of 6.1 for the most active plasma buffer, bicarbonate.

$$pH = pK' + \log \frac{[HCO_3^-]}{[H_2CO_3]}$$ (Eq. 11-4)

where $[H_2CO_3] = 0.03 \, PCO_2$. The symbol [Ⓜ] refers to the concentration of the ion or compound within the brackets.

Indicator Electrode: The electrode designed to respond to a change in the concentration of some substance in solution; also called the *sensing,* or *working,* or *measuring electrode.*

Indirect-Reading Electrode: An electrode that is exposed to a diluted serum specimen as the sample. It is usually applied to sodium and potassium electrodes.

Ion-Selective Electrode: An electrode whose potential varies with the concentration of some ion in solution. The *p*H electrode is a hydrogen ion-selective or ion-specific electrode.

Isopotential Point: The *p*H at which the combined potential of the *p*H and reference electrode is 0 mV and at which the response is relatively insensitive to changes in temperature. For most *p*H meter-electrode combinations, the isopotential point is approximately *p*H 7.

Liquid-Junction Potential: The electrical potential developing at a junction between solutions composed of different ions, not necessarily related to *p*H. Factors affecting the liquid-junction potential include physical structure of the junction, types of salts in solution (ionic strength), temperature, and colloidal particles. For reproducibility, the two solutions should be brought together under the same conditions on each occasion. Apparent *p*H drift may be caused by diffusion of the two electrolyte solutions, one into the other.

Nernst Equation: An expression relating the electrode response to the activity (or concentration) of an ion in solution.

$$E = E^0 + \frac{2.3\,RT}{n F} \log a \qquad\qquad \text{(Eq. 11-5)}$$

See text for explanation.

Oxidation: The process of losing electrons.

Partial Pressure: For a mixture of gases, the pressure contribution by any single gas will be equal to the mole-fraction of the gas times the total pressure. For example, for a gas at 760 mmHg and containing 5% CO_2, the partial pressure of the CO_2 (PCO_2) will be 38 mmHg.

pH: The negative common (base 10) logarithm of the hydrogen ion concentration or activity. In practice, hydrogen ion concentration $[H^+]$ and activity are used interchangeably because in dilute solutions the activity coefficient approaches 1.

pK: The negative common (base 10) logarithm of the dissociation constant (q.v.).

pK' (6.1):   The empirically determined *p*K for the bicarbonate buffer system of whole blood at 37°C. In practice, the actual *p*K' has been found to vary in patients from 5.8 to 6.4. It is unclear whether this variation is prevalent enough to introduce errors in parameters derived from the Henderson–Hasselbalch equation.[3]

Polarization: In an electrochemical cell, the departure from the linear relationship between the cell voltage and the current. Small electrodes are more easily polarized than large ones. Some electrochemical methods take advantage of electrode polarization while others guard against it.

Polarography: A voltammetric technique for determining the concentration of a substance in solution by measuring the current produced from a dropping-mercury polarized electrode when the substance undergoes oxidation or reduction at the electrode.

Potentiometry: An electrochemical technique for determining the concentration of a substance in solution by measuring the potential of an electrode in response to changes in concentration under conditions of no net current flow and at equilibrium.

Reference Electrode: The electrode against which the potential change created in an ion-specific electrode is measured. These electrodes are generally silver-silver chloride (Ag/AgCl) or calomel (Hg/Hg_2Cl_2). The potential of the reference electrode remains constant in the face of changing ion concentrations of the test solutions.

Salt Bridge: That solution used to connect the reference electrode with the test electrode and the intervening unknown solution. The salt bridge most commonly used is saturated potassium chloride (KCl), although 0.1 N, 3.0 N, 3.5 N, and 4.5 N solutions of KCl, 0.15 N NaCl, and other concentrations of NaCl have also been used.

Temperature Coefficient: The measurable millivolt change per *p*H unit at the various temperatures utilized for *p*H measurement (mV/*p*H unit). It is predicted by the Nernst equation to be equal to 2.3 RT/*n*F, or 59.16 mV for the hydrogen electrode at 25°C. This is not to be confused with the temperature coefficient of buffer solutions, in which their measurable *p*H changes with temperature (*p*H/°C). (For example, whole-blood *p*H changes 0.015 *p*H unit/°C, whereas plasma changes 0.01 *p*H unit/°C.)

Voltammetry: Electroanalytical methods that measure the current, when the indicating electrode is polarized, as a function of applied voltage and relate this current to the composition of a solution.

Introduction

The principles of electrochemistry have been used to develop several analytical techniques used in the modern clinical laboratory. The first major clinical electrochemical methods include the measurements of blood *p*H, PCO_2, and PO_2. Since the 1970s, refinements in electrode manufacturing have caused changes resulting in an increased use of analytical techniques based on measuring the flow of electricity. Now the electrolytes and some trace metals, as well as other analytes (e.g., glucose), are routinely measured using electrochemical methods. In this chapter we describe the clinical laboratory use of potentiometry, voltammetry, coulometry, amperometry, conductometry, and anodic stripping voltammetry.

Principles

ELECTROCHEMICAL CELLS

A metal rod, inserted into a solution of its own metallic ions, will develop an electrical potential (voltage) between the metal and the solution. This voltage results from the production of electrons as some of the metal atoms become dissolved in the solution. Free electrons are produced by this reaction.

$$M^0 \rightarrow M^+ + e^- \qquad \text{(Eq. 11-6)}$$

where

M^0 = metal atom
M^+ = metal ion
e^- = electron

This system is a half-cell, and the metal rod can be considered the electrode. Because oxidation is occurring at this electrode, it is also the anode.

The ions of another metal in solution and in contact with their metal atom may favor formation of metal atoms with acceptance of an electron.

$$M^+ + e^- \rightarrow M^0 \qquad \text{(Eq. 11-7)}$$

This second electrode would then be the cathode because reduction is taking place. This, too, is a half-cell. The two half-cells can be connected by means of a conducting solution (salt bridge). This establishes the circuit and enables a current to flow. Thus, a complete cell is formed.

An electrochemical cell may be used to determine the quantity of an analyte. This electrochemical device must consist of at least two electrodes (cathode and anode) and an electrolyte solution. Between the electrodes and the electrolyte there is a movement of charge, electronic at the electrode and ionic in the electrolyte solution. One electrode is the indicating electrode. At this electrode the electrochemical measurement of interest takes place. The second electrode is the counterelectrode, completing the redox reaction and current flow. It may either be the source of electrons or may use electrons. The counterelectrode may also serve as the reference electrode, maintaining a constant potential against which the potential of the indicating electrode can be measured.

A comparison of the voltage of one half-cell to another half-cell can be made. The International Union of Pure and Applied Chemistry in 1953 adopted the method of comparing all half-cell potentials to the standard hydrogen electrode, the potential of which they arbitrarily assigned as 0.0000 V. The standard electrode potential (E^0) for each half-cell is determined by a comparison to the standard hydrogen electrode. This standard electrode potential is defined as the emf or voltage (V) of the half-cell when all activities are unity and is usually given at 25°C. A few examples follow:

Half-cell	*Reaction*	*emf*
$\frac{1}{2}H_2$	$H^+ + e^-$	0.0000 V
Ca	$Ca^2 + 2e^-$	+2.87 V
Fe	$Fe^2 + 2e^-$	+0.441 V
Cu	$Cu^2 + 2e^-$	−0.337 V

If the ions in the cells are not at unit activity, the potential E is given by the Nernst equation.[4]

$$E = E^0 + \frac{RT}{nF} \ln a \qquad \text{(Eq. 11-8)}$$

where

E = observed potential (emf)
E^0 = standard electrode potential (emf)
R = molar gas constant (8.314 J/mole per °K)
T = absolute temperature in °K (25°C = 298°K)
n = number of electrons transferred
F = Faraday's constant (96,478 Q/Eq weight)
ln = log to the base e (natural log)
a = activity of the ion

At 25°C, with conversion of the natural $\log_e$ to $\log_{10}$ and insertion of the values for R and F, this equation simplifies to

$$E = E^0 + \frac{0.0591}{n} \log_{10} a \qquad \text{(Eq. 11-9)}$$

From this equation, it can be seen that voltage depends on the activity of the ion. A change in ion activity will change the measurable voltage. The activity of an ion can be determined by a difference in voltage. From the definitions at the beginning of this chapter, we see that activity (a) is equal to concentration (C) times an activity coefficient (γ) and that in dilute solutions this activity coefficient approaches 1. In most biological systems (dilute solutions), activity is a workable approximation of concentration. Thus, the concentration of an ion can be determined by a difference in voltage with the proper selection of electrodes.

REFERENCE ELECTRODES

There is no method for measuring the absolute potential of an electrode. One can only measure differences in potential between two electrodes. The measuring electrode, responding to the analyte of interest, is compared to a reference electrode. A reference electrode consists of three parts: an elemental wire or foil, a filling solution that forms a electrolyte salt bridge, and a fluid junction at the tip of the electrode through which a small amount of filling solution can flow so that contact can be made with the sample solution to complete the circuit.

The standard reference electrode is the *hydrogen electrode* that has arbitrarily been assigned a potential of 0.0000V when the hydrogen ion activity is 1 and the partial pressure of hydrogen is 1 atmosphere. This electrode is created by bubbling pure hydrogen gas through a solution in which a platinum electrode is immersed and establishing an equilibrium between the hydrogen ion and the hydrogen gas in that solution.

$$H^+ + e^- \rightleftharpoons \tfrac{1}{2}H_2(g) \qquad\qquad \text{(Eq. 11-10)}$$

The platinum electrode is covered by a surface catalyst such as platinum or palladium black, which reduces the energy barrier, increases the equilibrium pressure of hydrogen, and makes the electrode reversible in response to the hydrogen ion. It has better thermal stability than the calomel electrode, so it is used when measurement must be made at elevated temperatures. This electrode is not used in any clinical laboratory instruments for it has several disadvantages, such as equilibrating slowly, requiring large volumes of solutions, and requiring a source of hydrogen gas.

A *calomel reference electrode* consists of a combination of mercury (Hg) and a paste of mercurous chloride (Hg_2Cl_2) in a saturated KCl solution. The chloride ions become saturated with mercury at the surface of the mercury. Under these conditions, a typical calomel electrode will produce a constant reference potential of 224 mV to which other electrodes may be compared.

The saturated KCl solution is the salt bridge solution. A small hole in the tip of the electrode lets some of this solution flow very slowly into the sample solution. This flow establishes the electrical contact between sample and reference electrode. It is best to have the electrode's electrolyte solution and the salt bridge solution identical. Saturated KCl is often used because it is easy to make. Other solutions of KCl have been used but are less satisfactory. With dilute salt bridge solutions, liquid-junction potentials are much less predictable. The calomel electrode should be separated from the KCl salt bridge by a porous ceramic plug, which will reduce the chance of back diffusion and contamination.

The electrode potential of the calomel reference electrode system depends significantly on temperature, especially when saturated KCl is used as the fill solution. Thermal stability with $\pm 0.05°C$ is necessary. Equilibration at another temperature is also slow because of solubility factors with saturated KCl. The calomel electrode provides a potential independent of pH when connected to a glass electrode by a KCl bridge whenever the pH is greater than 1.5 and less than 12. For best operation, the calomel electrode should be intact, appear silver-gray, and have an open air vent during the time of use. The electrolyte level should be kept full using the fill hole on the side.

The most widely used reference electrode is the *silver-silver chloride electrode.* This electrode usually consists of a silver wire coated with a layer of silver chloride and immersed in a solution of potassium chloride (KCl) saturated with silver chloride. The potential developed at the electrode surface can be described by the following equation:

$$AgCl + e^- \leftrightharpoons Ag^0 + Cl^-$$

(Eq. 11-11)

The silver-silver chloride electrode has a better thermal stability than the calomel reference electrode, and there are less problems with hazardous chemicals (i.e., Hg and Hg_2Cl_2) if an electrode breaks. However, the silver chloride is soluble in the KCl electrolyte solution. Care must be taken to follow the manufacturer's directions about the concentration of KCl added as the fill solution.

Types of Electrochemical Methods

Six different electrochemical phenomena are commonly used in the clinical laboratory: potentiometry, voltammetry, coulometry, amperometry, conductometry, and anodic stripping voltammetry.

POTENTIOMETRY

Potentiometric principles are used to determine the concentration of several ionic species in biological samples. Potentiometry measures the electrical difference between two electrodes in a cell. One electrode is the sensing or indicating electrode, and the other is the reference electrode. The sensing electrode is composed of an *ion-selective membrane* that separates the test sample from the internal filling electrolyte solution that has a known concentration. A potential difference develops at the ion-selective membrane because of the difference in ion activity between the test solution and the internal electrolyte solution. The potential difference that develops at the indicating electrode is read against the constant potential of the reference electrode. As long as the current flow is zero, the potential is constant. When all potentials but the indicating electrode are held constant, the potential difference can then be related to the activity of a specific ion. Potentiometric methods are commonly referred to as determinations by *ion-selective electrodes.* Specificity to a particular ion is determined by the ion-selective membrane. Various types of ion-selective membranes are available including glass, precipitate, solid-state, liquid-liquid, and liquid membrane. Clinical applications of potentiometry include determination of *p*H, PCO_2, and ion-selective electrode measurements of Na, K, Cl, Li, and ionized calcium.

*p*H Electrode and *p*H Measurement

As noted in the definition section, *p*H is the negative log of the hydrogen ion activity or in dilute solutions, the negative log of the hydrogen ion concentration ($-\log [H^+]$). This concentration can be determined by measuring a change in potential between an electrode responding to $[H^+]$ and a reference electrode. The Nernst equation for this reaction at 25°C would be

$$E = E_0 - 0.0591 \, pH \qquad \text{(Eq. 11-12)}$$

This equation is a straight line with a negative slope of 0.0591 and an intercept at E_0.

The *p*H meter (Fig. 11-1) is the instrument that does the potentiometric comparison for determining *p*H and is composed of four parts: an indicating electrode, a reference electrode, a voltmeter, and the test solution. An indicating electrode is responsive to the activity of the hydrogen ion. These ions move across a membrane in the direction of lesser concentration; this movement creates a potential due to charge separation. The reference electrode is the stable potential to which the indicating electrode potential is compared. A voltmeter compares the voltage from the indicat-

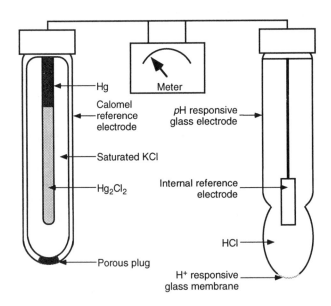

Figure 11-1.   System for measuring *p*H.

ing electrode to the voltage from the reference electrode and displays this measurement. The solution of unknown hydrogen ion activity completes the circuit.

The *indicating electrode* has a thin glass membrane, permeable to hydrogen ions, sealed to a glass or plastic tube that contains a silver wire. The tube is filled with a solution of saturated AgCl, a specific concentration of KCl, and a fixed concentration of HCl for a constant *p*H. This silver wire/silver chloride solution forms an internal reference electrode that is part of the glass electrode, but it is the glass membrane that responds to changes in hydrogen ion activity. This indicating electrode is connected to one terminal of the voltmeter.

The *reference electrode* is a second silver-silver chloride reference electrode and is connected to the opposite terminal of the voltmeter. A calomel electrode can also be used as the reference electrode.

The *voltmeter* must be capable of measuring emf to 0.1 mV (equivalent to 0.002 *p*H units). At this millivoltage an extremely small current will flow, in the neighborhood of 10^{-8}A, because of the high internal resistance of the glass electrode. In a direct-reading instrument, the actual emf produced by a change in *p*H is amplified and displayed digitally or on a meter.

The *test solution* completes the electrochemical cell. Both the indicating and the reference electrodes are immersed in the solution to be tested; each electrode is connected to the appropriate terminal of the voltmeter. If the test solution is continually mixed while the *p*H is being determined, the results will be more accurate.

At any given temperature, the change in voltage resulting from a change in $[H^+]$ will be directly proportional to the change in the $\log[H^+]$. Thus, the change in voltage is linear with respect to a change in *p*H. The Nernst equation shows that measured voltage also depends on temperature. The instrument converts a change in millivoltage to a change in *p*H units at the various electrode temperatures. The instrument's temperature control knob alters the constant proportionally between voltage and scale reading. For example, an electrode that would reflect a change of 59.1 mV for a change of 1.00 *p*H units at 25°C would show a change of some 74 mV for the same change in *p*H, 1.00, at 100°C. In other words, the instrument's temperature control knob will correct for temperature changes by altering the slope of the relationship between changes in *p*H and changes in millivolts.

Newer *p*H meters have built in automatic temperature compensators (ATCs). The ATC circuit consists of a temperature probe such as a platinum resistance thermometer, which is immersed into the test solution along with the reference and indicator electrodes. The resistance of the platinum element changes with temperature, and the output of the probe is used to modify the gain of the *p*H meter's amplifier. Some *p*H meters compensate directly for changes in temperature by measuring the change in resistance of the *p*H electrode's glass membrane. This resistance, like that of the platinum thermometer, varies with temperature. This eliminates the need for an extra ATC probe. This technique is termed *log R compensation*.[1]

The mineral composition of the glass membrane is critical, for minor changes in composition will produce major changes in electrode selectivity. Corning 015 glass, widely used for membranes, has a composition of approximately 72% SiO_2, 6% CaO, and 22% Na_2O.[5] Membranes of this composition are responsive to hydrogen ions up to a *p*H of 9, then other univalent cations, especially sodium, also become responsive. One percent Al_2O_3 produces a good *p*H-sensitive membrane with little other cation response. Changing the concentration of oxides to 68% SiO_2, 5% Al_2O_3, 27% Na_2O makes membranes with a general cation response.

The glass surface must be hydrated before alkaline metal ions in the membrane lattice will exchange for hydrogen ions in solution. Hydration is accomplished by soaking the electrode in water. Each surface of the glass membrane develops a hydrated glass lattice consisting of a network of oxygen atoms held together in an irregular three-dimensional network of silicon atoms. This lattice contains anionic sites capable of attracting cations of a certain size-to-charge ratio. The hydration process causes swelling of the glass, but constant dissolution of the surface of the hydrated area maintains the glass membrane's total thickness at a steady state. The glass needs to be of relatively high chemical durability, or alkaline earths within the glass will dissolve too rapidly and, in solution, will erode glass and electrode alike over a period of months. The rate of dissolution of glass is one major factor determining the electrode's life.

A combination glass electrode (Fig. 11-2) that contains the glass electrode with its internal reference electrode as well as the reference electrode can determine the *p*H of small-volume solutions.

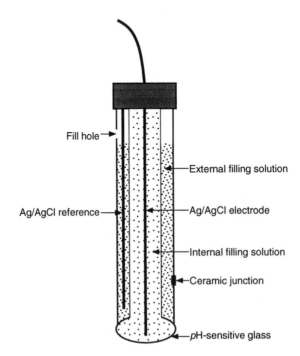

Figure 11-2.   Combination *p*H electrode.

All *p*H meters must be standardized before use so that the response and meter scale coincide. The first step is to immerse the electrodes into a *p*H 7.00 buffer and to adjust the meter to this value using the "zero," "standardize," or "calibrate" knob. For most *p*H meter-electrode combinations, *p*H 7 is the isopotential point so the output of the electrode pair should be 0 mV. The zero knob allows imposition of a small offset so the meter will read 7.00. This is roughly equivalent to a blank in a spectrophotometric assay.

The electrodes are then immersed in a second buffer to adjust the slope. The second buffer is chosen so the *p*Hs of the buffers bracket the *p*H of the unknown solution. The meter is adjusted to the second *p*H by using the "slope" knob. If all electrodes behaved as predicted by the Nernst equation, there would be no need for a slope adjustment. In the real world this is not the case; therefore, a slope correction is necessary for maximum accuracy. If no slope control is provided, the temperature control can be used for the same purpose (provided the electrodes, buffers, and samples are all at the same temperature).

Microprocessor-controlled *p*H meters modify the digital display so that it matches the values of the standardization buffers. To standardize these instruments successfully, the calibration algorithm provided by the manufacturer must be followed exactly.

Glass electrodes operate best at *p*H between 2 and 12 and ionic strength between 0.01 and 0.1. Proper *p*H measurements require the following: (1) sample and standard buffers must be treated identically, (2) the electrode must reflect the correct voltage-to-*p*H ratio at all times, and (3) the *p*H meter must translate millivolts to *p*H units correctly regardless of the temperature at which the measurements are taken. Meter standardization is best with buffers covering the entire useful range. Using a buffer with temperature, *p*H, and ionic strength similar to that of the unknown will reduce the variables created by liquid-junction potential difference and thermal effects.

Carbon Dioxide Partial Pressure Measurement

Carbon dioxide partial pressure (PCO_2) is measured as the change in *p*H of a weak bicarbonate buffer after it has reached equilibrium by dialysis across a semipermeable membrane with the CO_2 physically dissolved in an unknown solution, usually blood. The PCO_2 electrode takes advantage of the fact that *p*H has a linear relationship to the log PCO_2 over the range of 10 to 90 mmHg (1.4%-11.4%). The following equilibrium exists in blood as well as in bicarbonate buffer.

$$H_2O + CO_2 \rightleftharpoons H_2CO_3 \rightleftharpoons HCO_3^- + H^+ \tag{Eq. 11-13}$$

The dissociation equation can be written as follows:

$$K = \frac{[H^+][HCO_3^-]}{[H_2CO_3]} \tag{Eq. 11-14}$$

or since $[H_2CO_3]$ equals some constant (k) times PCO_2, then equation 11-14 becomes

$$K = \frac{[H^+][HCO_3^-]}{[k \times PCO_2]} \tag{Eq. 11-15}$$

Taking the log of Equation 11-15,

$$\log[H^+] + \log[HCO_3^-] = \log K + \log k + \log PCO_2 \qquad \text{(Eq. 11-16)}$$

Because pH equals the negative log of the hydrogen ion concentration and pK equals the negative log of the dissociation constant K,

$$pH - \log[HCO_3^-] = pK - \log k - \log PCO_2 \qquad \text{(Eq. 11-17)}$$

But pK and $\log k$ are constants. Therefore, pH is proportional ($\propto$) to:

$$pH \propto \log[HCO_3^-] - \log PCO_2 \qquad \text{(Eq. 11-18)}$$

If the concentration of $[HCO_3^-]$ in the weak bicarbonate buffer is relatively high compared to the small addition of $[HCO_3^-]$ formed from the dissolved CO_2, then log $[HCO_3^-]$ is also a constant and pH *has a linear dependence on log* PCO_2 when equilibrium has been established. The electrode is calibrated with known calibrating gases, and PCO_2 of the unknown sample is calculated from this linear calibration.

The PCO_2 electrode (Fig. 11-3)[6,7] interposes a semipermeable (to CO_2 dissolved as a gas only) membrane between the unknown solution (usually blood) and a weak bicarbonate buffer into which is immersed both a pH-sensitive glass electrode and a reference electrode (usually silver-silver chloride). After the CO_2, physically dissolved in the sample or as a calibrating gas or solution, reaches equilibrium with the bicarbonate buffer across the semipermeable membrane, some hydrogen ion concentration change within the buffer occurs (Fig. 11-3). This is detected by the pH-sensitive glass electrode. A potential difference then exists between the glass electrode and the reference electrode and is measured on the meter. The meter's scale is usually calibrated for PCO_2 in a semilogarithmic fashion, conforming to an observation that pH is inversely proportional to the log of the PCO_2 concentration.

The semipermeable membranes are either tetrafluoroethylene resin (Teflon) or silicon rubber. They are permeable to physically dissolved CO_2 but impermeable to

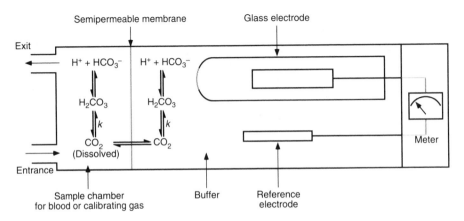

Figure 11-3. PCO_2 electrode.

anions and cations. The electrode's response time is directly proportional to the type and thickness of the semipermeable membrane, the strength of the bicarbonate buffer, the depth of buffer layer separating the glass electrode from the semipermeable membrane, and the temperature. Teflon measuring 0.1 mm thick will respond to 99% of equilibrium within 120 seconds, silicon rubber membranes are generally thinner (0.01 to 0.03 mm) and have slightly faster response times.

Sodium chloride is added to the bicarbonate buffer to increase conductivity and thus facilitate the measurement. If KCl were added, the conductivity would be increased, but great drift would occur as a result of the silver chloride surface of the reference electrode dissolving into the buffer.

A chemically inert spacer is placed in the buffer between the membrane and the glass electrode's surface to prevent direct contact between the two, which could produce irregular readings. Nylon, fine glass paper, or porous ("Joseph") paper may be used. Air bubbles at this point produce irregular equilibrium development and irregular readings.

The calibration response of the PCO_2 electrodes appears identical for gas and liquid of the same PCO_2, provided the gas has been saturated with water vapor prior to the introduction into the PCO_2 cell. The equilibration gases (low and high) should flow slowly so as to produce a slow, steady, regular stream of bubbles. Because the temperature of the electrode must remain constant, the flow of gases should be slow enough to allow thermal equilibrium as well as vapor saturation.

Total CO_2 can also be measured using a PCO_2 electrode by mixing a serum sample with a suitable acidic buffer before analysis. The addition of acid will force all of the ionic species toward the direction of CO_2, which will diffuse across the semipermeable membrane. The rate of the pH change in the PCO_2 electrode is directly proportional to the CO_2 concentration in the sample.

Sodium Electrode

Sodium electrodes are similar in design to pH electrodes. By increasing the aluminum content of the glass at the tip, the indicating electrode will show a preferential response to sodium over hydrogen ions. Actually, pH electrodes do respond to sodium ions to some extent, and at very high sodium concentrations, an appreciable pH error is induced. For measuring sodium potentiometrically, the only difference from a pH meter is the composition of the glass electrode's membrane to make it specific for Na^+.

Sodium ion-selective electrode (ISE) systems are of two kinds: direct-reading and indirect-reading. Direct-reading electrode systems use whole blood or serum as the sample, and the electrode is exposed to the undiluted sample. The electrode response is directly proportional to the sodium ion activity in the aqueous phase of the sample. In indirect-reading systems, a given volume of sample is first diluted before being introduced into the measuring system. The electrode response is then proportional to the quantity of sodium ions delivered to the diluent.

The differences in these systems can have important implications for the interpretation of the results in clinical situations. In situations of high lipid content, such as severe lipemia, or high protein content, such as multiple myeloma, the lipid or protein will displace some water from the aqueous phase of the sample. In direct-reading systems, this makes no difference, because the electrode responds only to the ion activity of the aqueous phase, regardless of how much lipid or protein there is. The indirect-reading electrode will see fewer sodium ions and will report a falsely lowered concentration. The biological activity of sodium ions is related only to the concentration in the aqueous phase. The condition of a falsely lowered sodium concentration in the face of elevated lipid or protein is termed *pseudohyponatremia.*[8]

Potassium Electrode

For a potassium electrode, the indicating electrode is a liquid-membrane design with a potassium ion exchanger incorporated into a solid plastic membrane. The ion exchanger is usually valinomycin, an ionophore with a particular affinity for monovalent cations with the ionic radius of potassium. These electrodes may be either of the direct-reading types and are usually included on instruments along with a sodium electrode.

Chloride Electrode

When chloride is measured by a potentiometric technique, the indicating electrode is a precipitate electrode. These anionic-sensitive electrodes exchange anions through a membrane containing cationic sites. One type uses polymerized silicon rubber diffusely permeated with small grains (5-10 μ) of a silver halide such as AgI. Each electrode exchanges best for the anion in common with its precipitate; that is, I^- for AgI-impregnated electrodes, Cl^- for AgCl, and Br^- for AgBr. The electrodes are relatively insensitive to redox interferences, surface poisonings, and to a cation effect.

Ionized Calcium Electrode

Ionized calcium (Ca^{++}) can also be measured by an ion-selective electrode.[9] The indicating electrode uses a liquid-membrane electrode. An ion exchanger is incorporated into the membrane itself. The membrane usually consists of polyvinylchloride. In the calcium electrode (Fig. 11-4), calcium organophosphorous is used as the ionic exchange compound. It is active between pH 5.5 and 11. Higher pH levels cause interference by calcium hydroxide formation. Reagents that complex calcium and prevent ionization, such as phosphate buffers, EDTA, and the like, cannot be used. A calomel reference electrode is used to develop a circuit. Standard solutions of ionic calcium (which have sodium, potassium, and magnesium ions added at levels approximately those of the unknown) establish the standard curve.

Lithium Electrode

Potentiometric measurement of lithium is widely available and has become the favored technique over flame photometry. The ion-selective membrane is a liquid membrane containing a lithium selective ionophore, dodecylmethyl-14-crown-4, to which trioctylphosphine oxide has been added to improve lithium selectivity over other alkalai metal ions.[10]

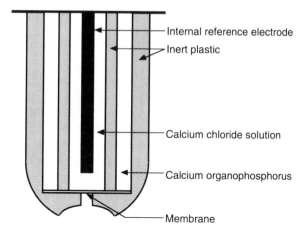

Figure 11-4. Calcium ion-specific electrode.

VOLTAMMETRY

Voltammetry is an electrochemical analysis that measures current flow through a cell that has a polarized electrode and an applied potential from an outside source. As a potential is applied to a cell, current is not immediately generated. The cell must first have enough potential applied to be completely polarized. The amount of voltage applied for complete polarization depends on the cell, the concentration, and the composition of the solution. At complete polarization, reduction begins at the cathode, oxidation at the anode, electrons flow, and current is generated. When the indicating electrode is small, the *amount of current generated* depends on the potential applied and on the *rate of diffusion* of the analyte through the solution. The rate of diffusion of the analyte is the rate at which the analyte can move through the supporting electrolyte to the surface of the small electrode. This *rate of diffusion* depends on the *concentration of the analyte in the solution.*

$$i = kC$$

(Eq. 11-19)

where

i = current in amperes
k = constant obtained from electrode area, diffusion coefficient of ion, and thickness of diffusion layer
C = concentration of the analyte

Standards of known concentrations are used for the linear standard curve, and the concentration of the unknown analyte is determined from this curve.

One particular type of voltammetry, *polarography,* was widely used for the determination of trace metals before the advent of atomic absorption. Polarography uses a dropping mercury electrode as the small indicating electrode. You might see the term polarography used more generally, i.e., for all voltammetry even when the electrode is not a dropping mercury electrode.

Clark Oxygen Sensor

The Clark oxygen sensor[11,12] is one of the voltammetric methods used in the clinical laboratory. Oxygen partial pressure (PO_2) is measured as the current flowing between a very small platinum electrode and a reference electrode to which a potential has been applied. Dissolved oxygen in the unknown solution diffuses across a semipermeable membrane into the buffer (phosphate with added KCl) in which the electrodes are immersed. The current results from oxygen reduction at the platinum electrode's surface after the electrode is polarized using a standard DC voltage, usually a mercury battery. This electrode differs from the ion-specific electrodes previously described. The specificity of the electrode results from the membrane's permeability to dissolved oxygen and the potential applied. The indicating electrode has been polarized, and current flow is measured. This is a voltammetric measurement, in contrast to the potentiometric measurements previously described. With ion-specific electrodes and potentiometry, the analyst avoids polarization of the electrode, keeps the current at zero, and measures the difference in potential.

The Clark-type electrode (Fig. 11-5) utilizes a silver-silver chloride reference electrode (anode) and a glass-coated small platinum electrode (cathode) connected to a small external voltage source, such as a 1.35-V mercury cell, to charge the circuit with a potential difference of 500 to 800 mV. This is called the *polarizing voltage*. The electrodes are connected by a buffer, generally saturated KCl with phosphate or sodium hydroxide added.

When the dissolved oxygen (PO_2) in the blood sample, or calibrating gas, permeates the oxygen-permeable membrane and is equilibrated with the buffer, the

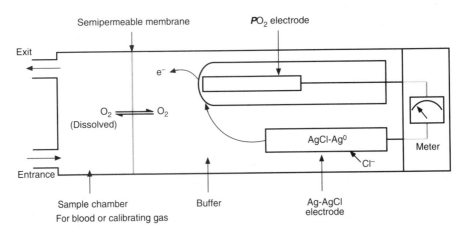

Figure 11-5. PO_2 electrode.

following reaction occurs. At the platinum electrode (cathode) electroreduction occurs.

$$O_2 + 4e^- \rightleftharpoons 2\,O^{-2} \tag{Eq. 11-20}$$

where the $2\,O^{-2}$ ions combine with $4\,H^+$ ions to form $2\,H_2O$. The electrons necessary for this electroreduction are produced at the reference electrode (anode) as follows:

$$4Ag + 4Cl^- \rightarrow 4\,AgCl\downarrow + 4e^- \tag{Eq. 11-21}$$

The reaction is both voltammetric and consumptive. The current through the system is directly proportional to the PO_2 in the blood sample outside the membrane.

Solutions of high viscosity and low oxygen solubility may have difficulty reaching equilibrium with the buffer or may have a residual oxygen gradient between the sides of the membrane leading to faulty readings.

Equilibrium depends on membrane permeability. Examples of membranes are Teflon, which is highly permeable but responds differently to a gas from a liquid or Mylar, made of polypropylene and polyethylene. Mylar is less permeable but shows little difference in response between liquid and gas. Dissolved O_2 diffuses more rapidly across polyethylene than polypropylene but the system is less stable with polyethylene membranes.[13]

A background current can develop within the system even when no oxygen is presented to the electrode. The background current is usually independent of the membrane but becomes important especially if Mylar is used. It is important to adjust the PO_2 meter to zero value with the calibration control when a solution of gas of known zero PO_2, such as CO_2 or N_2, is in equilibrium within the chamber. This cancels out the residual background current.

Oxygen utilization is proportional to the area of the platinum electrode (usually held to a diameter of $20\,\mu$) available for electroreduction and the applied voltage. The current flow is low (10^{-11} A/mmHg at $37°C$), when using a thin polyethylene or polypropylene membrane and a small platinum electrode.

Glucose Electrode

Electrochemical measurement of glucose is based on the glucose oxidase reaction.

$$\text{Glucose} + \text{oxygen} \xrightarrow[\text{oxidase}]{\text{glucose}} \text{gluconic acid} + H_2O_2 \tag{Eq. 11-22}$$

The rate of this reaction may be measured by two different electrochemical methods or by a colorimetric method. One electrochemical method measures the rate of oxygen consumption with a voltammetric electrode system. The electrode measures a current that is limited by the diffusion of O_2 across a gas-permeable Teflon membrane. The rate of O_2 consumption is directly proportional to the glucose in the test sample. Another electrochemical method uses an amperometric electrode (see the section on amperometric detection under Coulometry and Amperometry) to measure the amount of H_2O_2 produced during the enzymatic reaction. The enzyme glucose oxidase is immobilized on the electrode membrane. H_2O_2 is oxidized at the surface of the platinum anode.

$$H_2O_2 \rightarrow 2H^+ + O_2 + 2e^- \tag{Eq. 11-23}$$

The current generated by the flow of electrons is proportional to the glucose concentration of the sample.

COULOMETRY AND AMPEROMETRY

Coulometry is one form of titration. In this, like all titration methods, the basic principle is that equivalents of titrant react with equivalents of sample to produce equivalent amounts of product. In order to derive the number of equivalents of an unknown, one must know the number of equivalents of titrant produced. In coulometry the number of equivalent weights of titrant produced is calculated by application of the formula stated in Faraday's law. Faraday showed that 96,487 Q of electricity always liberated one equivalent weight of a compound or ions at each electrode. This law is stated in the formula

$$X = Q/F \tag{Eq. 11-24}$$

where

> X = number of equivalent weights of titrant generated at the electrode
> Q = number of coulombs of electricity used to generate the titrant
> F = Faraday's constant (96,487 Q/equivalent weight)

Q can also be derived by a second equation

$$Q = iT \tag{Eq. 11-25}$$

where

> i = electrical current (in amperes) that flows through the cell
> T = time (in seconds) during which the current flowed

By combining Equations 11-24 and 11-25, it is possible to relate the equivalents of titrant to current and time:

$$X = iT/F \tag{Eq. 11-26}$$

Using this formula, the number of equivalent weights of titrant generated is calculated. If the current is kept constant while titrating standard solutions and unknowns, and because F is a constant, a linear relationship exists between the equivalents of titrant and time.

Amperometry is used in clinical chemistry as an electrochemical titration. The potential between two electrodes is held constant, and current is measured as a function of analyte concentration. If time is held constant and F is a constant, then current generated is proportional to the number of equivalents oxidized or reduced per unit time.

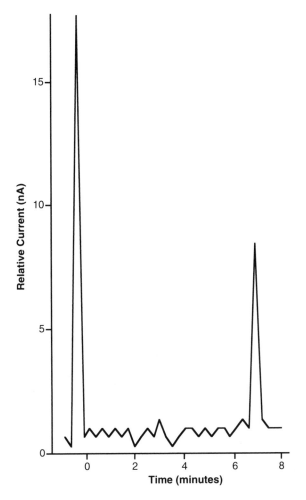

Figure 11-6.   Chromatograph from an electrochemical detector.

The sensitivity of amperometric measurement makes it practical as a detector for high-pressure liquid chromatography (see Chapter 14). If the analyte in the eluate stream can be either oxidized or reduced, an electrochemical detector can be the sensor that determines concentration. As analyte in mobile phase passes by the electrodes, current increases or decreases depending on the analyte concentration. This current is amplified and recorded to give a chromatogram (Fig. 11-6).

In another type of amperometric titration, measured current is plotted on the *y* axis with volume of titrant added on the *x* axis. Several values in excess of the equivalence point are also plotted. Extrapolation of the lines to where they intersect identifies the endpoint of the titrant, and concentration can be determined from this (Fig. 11-7).

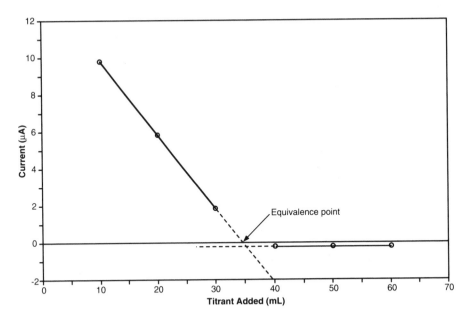

Figure 11-7.   Titration curve in an amperometric titration.

Chloride Detection by Coulometry and Amperometric End-Point Detection

Amperometry is also used to detect the endpoint of a coulometric reaction. Coulometric titration is one method of determining the concentration of chloride ion in biological samples. Chloride ions are titrated with silver ions generated at the silver anode. This is accomplished by applying a direct current (dc) voltage across a pair of silver electrodes.

$$Ag^0 \rightleftharpoons Ag^+ + e^- \tag{Eq. 11-27}$$

$$Ag^+ + Cl^- \rightleftharpoons AgCl\downarrow \tag{Eq. 11-28}$$

When the coulometric circuit is activated so that silver ions are generated, an automatic timer is also initiated. Chloride ions present in the sample combine with the silver ions to form insoluble silver chloride. As in any titration, an indicator of some type must be used to signal the end of titration. Amperometry is commonly used as the indicator system. The amperometric system consists of a second pair of silver electrodes that are placed in the solution and are charged with a small, constantly applied potential. When sufficient silver ions have been generated to react with all the chloride ions present, any additional generation of silver ion will result in a sharp increase in the silver ion concentration and, consequently, the conductivity of the titration solution. The current across the pair of amperometric electrodes increases because of the silver ions being reduced. A relay is activated by this increase in current, and this in turn will stop the automatic timer and the additional generation of silver ions.

The constant rate systems[14] produce silver ions at a steady rate because a constant current is applied across the generating electrodes. When this is accomplished, chloride ions are titrated at a set rate, and concentration is directly proportional to the time of reaction. When one analyzes standard and unknown solutions in a like manner, the time needed to reach the titration endpoint can be equated to the chloride concentration.

In the proportional systems, the electrode potential and, consequently, the silver ions generated are regulated by a proportional control circuit. When a sample containing chloride is added, a difference of potential is detected by the silver detector electrodes, and the coulometric generator is started. As the endpoint of the reaction is approached, the proportion control circuit reduces the generation rate of silver ions, lessening the chances of overtitration. In this system, the total current that flows in the anode-to-cathode circuit of the coulometric generator is integrated electronically and displayed digitally in a direct conversion to chloride concentration in the sample.

CONDUCTOMETRY

Conductometry is a measurement of the cumulative ability of all the ions in a solution to carry a charge. The conductivity of a solution depends on the applied voltage and the nature of ions present as well as their concentration. Conductivity equals the reciprocal of the resistance ($ohm^{-1}\ cm^{-1}$, or mho).

$$S = 1/R \qquad \text{(Eq. 11-29)}$$

where

S = conductivity
R = resistance

In conductance measurements, it is important that the electrodes do not become polarized. Thus, the voltage applied is usually alternating (AC). Multiple ions represent an additive increase in conductivity; therefore, the measurement is very nonspecific. However, it is easy to measure conductance because the meter is a modification of a Wheatstone bridge. The method's nonspecificity has been exploited as a way to monitor water purity. Very pure water has a specific conductance of 5×10^{-8} mho.

The Coulter principle for cell counting takes advantage of the fact that the conductivity of a blood cell is less than the conductivity of the electrolyte solution in which the cells are suspended (see Chapter 20 under *Principles* for further explanation).

ANODIC STRIPPING VOLTAMMETRY

Anodic stripping voltammetry (ASV) is an electrochemical technique that offers an alternative to atomic absorption spectrophotometry for the determination of heavy metals. Anodic stripping voltammetry is similar to the principle of the Clark PO_2 electrode, except that in ASV the applied potential is varied over time. Anodic stripping voltammetry is most often applied to the analysis of lead in biological samples.

The apparatus for performing an ASV experiment consists of a working electrode, a reference electrode, a sample chamber, a variable DC voltage source, a voltmeter, and a microammeter. In ASV, a large, negative (cathodic) potential is first applied to the working electrode. This causes the metal ions in solution to be reduced on to the surface of the working electrode. (The current is not recorded in this step.) The purpose of this step is to concentrate and purify the metals from the solution. The metals are concentrated from a volume of several milliliters down to the volume that covers the surface of the electrode, perhaps 10^{-3} to 10^{-4} cm^3. Then the potential is increased in the positive direction (anodic) in a linear fashion (sweep). The metals are reoxidized (stripped) in the order of their characteristic potentials (Fig. 11-8), and currents flow because of the oxidation reactions of the metals that were plated on to the surface of the electrode. The heights (or areas) of the current-versus-voltage peaks are directly proportional to the amounts of the metals originally present in the solution.

The working electrode consists of mercury plated on to a wax-impregnated carbon rod. A silver-silver chloride reference electrode is used. The sample, either blood or urine, is first treated with an exchange reagent that lyses the red blood cells and releases the metals from any complexes. The exchange reagent contains chromium (III) and is an acidic, oxidative medium. Even small amounts of EDTA can be used as an anticoagulant if sufficient equilibration time with the exchange reagent is allowed. Only 100 μL of blood sample is required.

An example of an ASV is the Environmental Science Associates' (ESA, Inc., Bedford, MA 01730) Model 3010A Trace Metal Analyzer, which can determine lead, arsenic, cadmium, copper, or zinc.[15] A typical reaction requires 90 sec per sample. Standards are run to determine both the oxidation potential and the standard curve relationship for each metal. The potentials for some metals can lie close to one another, so large amounts of copper, for example, in a sample can interfere with the

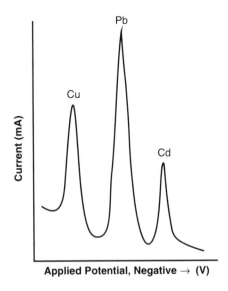

Figure 11-8.   Recorder tracing for anodic stripping analysis of blood.

determination of lead if the peaks are not carefully identified. The starting and stopping points and the rate of the voltage sweep are selected, and the current peaks are recorded on a strip chart recorder. Because the voltage sweep rate is known, the chart speed can be related to voltage. The Model 3010A automatically integrates the current peak and expresses the result in terms of the lead (or other metal) concentration directly.

Semiautomated/Automated Instruments

Multipurpose instruments have been developed that will provide greater instrument stability, faster throughput, and additional calculated data important to the physician. A variety of them exist, varying in sophistication and cost. Instruments are available that measure only pH and blood gases, and others offer a combination of pH, blood gases, various electrolytes, and glucose measurements. Lithium analyzers will also routinely measure sodium and potassium. These instruments have part or all of the following configurational characteristics.

Sample

Whole-blood or serum samples may be used depending on the analytes being measured. Sample sizes vary depending on the instrument and the number of analytes being measured. Sample volumes may range from 70 to 500 μL. In most instruments, the sample chamber (Fig. 11-9) is located to permit visual inspection and

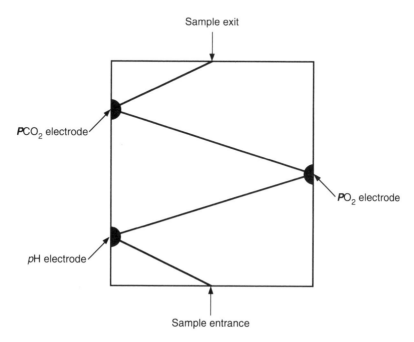

Figure 11-9.   Sample chamber for a pH, blood gas instrument.

identification of bubbles, clots, dirt, and so forth, that could invalidate the results. Some instruments have a sample error detector, an electronic sensor in the postelectrode sample line, to ensure that the electrode chamber is completely filled.

Measurement

These instruments use standard electrode systems (i.e., pH-sensitive glass, Clark-type voltammetric PO_2, Severinghouse PCO_2, and potentiometric measurement of Na, K, Cl, iCa) with configurational changes to facilitate automatic calibration, sample introduction, and flush. The pH electrode is connected to the calomel reference electrode by a flowing open KCl liquid junction. Some instruments measure total hemoglobin, using a spectrophotometric system following lysis of the erythrocytes.

Additional Data Input

Instrumental requirements are quite varied. The whole-blood hemoglobin level can be entered electronically if it is not measured by the system. The patient's current body temperature may be entered if "corrected" values are to be automatically determined. The barometric pressure is entered, if not automatically measured, so that the current values of the calibrating gases may be established.

Derived Data

A wide variety of data helpful to the physician are often provided automatically, including standard bicarbonate, bicarbonate content, total CO_2 content, base excess, oxygen saturation, as well as pH, PCO_2, and PO_2 corrected from $37°C$ to the patient's body temperature. The derivations are computed using programs that have been developed from equations containing constants that are empirically established. One should be familiar with the instrument's instruction manual to know the nature of the equations and constants used.

Calibration

Calibration is performed manually or on a predetermined periodic cycle. Humidified gases or buffers equilibrated with CO_2, oxygen, and nitrogen are introduced into the chamber, usually with a peristaltic pump; pH calibration is performed with a pair of standard buffers. These usually have values of 7.384 for the zero calibration and 6.840 for the slope calibration. Electrolytes and other analytes are calibrated with a pair of standards. The calibration standards (and samples as well) are usually automatically preheated to $37°C$ prior to introduction into the electrode chamber.

Microprocessor-controlled blood gas instruments perform the calibration sequence automatically at fixed intervals. The instruments are programmed for the composition (in volume percentage) of the calibration gases. Most instruments can also measure barometric pressure and will calculate the partial pressures of oxygen and CO_2. The results for patient samples are then calculated based on the responses of the electrodes, and factors are derived from the calibration sequence. The instruments are capable of performing one-point and two-point calibrations. Generally, the one-point calibration is performed twice as frequently as the two-point. Instrument stability is required before patient samples are introduced. Most microprocessor-controlled instruments have diagnostics packages that monitor for faults such as electrode drift, out-of-range sensitivity, and unstable readings.

Flushing

The electrodes are automatically flushed following each use as well as periodically when not in use, using humidified "low" calibrating gas, buffer, or wash solutions such as polyethylene glycoloctylphenyl ether. This process automatically cleans the sample lines and keeps the electrodes humidified and equilibrated to some degree as well. Most instruments flush the sample out in the reverse direction from which it was introduced. This prevents the pump tubing from being contaminated with sample.

Maintenance

Daily maintenance involves injecting a cleaning solution through the system and checking the levels of the solution reservoirs and gas tanks. Electrode membranes and electrolyte solutions must be replaced periodically. Refer to specific instrument manuals for recommendations on electrode maintenance.

Transcutaneous Blood Gas Measurement

Noninvasive techniques to estimate the partial pressure of arterial blood gas are becoming more popular because they seem to offer the opportunity for continuous monitoring without expenditures of large volumes of whole blood. This technique has been applied most frequently to neonates, especially those receiving oxygen therapy. The stability and accuracy of transcutaneous blood gas instruments is satisfactory for the purposes suggested. The results should be confirmed by standard whole-blood measurements before definitive therapeutic decisions are made.

Skin is resistant to the diffusion of gas out of the vascular walls. Infants' skin is much less resistant than adults'. If the skin is heated externally to 43°C, skin capillary blood temperature is raised to 41°C, and transcutaneous PO_2 closely approximates the arterial PO_2. Transcutaneous PCO_2 values tend to be higher than arterial PCO_2 values.

The transcutaneous electrode system is held closely to the depilated skin surface by an airtight bond. A polypropylene membrane separates the heated skin surface from the electrode assembly, which consists of a polarized platinum monocathode surrounded by a silver ring-type anode held at a constant temperature, usually 43°C. Oxygen in the blood can diffuse from the capillary through the skin and electrode membrane and actuate the Clark-type electrode to produce the reading.

Maintenance and Quality Assurance

Standard systems for quality control in the clinical chemistry laboratory are generally applicable to electrochemical analysis. The periodicity of the assay of the control materials should be varied to meet the individual instrumental needs, depending on the instrument's stability, volume of use, time of day, number of persons performing the tests, and so on. Some of the most important factors affecting quality are preanalytical variables. Obviously, proper sample handling is essential for reliable results. Handling without contact with air is desired, because samples exposed to the atmosphere will lose CO_2 and the pH will rise. Some ionized calcium analyzers can add CO_2 to the sample before analysis. Others correct the ionized calcium concentration to pH 7.4. It should be remembered that this value will not be true in patients who have an acid-base disturbance. Clearly, specimens should not be collected in ethylene-diaminetetraacetate (EDTA) or oxalate anticoagulants, because these will bind calcium. Heparin will also bind calcium if there is an excess amount in the blood collection tube. It is absolutely imperative to completely fill all evacuated, heparized specimen containers with blood if ionized calcium is to be determined on that sample. If the containers are completely full, there is no excess heparin to bind the ionized calcium and falsely decrease the results. The reader is referred to the National Committee for Clinical Laboratory Standards guidelines[16] for further information.

Calibration and control materials for blood gas and electrolyte measurement by ion-specific electrodes have been a controversial topic for many years.[17] Most manufacturers recommend their own controls and calibrators for their instrument. Usually, trilevel controls are used, with parameters designed to simulate acidemic, normal, and alkalemic conditions. These controls consist of aqueous buffers or perfluorocarbon synthetic oxygen carriers equilibrated with gas to produce the desired pH, $P$$CO_2$, and $P$$O_2$ values. These materials should be opened and used immediately because of the small but significant rise in pH and $P$$O_2$ that occurs rather rapidly after exposure to room air. Microprocessor-controlled instruments have quality control routines that store the data, calculate means and data limits, identify outliers, and provide Levy-Jennings charts.

In potentiometric measurements, it is essential to maintain constant temperature, for the Nernst equation depends on temperature. The ion-selective electrodes must be sloped at regular intervals. In automated pH and blood gas analyzers, the slope is determined automatically, usually every 2 hours. Other functional characteristics, such as drift, noise, response time, and linearity, should also be periodically determined. Blood gas calibrations and determination of unknowns must be corrected for changes in barometric pressure. The reader is referred to the specific instrument manuals for routine quality control of specific instruments.

Summary

The six electrochemical methods of analysis described in this chapter are potentiometry, voltammetry, coulometry, amperometry, conductometry, and anodic stripping voltammetry. Varied clinical applications of these methods have employed either a single method or a mixture of methods. See Table 11-1 for a summary of electrochemical methods that have clinical applications.

Potentiometry is the measurement of the electrical difference between two electrodes in an electrochemical cell. With proper selection of electrodes, the potential difference is proportional to the concentration of the analyte of interest.

Table 11-1
Electrochemical Methods of Detection

Method	Equation	Potential E	Current I	Indicating Electrode	Clinical Applications
Potentiometry	$E = E^0 + \dfrac{RT}{n\text{F}} \ln a$	measure difference	zero	ion-selective	pH, Na^+, K^+, Cl^-, CO_2, Ca^{++}, Li^-, PCO_2 PO_2, glucose
Voltammetry	$i = kC$	applied from outside source	measure	small, polarized	
Coulometry	$X = Q/\text{F}$, where $Q = iT$	small, constant	constant	silver	Cl^-
Amperometry	$X = Q/\text{F}$, where $Q = iT$	constant	measure	small, polarized	Detector for HPLC
Conductometry	$S = 1/R$	alternating	measure	nonpolarized	water purity, cell counting
Anodic-stripping voltammetry		applied from outside source	measure	thin-film of mercury	metals, especially Pb

The electrolytes, *p*H, and therapeutic drug, Li, can all be determined by this method with ion-selective electrodes. Measurement of the partial pressure of CO_2 is also a potentiometric application.

Voltammetry is the dual measurement of the current flowing through an electrochemical cell and the electrical potential between two electrodes when the potential is gradually increased at a constant rate. The two electrodes consist of a polarizable indicator electrode and a nonpolarizable reference electrode. The partial pressure of oxygen in blood and the concentration of glucose by the glucose oxidase method can be measured by voltammetry.

Coulometry is the measurement of charge passing between two electrodes in an electrochemical cell. The amount of electricity generated is proportional to the amount of substance produced or consumed by the redox process at the electrodes. This method is commonly used in conjunction with amperometry as in the measurement of chloride.

Amperometry is the measurement of a current flowing through an electrochemical cell when a constant potential is applied to the electrodes. This current is directly proportional to the concentration of the analyte being measured. Electrochemical detectors for HPLC are based on this procedure.

Conductometry is the measurement of the current flow between two nonpolarized electrodes between which a known electrical potential is established. Conductivity of an aqueous solution depends on the concentration of the electrolytes in the solution. Although nonspecific, a measure of conductance is a sensitive method, and applications include determination of water purity and the Coulter principle of counting blood cells.

Anodic stripping voltammetry is essentially the reverse of voltammetry. After the analyte has been deposited on to the surface of the indication electrode, the potential is reversed, and the metal is "stripped" from the electrode. Concentration of the metal is determined by calculating peak height or area when current is plotted versus voltage.

Questions and Problems

1. The *p*H of a solution was determined to be 5.5. What is the hydrogen ion concentration?
2. Draw a diagram of the instrumentation needed to determine Na^+ concentration by a specific ion electrode.
3. The following data were obtained in the measurement of serum chloride by a coulometric technique. The 100 mEq/L standard was titrated in 121.3 seconds. The serum sample was titrated in 126.2 seconds. What is the concentration of chloride ion in the serum sample?
4. Describe the electrode for measuring PO_2.
5. Compare and contrast potentiometry and voltammetry.
6. How is glucose determined by an electrochemical method?
7. A 15-year-old boy in the pediatric ICU had a cholesterol of 844 mg/dL and triglycerides of 5520 mg/dL. Sodium results that day, determined by a direct-

reading potentiometric method, were 126 and 132 mmol/L. A pediatrics resident called the lab to ask if the low sodium results were due to plasma displacement by lipids (pseudohyponatremia). How would you answer this question?

8. A nurse in the neonatal ICU called because the laboratory has just requested another sample for the determination of ionized calcium on a neonate. The nurse questions the necessity of drawing another tube just because the last specimen container was not completely filled. What should you reply?

References

1. Orion Research. Handbook of electrode technology. Cambridge, MA: Orion Research, 1982.
2. Willard HH, Merritt LL Jr, Dean JA, Settle FA Jr. Instrumental methods of analysis, 7th ed. Belmont, CA: Wadsworth Publishing, 1988:748.
3. Siggard-Andersen O. Factors affecting the liquid-junction potential in electrometric blood pH measurement. Scand J Clin Lab Invest 1961, 13:205.
4. Nipper HC. Electrochemistry introduction. In: Nipper HC, ed., Selected papers on clinical chemistry instrumentation. Washington, DC: AACC Press, 1985:99-100.
5. Skoog DA, Leary JJ. Principles of instrumental analysis, 4th ed. Fort Worth: Saunders College Publishing, 1992:496.
6. Severinghaus JW. Electrodes for blood and gas PCO_2, PO_2 and blood pH. Acta Anaesthesiol Scand (Suppl) 1962, 11:207-20.
7. Severinghaus JW, Bradley AF. Electrodes for blood PO_2 and PCO_2 determination. J Appl Physiol 1958, 13:515-20.
8. Ladenson JH, Apple FS, Koch DD. Misleading hyponatremia due to hyperlipidemia: A method-dependent error. Ann Intern Med 1981, 95:707-08.
9. Bowers GN, Brassard C, Sena SF. Measurement of ionized calcium in serum with ion-selective electrodes: A mature technology that can meet the daily service needs. Clin Chem 1986, 32:1437-47.
10. Osorodudu AL, Burnett RW, McComb RB, Bowers, GN Jr. Evaluation of three first-generation ion-selective electrode analyzers for lithium: Systematic errors, frequency of random interferences, and recommendations based on comparison with flame atomic emission spectrometry. Clin Chem 1990, 36:104-10.
11. Clark LC. Monitor and control of blood and tissue oxygen tensions. Trans Am Soc Artif Intern Organs 1956, 2:41-48.
12. Clark LC, Lyons C. Electrode systems for continuous monitoring in cardiovascular surgery. Ann NY Acad Sci 1962, 102:29.
13. Sykes MK, Vickers MD, Hull DJ. Principles of measurement and monitoring in anaesthesia and intensive care, 3rd ed. Oxford: Blackwell Scientific Publications, 1991:258.
14. Cotlove E, Trantham HV, Bowman RL. An instrument and method for automatic, rapid, accurate, and sensitive titration of chloride in biological samples. J Lab Clin Med 1958, 51:461-72.
15. ESA, Inc. The Model 3010A trace metals analyzer: Methods manual. Bedford, MA: ESA, Inc. 1988.
16. National Committee for Clinical Laboratory Standards. Blood gas pre-analytical considerations: Specimen collection, calibration, and controls. Document C27A. Villanova, PA: NCCLS, 1993.
17. Burritt M. Current analytical approaches to measuring blood analytes. Clin Chem 1990, 36:1562-66.

Suggested Readings

Bender GT. Principles of chemical instrumentation. Philadelphia: WB Saunders, 1987:139-72.
Skoog DA, Leary JJ. Principles of instrumental analysis, 4th ed. Fort Worth: Saunders College Publishing, 1992:489-567.
Willard HH, Merritt LL Jr, Dean JA, Settle FA Jr. Instrumental methods of analysis, 7th ed. Belmont, CA: Wadsworth Publishing, 1988:656-760.

12

ELECTROPHORESIS

Judy M. Anderson
Gregory A. Tetrault

Objectives

After completing this chapter, the reader will be able to:

1. Explain the principle of electrophoresis.
2. Understand the factors affecting electrophoretic mobility.
3. Calculate the heat generated during electrophoresis.
4. Describe the process of electroendosmosis.
5. Explain the significance of isoelectric points to electrophoresis.
6. List common clinical uses for electrophoresis.
7. Describe the component parts of an electrophoresis system.
8. Compare automated plate electrophoresis to capillary electrophoresis.
9. Describe three variants of electrophoresis: isoelectric focusing, rocket immuno-electrophoresis, and polyacrylamide gel electrophoresis.
10. List common problems in electrophoresis and their causes.

Definitions

Amperes (amp): A measure of current equal to a flow of one coulomb per second.

Amphoteric: Able to be positively or negatively charged, depending on *p*H and other conditions.

Anode: The positively charged electrode in an electrophoretic system.

Cathode: The negatively charged electrode in an electrophoretic system.

Densitometer: Instrument commonly used to measure optical density of a solid substance such as an electrophoresis plate.

Electroendosmosis: The movement of weakly or neutrally charged particles due to the flow of ions (and buffer) to one of the electrodes in an electrophoretic system.

Electrophoretic mobility: The average velocity of a particle in an electrophoretic system at a given voltage.

Electrophoresis: The movement of charged particles due to an external electric field.

Isoelectric point: The pH at which a substance has a net charge of zero.

Sucking flow: The process in which solvent evaporation from an electrophoresis plate results in flow of buffer toward the center of the plate.

Volt (V):   Measure of electrostatic potential equal to one joule (J) per coulomb (Q).

Introduction

Tiselius revolutionized the study of serum proteins by his development of protein electrophoresis in 1937. Electrophoresis is the movement of charged particles by an electric current. Tiselius discovered that by placing positive and negative electrodes in a solution, proteins could be separated into groups based on their charges. This methodology has been refined and used in clinical and research laboratories since the late 1930s for the separation of proteins and other macromolecules such as DNA and RNA. Many advances in electrophoresis have taken place since the original method of Tiselius was introduced.

The earliest apparatus for electrophoresis used electrodes placed in an aqueous buffer containing dissolved proteins.[1] This crude methodology allowed only the slowest and fastest migrating proteins to be separated in pure form. Expensive instrumentation and a large amount of sample were needed. Zone electrophoresis, which uses a stable support medium, allows greater resolution of proteins or other large molecules. Paper was the original support medium. Inexpensive equipment sufficed for paper electrophoresis, which produced a more complete separation of proteins or other large molecules. The major disadvantage of paper as a support medium is protein adherence to cellulose.

Cellulose acetate replaced paper as a support medium in the 1950s. It provides better separation because proteins adhere less readily when hydroxy groups are converted to acetate groups. Another advantage is that cellulose acetate, when treated with organic solvents, dries to a clear film for easy visualization and densitometric quantitation. More recently, agarose gels were found to give better resolution than cellulose support media. Today, most clinical laboratories perform electrophoreses on a plastic support coated with a thin layer (1 mm or less) of agarose gel. Agarose gel electrophoresis plates may be purchased or prepared in the laboratory.

Equipment needed for electrophoresis includes a power source, a positive electrode (anode), a negative electrode (cathode), and an electrophoretic cell to contain buffer and support (plate). Electrophoresis procedures also require a means of visualizing, and sometimes quantitating, separated molecules.

Principles[1-4]

ELECTROPHORETIC MOBILITY

An electrophoretic system is illustrated in Figure 12-1. The power source provides constant voltage or constant current. The anode is the positive electrode that

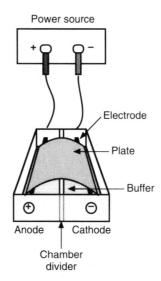

Figure 12-1.   Some components of an electrophoresis system. The power supply is connected to a cathode and an anode that lie horizontally in separate buffer chambers. The support medium (plate) bridges the buffer chambers and completes the electrical circuit.

attracts negatively charged anions. The cathode is the negative electrode that attracts positively charged cations. The plate (paper, cellulose acetate, or agarose gel-coated plastic) provides the connection between the two electrodes that are submerged in an aqueous buffer. The electrophoretic mobility rate of a charged macromolecule such as a protein depends on buffer composition, pH, and ionic strength; choice of support medium; temperature; and voltage. Under controlled conditions, measurement of electrophoretic mobility rate can help to identify a protein. This mobility rate is represented mathematically by Equation 12-1.

$$\mu = d/Et \qquad \text{(Eq. 12-1)}$$

where

μ = electrophoretic mobility (cm/V-sec)
d = distance traveled from the origin (cm)
E = electrical field strength (V/cm)
t = time of electrophoresis (sec)

The mobility or rate of migration of an ion can also be expressed by Equation 12-2.

$$\mu = Q/f \qquad \text{(Eq. 12-2)}$$

where

Q = net charge of ion (coulombs)
f = frictional coefficient of the ion in a specific electrophoresis system (J-sec/cm)

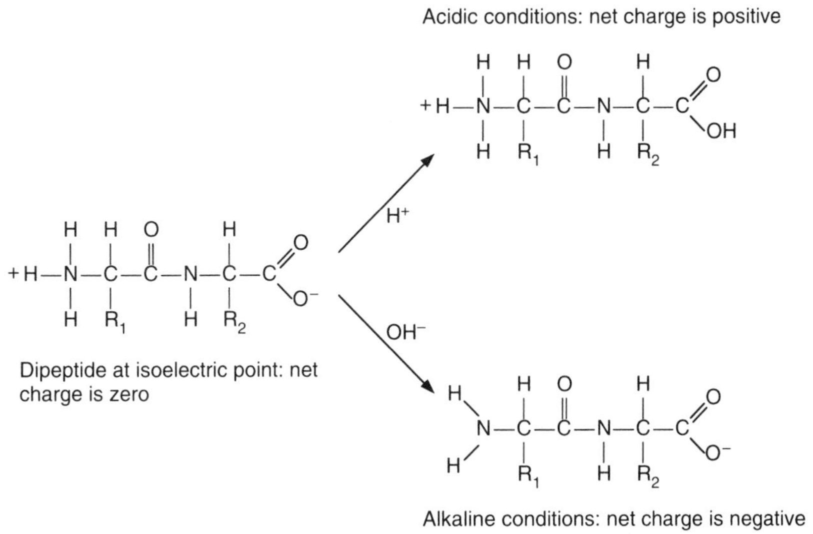

Acidic conditions: net charge is positive

Dipeptide at isoelectric point: net charge is zero

Alkaline conditions: net charge is negative

Figure 12-2. Net charges of a dipeptide at different *p*Hs. All amino acids, as well as all peptides and proteins, are amphoteric compounds.

The original charge of the particle depends on the composition of the molecule itself. The net charge, which gives the molecule its mobility, results from the effects of the buffer system on the molecule. Proteins are amphoteric, which means they will be positively charged in an acidic buffer and negatively charged in an alkaline buffer (Fig. 12-2).

The frictional coefficient of a molecule is determined by its size, shape, composition, and by the viscosity of the buffer and the support medium. A large, asymmetrical particle will travel slower than a small globular one. Molecular size is a major factor in paper electrophoresis. The combination of size and net charge is the basis of separation in polyacrylamide gel electrophoresis (see that subsection under Variations in Electrophoresis). The thin agarose gels used in clinical laboratories today typically have large pore sizes that allow proteins to migrate easily. This minimizes the effects of molecular size and shape. However, very large particles, such as immune complexes and chylomicrons, will not pass through the pores.

The frictional coefficient is also affected by the resistance of the system. The resistance is directly proportional to electrophoretic voltage and indirectly proportional to the current (Eq. 12-3).

$$R = V/i \qquad \text{(Eq. 12-3)}$$

where

R = resistance (Ω)
V = voltage (V)
i = current (A)

The resistance in an electrophoretic system is related to the concentrations of all charge-carrying species: buffer ions and charged macromolecules. Resistance can be decreased by increasing the ionic strength of the buffer, using a large sample size or altering *p*H to increase the net charges of the macromolecules. When resistance is decreased, current increases (assuming voltage is held constant). Increased current produces increased electrical heat. The amount of heat generated is calculated using Equation 12-4.

$$H = (E)(i)(t) \qquad\qquad\qquad \text{(Eq. 12-4)}$$

where

H = heat (J)
E = electromotive force (V)
i = current (A)
t = time (sec)

Increased voltage, current, or time of electrophoresis will produce more heat. Uncompensated heat generation reduces the frictional coefficient and increases migration rates. However, the rise in temperature creates convective disturbances that adversely affect electrophoretic separations. Higher temperatures also produce increased sucking flow.[5] Sucking flow is caused by evaporation of solvent from the support medium, causing a capillary flow of buffer from the buffer chambers to the center of the plate. This flow of solvent, charged ions, and macromolecules produces

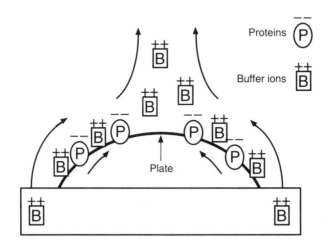

Figure 12-3.   Sucking flow in electrophoresis. Evaporation of solvent results in migration of buffer from the buffer chambers to the middle of the plate. This sucking flow affects the migration of macromolecules. Evaporation, when not too intensive, occurs uniformly over the surface of the plate. If evaporation is intense, the center of the plate becomes driest, and a moisture gradient occurs. This results in greater migration of water molecules toward the center of the plate.

a current that disrupts the orderly migration of macromolecules (Fig. 12-3). If evaporation is intense, the plate starts to dry in the middle, and a moisture gradient occurs. This results in the flow of water molecules toward the center and flow of buffer ions away from the center of the plate. Finally, if temperatures rise above 40°C, proteins begin to denature.

ISOELECTRIC POINTS AND ELECTROENDOSMOSIS

Barbital and Tris buffers are commonly used for the electrophoretic separation of proteins at *p*H 8.6. Most proteins have isoelectric points between 4 and 7.5 and, therefore, have a negative net charge. These proteins will all migrate toward the anode. Given two proteins of equal size and similar shape, the one with the lower isoelectric point will have a higher net charge in an alkaline buffer and will migrate more rapidly toward the (positively charged) anode. Proteins with isoelectric points greater than 6 will have a small net charge. These proteins are most susceptible to the effects of *electroendosmosis* (Fig. 12-4). In electroendosmosis, the flow of positively charged buffer ions toward the cathode creates a positive ion cloud. The moving ion buffer cloud drags weakly charged and neutral macromolecules toward the cathode. Although electroendosmosis interferes with the orderly separation of macromolecules strictly by net charge, it can actually assist in their separation. In serum, urine, and body fluid samples, gamma globulins are most affected by electroendosmosis.

After electrophoretic separation, the plates are dried and stained with an appropriate dye (if necessary). Coupled enzyme reactions may be used before staining to identify a specific group of enzymes. The type of dye and chemical reactions used determine which components will be visualized. Table 12-1 lists a variety of stains and their normal wavelengths for densitometer readings.[3] If resolution is high enough, proteins or macromolecules appear as discrete bands.

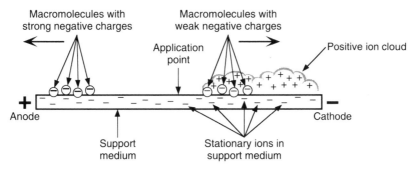

Figure 12-4. Electroendosmosis. In this setup, many of the macromolecules have a negative charge and are pulled toward the anode. A countermigration by positively charged buffer ions and their solvent drags neutral or weakly charged macromolecules toward the cathode. In this example, electroendosmosis would also accelerate the migration of positively charged macromolecules toward the cathode.

Table 12-1
Analyte Specificities and Optimum Wavelengths for Common Stains

Analyte	Stain	Wavelength (nm)
Proteins	Amido Black	640
	Coomassie Brilliant Blue	595
	Ponceau S	520
Enzymes	Nitrotetrazolium Blue	570
Lipids/lipoproteins	Oil Red O	520
	Sudan Black B	600

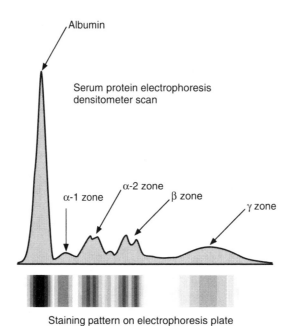

Figure 12-5. Staining pattern and densitometer scan of serum protein electrophoresis. Albumin is at the far left, and gamma globulins are at the far right. The application point is near the center of the plate.

CLINICAL USES OF ELECTROPHORESIS[1-4,6,7]

Electrophoresis can separate any class of macromolecule, but in clinical laboratories it is used almost exclusively to separate proteins. The most common use is *serum protein electrophoresis.* All methods of electrophoresis can separate serum proteins into five major bands: albumin, α-1, α-2, β, and γ (Fig. 12-5). High-resolution techniques can resolve individual proteins within the latter four bands. After concentration procedures, similar methods can be used to separate proteins in urine, cerebro-spinal fluid, and other body fluids.

Hemoglobin electrophoresis is another common technique. A hemolysate of red blood cells is applied to a plate. Hemoglobins are readily separated. No staining is required, although protein stains allow better visualization of faint bands. Traditionally, hemoglobin separations are performed under both mildly acidic and mildly alkaline conditions. This allows identification of hemoglobin variants that may comigrate under one set of conditions.

Isoenzymes of creatine kinase (CK), lactate dehydrogenase (LD), alkaline phosphatase (ALP), and other enzymes can be separated and quantitated electrophoretically. After separation, substrates are added to the plates. The enzymes convert substrate to a colored product (or one that can be stained).

Immunofixation electrophoresis (IFE) allows accurate identification of separated proteins. The electrophoresed agarose gel plate is coated with an antiserum that binds a specific protein antigen. An antibody-antigen complex precipitates. Nonprecipitated proteins and antibodies are washed away before staining. This method is often used to identify clonal bands in the gamma zone seen in multiple myeloma, Waldenstrom's macroglobulinemia, and monoclonal gammopathy of undetermined significance.[8]

Component Parts of Electrophoretic Systems

All electrophoretic systems require a support medium, a power supply, positive and negative electrodes, a chamber for the buffer and support medium, a dryer, and a means of identifying separated macromolecules. A densitometer is usually employed if quantitation of individual bands is required.

SUPPORT MEDIA

Typical support media include cellulose acetate and agarose gel-coated plastic plates. Paper or starch gel plates are rarely used. Most plates are held in a horizontal or an arched position (see Fig. 12-1). A holding device secures the plate so that each end stays in contact with buffer overlying the anode and cathode.

POWER SUPPLY

Power supplies for electrophoresis are usually designed to provide a constant voltage across the plate. Some power supplies also have the option of providing constant current or constant power. Electrophoreses are typically performed between 50 and 200 V. The voltage is selected by adjusting a rheostat or activating a switch selector. Higher voltages improve resolution and decrease the time needed for separation. As discussed, voltage can't be increased too much, though, or excessive heating will occur. Some electrophoresis systems include a cooling device for the plate. Such systems can be run at much higher voltages. Power supplies for these systems can deliver up to 2000 V.

ELECTRODES AND CHAMBER(S)

These components are often combined into a single unit. The anode and cathode lie within a divided buffer chamber (or two separate chambers). The electrodes are made of graphite or metal. The divided buffer chamber prevents completion of the electrical circuit until each end of the plate is immersed in buffer. The chambers should hold a sufficient volume of buffer to cover the electrodes and to act as a heat reservoir. Most systems provide covers for the buffer chambers and for the support medium to minimize evaporation.

DRYER

Most electrophoresis methods require that the plate be dried before visualization and quantitation. Plates can be allowed to dry under ambient conditions, but this process is slow. Two types of dryers are available: presses and ovens. *Press dryers* can be used alone or in conjunction with ovens. Press dryers work by placing the plate between layers of absorbent paper. Heavy weights are applied to squeeze moisture out of the plate. The water-saturated absorbent papers can be replaced, and the process can be repeated. Press dryers will not remove all moisture from the plate. Small *ovens* are used for complete drying. Oven temperatures are typically kept between 60 and 90°C. This allows rapid evaporation of water without disruption of the support medium. Humidity is kept low by venting the heated air. Drying is fastest if the plate is press-dried before it is oven-dried.

VISUALIZATION

A few macromolecules, such as hemoglobin, are intensely colored and require no special methods for visualization of bands on the dried plate. Most other proteins and macromolecules are colorless and require staining. Staining can be done on the native plate (e.g., lipid or protein stains) or can be deferred until chemical or enzymatic reactions produce a stainable compound. Some stains are fluorescent and are visualized under ultraviolet light in a darkened room. Visual inspection is used to identify and crudely quantify bands on the plate. Accurate quantitation requires densitometric measurements.

DENSITOMETER

A *densitometer* is a special type of spectrophotometer used to measure light transmittance through a solid sample such as an electrophoresis plate. The plate is positioned over or in front of the exit slit of the monochromator. Most densitometers can scan a plate. This is usually accomplished by moving the plate across the exit slit. Transmitted light is measured by the detector. Some densitometers can also measure fluorescence. A second monochromator is positioned between the plate and the detector to exclude wavelengths other than those of the fluorescent light.

Figure 12-5 shows an electrophoregram or densitometer tracing of a stained serum protein electrophoresis gel. The scanning densitometer is connected to a recording device. The optical densities $(2 - \log \%T)$ across the plate are plotted.

Each peak represents an individual band on the plate. The resolution depends not only on the resolution of the electrophoresis but also on the width of the exit slit. Quantitation is performed by measuring the areas of each of the bands and under the entire scan. In this example, the total serum protein has been determined by another method, and the concentrations of the individual bands are calculated by multiplying their relative areas by the total protein concentration. Most densitometers automatically determine the areas for each band. Three manual methods for determining areas are: cutting and weighing, one-half of peak height times width at half-height, and trapezoidal area estimation.[9]

Automated Electrophoresis

Automated electrophoresis systems are being used in clinical laboratories that perform large numbers of electrophoreses. Two types of automated systems are available. One type uses a modified agarose gel plate but otherwise simply automates standard electrophoresis. The other type is known as capillary electrophoresis and resembles a hybrid of electrophoresis and high-performance liquid chromatography (HPLC).

AUTOMATED PLATE ELECTROPHORESIS

No *plate electrophoresis* systems are fully automated. A number of manual steps are still required. The most automated electrophoresis system is Helena's REP (Rapid ElectroPhoresis) (Helena Laboratories, Beaumont, TX 77704). The REP consists of a sample rack containing disposable specimen cups; an automated pipettor for samples and reagents; a modified agarose gel plate; a refrigerated plate-processing compartment; a plate incubation, staining, and drying compartment; a high-voltage power supply; a densitometer; and a microcomputer with printer.

Samples are placed in two parallel rows of cups. Thirty samples can be applied to one plate. The plate is agarose gel-coated plastic with thick ridges of low-density gel at each end of the plate. These thick areas contain buffer—no liquid buffer chambers are required. Samples are automatically applied to the plate by the pipettor. Sample application takes only one minute. The plate lies in a special compartment with a cooling block. A film of water between the plate and the cooling block improves thermal conductivity. During electrophoresis the temperature of the cooling block drops below 0°C, and the plate is frozen to the block. This is necessary because electrophoreses are performed at very high voltages (1000–2000 V). Without adequate cooling, heat production would denature proteins and "melt" the gel. Electrophoresis times are reduced to about 2 minutes. The combination of high voltage, low temperature, and short electrophoresis time produces good resolution.

Substrate addition (if needed) is performed by the automated pipettor immediately after electrophoresis. The plate is moved to the gel processor for incubation (about 5 minutes). Staining is performed (if necessary), and the plate is dried. After drying, the plate must be removed manually and placed in the densitometer. The densitometer can measure light transmittance or sample fluorescence. Scans are performed automatically, and results are sent to the microcomputer. The analysis software automatically integrates peaks, reports percentages and concentrations for each band, and even interprets the results. Reports can be printed or downloaded to a laboratory information system. Total time for sample analysis on the REP is about 15 to 30 minutes.

CAPILLARY ELECTROPHORESIS

Capillary electrophoresis occurs within a thin capillary tube with each end connected to a buffer reservoir containing either the cathode or the anode. As in HPLC, one sample at a time is placed in the capillary. A capillary electrophoresis system consists of a power supply, a capillary tube, a sample injector, buffer reservoirs with electrodes, an on-line detector, and a readout device (Fig. 12-6).[10]

Capillary electrophoresis requires extremely high voltages (20,000 to 60,000 V). This is especially true with long tubes (>50 cm). Tremendous heat can be generated by these voltages, so many systems include a cooling fan, flowing liquid bath, or solid-state cooling device. The power supplies have safety devices that prevent handling the high-voltage electrode while the power is on.

Two types of capillary tubes are used for electrophoretic separations: fused silica tubing coated with a polyamide, and agarose gel tubes. Most capillary electrophoresis systems use polyamide-coated silica tubing. Polyamide coating is necessary because fused silica is strongly negatively charged at *p*H values above 3. Electro-

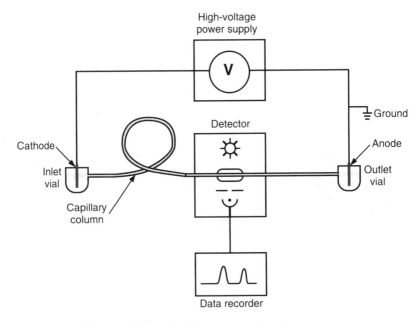

Figure 12-6.   Capillary electrophoresis system.

endosmosis is a great problem with uncoated fused silica. The polyamide coating also prevents protein adsorption to fused silica. Agarose gel-containing tubes are infrequently used. Polyacrylamide gel tubes are more common (see Polyacrylamide Gel Electrophoresis under Variations in Electrophoresis). Isoelectric focusing gels are also used with capillary electrophoresis (see Isoelectric Focusing under Variations in Electrophoresis).

Capillary electrophoresis can be performed on picomole analyte quantities and nanoliter sample volumes. There are three sample loading techniques: electrophoretic, electrokinetic, and displacement. For *electrophoretic loading,* the capillary inlet is immersed in the sample while high voltage is applied. Charged ions are drawn into the capillary tube in proportion to their electrophoretic mobility. *Electrokinetic loading* is similar to electrophoretic loading, except that electroendosmotic pumping is added to aid sample injection. *Displacement loading* uses pressure on the sample (pump or gravity) or vacuum on the capillary tube to force sample liquid into the capillary.

Typical buffers for capillary electrophoresis are phosphate, borate, and Tris. The electrodes must be stable under high voltage. Platinum is the substance of choice for these electrodes.

Detection techniques for capillary electrophoresis include spectrophotometry, fluorometry, conductivity, and electrochemistry. Most instruments use UV-visible spectrophotometry. These detectors are discussed in Chapter 14. The gel or coating of the capillary tube is removed at the site of detection. Some capillary electrophoresis devices can collect specific fractions of eluate after detection. This works best with uncoated tubes.

Common readout devices include strip chart recorders and microcomputer displays and printouts. Both methods can be used with integrators to calculate peak areas and quantitate each band.

Capillary electrophoresis is a versatile technique. It can be used to separate smaller molecules such as peptides, DNA fragments, vitamins, and organic acids.

Variations in Electrophoresis

Three major electrophoresis variations are possible by altering the composition of coating gels: isoelectric focusing, rocket immunoelectrophoresis, and polyacrylamide gel electrophoresis.

ISOELECTRIC FOCUSING

Isoelectric focusing uses a pH gradient to separate macromolecules by their isoelectric points. A pH gradient is established within an agarose gel by incorporating a mixture of numerous low-molecular-weight ampholytes (polyamino-polycarboxylic acids). The polyamino-polycarboxylic acids quickly migrate and separate at the start of the electrophoresis. Each different polyamino-polycarboxylic acid migrates to a single band on the plate and establishes a pH zone that corresponds to its isoelectric point (pI). A pH gradient is possible because the buffering capacities of the polyamino-

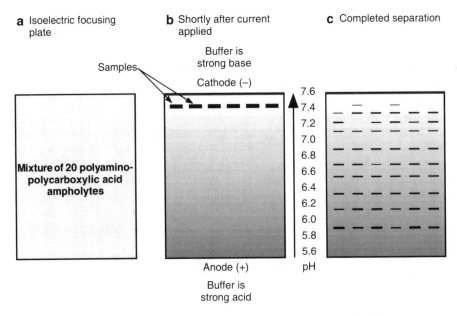

a Isoelectric focusing
plate

b Shortly after current
applied

c Completed separation

Figure 12-7.   Isoelectric focusing: (a) Agarose gel contains mixture of 20 different polyamino-polycarboxylic acids. Samples are applied (not shown), and current is turned on. The polyamino-polycarboxylic acids migrate quickly and establish 20 pH zones. (b) Macromolecules migrate (more slowly) to the pH zone closest to their isoelectric point. (c) Most isoelectric focusing applications use at least 50 different polyamino-polycarboxylic acids.

polycarboxylic acids are greater than that of the ions in the aqueous buffer. When the slower moving macromolecules are electrophoresed, they migrate until their isoelectric point matches the local pH (Fig. 12-7). At this point the charge on the macromolecule is zero, and it is unaffected by electric forces. Isoelectric focusing can resolve proteins with pI differences as small as a 0.02. Common applications include separating and identifying hemoglobin variants and α-1 antitrypsin variants (Pi typing).

ROCKET IMMUNOELECTROPHORESIS

Rocket immunoelectrophoresis uses an antibody-impregnated agarose gel to quantitate a specific protein. Conditions are established that confer a high charge to the protein of interest. At the sample application point, the protein of interest has a much higher concentration than its antibody (antigen excess). During electrophoresis the proteins diffuse laterally. As the protein migrates and diffuses, its concentration falls enough so that large, stable antigen-antibody complexes form (equivalence zone). These complexes precipitate and will no longer migrate. The result is a sharp arc of precipitated antigen-antibody complexes that resembles a rocket. The maximum height of the precipitation arc is proportional to the concentration of protein in the sample. Figure 12-8 demonstrates how standards are used to estimate the concentration of analyte in patient samples.

a

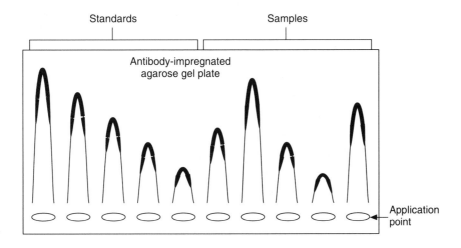

b Plot of Rocket Height vs. Standard Concentration

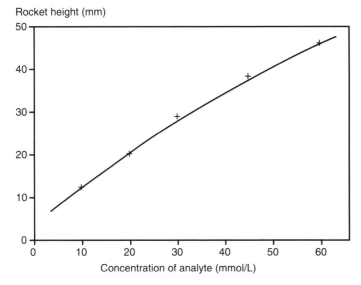

Figure 12-8. (a) A stained rocket immunoelectrophoresis plate. Standards are on the left; controls and patient samples are on the right. (b) A standard curve of rocket height versus concentration used to calculate the analyte concentrations of controls and samples. The standard curve may not be linear.

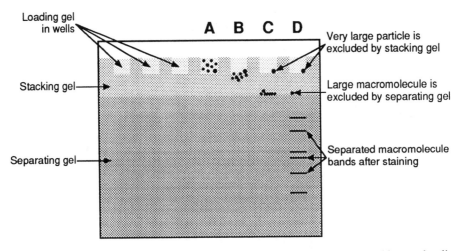

Figure 12-9.   Polyacrylamide gel electrophoresis plate. Left side: three gel layers: loading, stacking, and separating. Right side: movement of macromolecules. Macromolecules are mixed throughout the loading gel. (a) After current is applied, macromolecules are driven into the stacking gel. (b) Extremely large particles are excluded. Macromolecules stack up at the interface between the stacking and separating gels. (c) Macromolecules small enough to pass through the separating gel pores migrate at different rates based on their sizes, shapes, and net charges. (d) Final gel appearance after staining.

POLYACRYLALMIDE GEL ELECTROPHORESIS

Polyacrylamide gel electrophoresis (PAGE) uses three or more densities of polyacrylamide gel to separate macromolecules by a complicated combination of charge and size. The density and thus the pore size of the gel is altered by varying the concentrations of acrylamide and methylene bisacrylamide before polymerization. The typical PAGE method uses a separating gel (small pore size), a stacking gel (medium pore size), and a small amount of loading gel (large pores size) that contains the sample (Fig. 12-9). Once current is applied, sample macromolecules in the loading gel quickly move to the stacking gel. Here, the smaller pore size retards migration, and the macromolecules stack up (like traffic from a six-lane highway approaching a two-lane toll booth). Extremely large macromolecules will not even pass into the stacking gel. Macromolecules move through the stacking gel in a sharp band until they reach the separation gel. The pore size of the separation gel is chosen to exclude compounds with sizes greater than those of the analytes of interest. Macromolecules small enough to fit through the separation gel pores will be separated on the basis of size and charge—molecules of similar size are separated by charge, molecules of similar charge are separated by size. The smallest macromolecules move easily through the pores and are separated by charge alone. The PAGE technique is used to separate alkaline phosphatase isoenzymes and to type haptoglobins.

Table 12-2
Electrophoresis Problems and Their Causes

Electrophoresis Problems	Possible Causes
Inadequate resolution or altered migration	Decreased buffer ionic strength, increased temperature, incorrect power supply settings, or incorrect electrophoresis time. Applying too much sample can also decrease resolution.
Bands not straight and parallel	Wickflow, especially if the edges of the plate are more affected than the center. This can also occur if the plate was not stored correctly and has nonuniform hydration.
Bands too dark or too light	Staining or application problems: Stain too strong or too weak, staining or destaining times too short or too long; too much or too little sample applied or sample left in contact with plate for too short or too long a time. Some samples may require dilution or concentration to bring the analyte(s) into an appropriate range.
Quantitative results for the control too high or too low	Incorrect wavelength or slit width selection on the densitometer, incorrect alignment of the plate on the densitometer, incorrect calibration of the densitometer, deterioration or incorrect preparation of the control, or any of the problems in the preceding item.
Streaks perpendicular to bands	Seen on gel plates when the gel is poked during sample application.

Maintenance and Quality Assurance

Electrophoretic methods require rigid adherence to a well-documented procedure so that reliable, reproducible results will be obtained. Proper maintenance involves thorough cleaning of electrodes and buffer chambers between uses; frequent replenishment of staining solutions; and performance of linearity, wavelength and photometric accuracy, and stray light checks on the densitometer (see Chapter 6).

At least one control with known proportions of analytes should be included on each plate. The control should exhibit adequate resolution and quality. If quantitative electrophoresis is performed, control limits and rules should be established to identify problem runs.

Numerous problems can occur with electrophoresis. Some problems and their possible causes are listed in Table 12-2.

Summary

Electrophoresis is a powerful technique that separates charged proteins and macromolecules by using an electrical field. Resolution and migration rate can be optimized by altering the buffer system, voltage, type of support medium, or time of electrophoresis. Electrophoresis is used to identify and quantitate macromolecules and has many uses in the clinical laboratory.

An electrophoresis system is comprised of a support medium, a power supply, positive and negative electrodes, a chamber for the buffer and support medium, a dryer, a means of identifying separated macromolecules, and (if quantitation is desired) a densitometer. Automated systems exist for plate electrophoreses. Capillary electrophoresis resembles HPLC.

Three variants of electrophoresis are frequently used in clinical laboratories. Isoelectric focusing is based on the use of polyamino-polycarboxylic acids to establish a *p*H gradient across a gel plate. Macromolecules migrate to the zone corresponding to their isoelectric point. Rocket immunoelectrophoresis is based on impregnation of gel with antibody to the analyte of interest and allows visual quantitation. PAGE separates macromolecules by charge and by size.

Electrophoresis is subject to many variables. Reproducibility is impossible without strict adherence to written protocols and good quality assurance procedures.

Questions and Problems

1. An electrophoretic separation is performed for 30 minutes on a 10-cm plate using 150 V. The protein of interest migrates 4 cm. What is its electrophoretic mobility?
2. How much heat is generated when electrophoresis is performed under the following conditions: voltage = 120 V, current = 0.03 A, time = 1200 sec?
3. Assume that the rise in temperature of buffer, gelatin, and plate when heated is the same as that of pure water. If, in Problem 2, the mass of buffer, gelatin, and plate total 50 g, how much would their temperature increase (assuming that there is no transfer of heat away from the plate)? Hint: 1 calorie = 4.184 J.
4. Why will an uncharged macromolecule move away from the application point during electrophoresis?
5. What is the most common application of electrophoresis in clinical laboratories?
6. List the component parts of an electrophoresis system that can quantitate separated analytes.
7. What is the main disadvantage of capillary electrophoresis compared with automated plate electrophoresis?
8. What support media are used for each of the following: isoelectric focusing, rocket immunoelectrophoresis, and PAGE?
9. Visual inspection of an electrophoresis plate shows poor separation of bands and decreased migration of control macromolecules from the application point. What are the most likely causes of this problem?

References

1. Epstein E. Electrophoresis. In: Tietz NW, ed. Fundamentals of clinical chemistry. Philadelphia: WB Saunders, 1987:77-86.
2. Rilbe H. Basic theory of electrophoresis: Definitions, terminology and comparison of the basic

techniques. In: Simpson CF, Whittaker M, eds. Electrophoretic techniques. New York: Academic Press, 1983:1-26.

3. Brewer JM. Electrophoresis. In: Kaplan LA, Pesce AJ, eds. Clinical chemistry, 2nd ed. St. Louis: CV Mosby, 1989:140-52.

4. Kruger RL. Electrophoresis. In: Hicks MR, Schenken JR, Steinrauf MA, eds. Laboratory instrumentation, 2nd ed. Hagerstown, PA: Harper & Row, 1980:157-72.

5. Vacík J. Theory of electromigration processes. In: Deyl Z, ed. Electrophoresis: A survey of techniques and applications, part A: Techniques. Journal of Chromatography Library, vol. 18, New York: Elsevier Scientific Publishing, 1979:1-21.

6. Keren DF. High-resolution electrophoresis and immunofixation. Boston: Heinemann-Butterworth Publishers, 1987:131-83.

7. Rosenfeld L. Serum protein electrophoresis. Am J Clin Pathol 1974, 62:702-6.

8. Caron J, Penn GM. Electrophoretic and immunochemical characterization of immunoglobulins. In: Rose NR, deMacario EC, Fahey JL, Friedman H, Penn GM, eds. Manual of clinical laboratory immunology, 4th ed. Washington, DC: American Society for Microbiology, 1992:84-95.

9. Willard HH, Merritt LL, Dean JA. Instrumental methods of analysis, 5th ed. New York: D van Nostrand, 1974:533.

10. Karger BL, Cohen AS, Guttman A. High-performance capillary electrophoresis in the biological sciences. J Chromatography 1989, 492:585-614.

Suggested Readings

Costas M. Microcomputers in the comparative analysis of one-dimensional electrophoretic patterns. In: Bryce CFA, ed. Microcomputers in Biochemistry. Oxford: Oxford University Press, 1992:189-213.

Deyl Z, ed. Electrophoresis: A survey of techniques and applications, part A: Techniques. Journal of Chromatography Library, vol. 18. New York: Elsevier Scientific Publishing, 1979:1-21.

Mosher RA, Saville DA, Thormann W. The dynamics of electrophoresis. New York: VCH Publishers, 1992.

Simpson CF, Whittaker M, eds. Electrophoretic techniques. New York: Academic Press, 1983.

13

BASIC PRINCIPLES OF CHROMATOGRAPHY

Ulrike T. Otten

Objectives

After completing this chapter, the reader will be able to:

1. Define chromatography, and state the two basic components needed in a chromatographic system.
2. Explain the concept of polarity and how it influences the solubility of a substance.
3. List the general physical and chemical properties of molecules that influence their molecular interactions with other compounds and molecules.
4. Describe the four physiochemical properties used in chromatography by stating the basic principle used to achieve separation of compounds.
5. Classify chromatographic methods by the composition of their stationary and mobile phases.
6. Define the term R_f (retention factor), state the equation used to calculate this factor, and give a clinical application that uses R_f.
7. Formulate a maintenance program for planar chromatographic equipment.

Definitions

Adsorbent: A material that absorbs one substance preferentially to another from solution and usually serves as the stationary phase in adsorption chromatography.

Adsorption: The tendency for a molecule to attach itself to a finely divided solid.

Adsorption chromatography: The form of chromatography using an adsorbent, such as silica gel or alumina, as a solid stationary phase and a liquid or a gas as the mobile phase.

Anion exchanger: A molecule capable of exchanging anions. Two main categories are strong base and weak base exchangers.

Cation exchanger: A molecule capable of exchanging cations. Two main categories are strong acid and weak acid exchangers.

Chromatogram: In gas and liquid chromatography, it is a plot of the response of a detector device as a function of time or volume. Response is usually proportional to concentration. For paper and thin layer chromatography it is the developed surface on which the separate zones or spots have been revealed.

Chromatography: A technique for separating mixtures of compounds.

Column: A plastic or metal circular enclosure or tube containing the stationary phase.

Densitometer: A device that scans individual spots on a chromatogram by reflectance or absorption of a beam of monochromatic light.

Development: The movement of mobile phase over the stationary phase causing separation of components in a mixture.

Eluant: The mobile phase used to carry out chromatographic separation.

Eluate: The combination of mobile phase and solute after passage through the column; also referred to as the effluent.

Elution: The process of passing the mobile phase over the stationary phase while transporting the solutes.

Gel permeation chromatography: The separation process in which molecules are separated according to their differences in molecular dimensions such as size and shape; also referred to as filtration, exclusion, and gel chromatography.

Hydrophilic: Literally meaning "water loving," used in connection with substances that have an affinity for water and are capable of associating with water molecules through the formation of hydrogen bonds. Implies polarity of the substance.

Hydrophobic: Literally meaning "water hating," used to describe those substances that have little affinity for water molecules and will repel them. Compounds in this group usually possess few polar functional groups and have essentially a hydrocarbon or aromatic structure. Implies nonpolarity of the substance.

Ion exchange chromatography: An inclusive term for all chromatographic separations of ionic substances by using an insoluble ion exchanger as the stationary phase.

Mobile phase: The phase carrying the solutes that flows or percolates over the stationary phase, generally a liquid or inert gas.

Mobile phase velocity: The rate of migration of solute over the stationary phase, often referred to as the flow of the mobile phase.

Paper chromatography: Essentially a partition process in which the paper acts both as the support and, by virtue of the water held in its fibers, as the stationary phase.

Partition: The tendency of a molecule to distribute itself between two phases.

Partition chromatography: Any separation of compounds achieved by the partition process; includes liquid-liquid, gas-liquid, and paper chromatography.

Polarity: The ability of a compound to attract or bind to another compound or molecule. Refers to or implies associative bonding to molecules via hydrogen bonds.

Resolution: A measure of the degree of separation of a component in a mixture.

Reverse phase system: A liquid chromatography system with a hydrophilic (polar) mobile phase and a hydrophobic (nonpolar) stationary phase.

R_f (Retentive Factor) Value: A measure of the movement of a solute relative to the solvent front in paper chromatography and thin layer chromatography.

Solubility: The tendency of a molecule to dissolve in a liquid.

Solute: Any dissolved component of a mixture being separated.

Solvent: The liquid matrix of the mobile phase or equilibrating buffer.

Solvent Front: The top of the layer of solvent as it flows up through the chromatogram, representing the maximum height achieved by the solvent.

Stationary Phase: The nonmoving phase, generally a solid, liquid film, or liquid bonded to an inert solid.

Support: Inert material that serves as the support for a liquid film in partition chromatography, usually glass or plastic.

Thin Layer Chromatography (TLC):   Adsorption chromatography in which layers of adsorbent are adhered to or spread on an inert support (such as a glass or plastic plate).

Two-dimensional Chromatography: Separation by paper chromatography or TLC in which chromatograms are run sequentially in two different solvent systems at right angles (90°) to each other.

Volatility: The tendency for a molecule to enter the vapor state or to evaporate.

Zones: Individual substances separated on chromatographic columns or TLC plates.

Introduction

Chromatography is a separation technique primarily used to isolate components of a mixture. This technique has a high degree of resolving power in spite of the relative complexity of the separation processes used. Although the word implies color, there is no direct connection, except that the first compounds to be separated by the technique were plant pigments by the Russian scientist Michel Tswett in 1903.[1] Forty years elapsed before this separation technique was improved by Martin and Synge, who applied paper chromatography and the concept of partition chromatography to separate organic compounds.

The scope of chromatography today is diverse, and its applications cover many fields of study, particularly chemistry, biology, and medicine. Examples include the analysis of constituents in petroleum products, the separation of amino acids in proteins, the isolation and purification of components in antibiotics, and the identification and quantitation of suspected drugs of abuse. Chromatography is a flexible and powerful analytical procedure, yet it remains an efficient separation technique.

Basic System Design

All chromatographic separations are based on a common concept: the distribution of components in a mixture between two immiscible phases, one being a stationary phase, the other a mobile phase. In order for separation of compounds to occur, a dynamic, or "moving," situation must be initiated. This is accomplished by causing one of the phases (the mobile phase) to flow past the other (the stationary phase). This movement may be accomplished by way of capillary action, gravity forces, or application of pressure to the mobile phase.

The basic components needed in a chromatographic system are the stationary and mobile phases. The mobile phase may be a liquid, a gas, or a supercritical fluid. The stationary phase, however, may take on many forms. It may be a liquid supported by a porous, inert material, or it may consist of molecules chemically bonded to such a material. It may be an adsorptive or inert solid, usually porous, or it may be an ion-exchange resin or a gel. It may simply be a piece of filter paper!

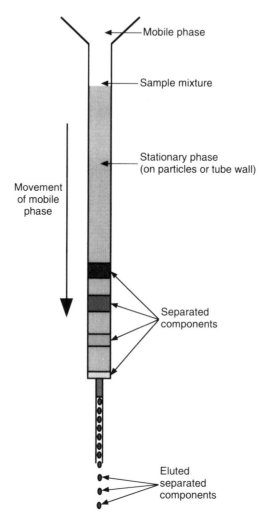

Mobile phase

Sample mixture

Stationary phase
(on particles or tube wall)

Movement
of mobile
phase

Separated
components

Eluted
separated
components

Figure 13-1. Chromatographic separation using a column chromatography technique.

The stationary phase may be arranged in a column or may constitute a planar layer. In column chromatography, a small volume of sample is introduced into the flowing mobile phase (eluent). After passage through the chromatographic column, the various components of the sample are observed as bands or zones separated in time (Fig. 13-1). In planar chromatography, the sample is applied in a small area or spot, and the mobile phase is allowed to pass through or over the stationary phase by capillary action. After development, observation of the physically separated components or spots is possible (Fig. 13-2).

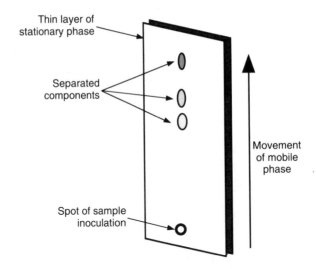

Figure 13-2.   Chromatographic separation using a planar chromatography technique.

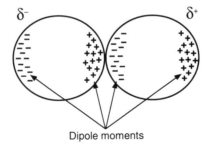

Dipole moments

Figure 13-3.   Dipole moment of two molecules and their subsequent interaction.

CONCEPT OF POLARITY

The polarity of a molecule means that the molecule possesses separate positive and negative centers, termed dipoles, arising from the atoms involved and their arrangement or configuration. Polar molecules are electrically dissymmetric molecules and will show dipole moments. A *dipole moment* occurs in a molecule whenever the electrons are arranged so that at any given instant, part of the molecule has a net negative charge and part has a net positive charge (Fig. 13-3). The extent of separation between the charged centers or poles determines the degree of polarity of the molecule and its relative attraction to another molecule. Highly polar molecules are strongly attracted to other polar molecules.[2]

In chromatography, the meaning of polarity is broadened to include such properties as hydrogen bonding. This type of dipolar interaction occurs when hydrogen is

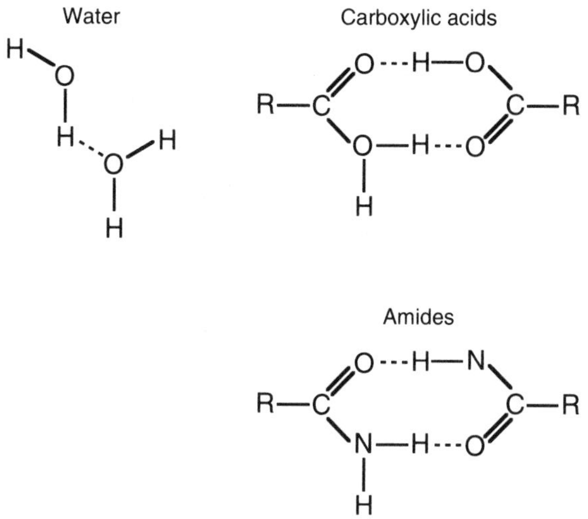

Figure 13-4.   Hydrogen bond (dotted lines).

bonded to an atom that is in close proximity to an electronegative atom such as oxygen, nitrogen, or a halogen. The hydrogen atom can interact with nearby electron-rich molecules, forming a second weaker bond in addition to the main covalent molecular bond. Examples of hydrogen bonding are between water molecules, carboxylic acids, and amides[3] (Fig. 13-4).

Polarity is a relative term applied to solvents, solutes, and adsorbents. Water has a strong permanent dipole by virtue of its molecular geometry, electron configuration, and hydrogen bonding. Thus, water is considered a very polar solvent. Polar molecules are termed hydrophilic because they are readily soluble in water. Oxygenated compounds (such as alcohols and ketones) have less strong dipoles, are less hydrogen-bonded, and are, therefore, less polar than water. The hydrocarbons are the least polar of all, because they have the least polar functional groups and a very rigid, symmetric geometric structure where the primary intermolecular interaction is dispersion. The hydrocarbons are not readily attracted to or bonded to another molecule. Nonpolar molecules are termed hydrophobic because they are not readily soluble in water.

The polarity of a molecule influences its degree of solubility in certain solvents or adsorbents. Based on the assumption that "like dissolves like," we can predict that a polar adsorbent will adsorb a polar solute more tightly than a nonpolar or less polar solute. The concept of polarity is more obviously extended to the liquid phase of chromatographic separations. Again, "like dissolves like," and we can predict that a polar solute will be more readily dissolved in a polar solvent compared to a less polar solvent. The degree of polarity of a molecule determines the extent of attraction of that molecule to the stationary or mobile phase and thus influence the degree of separation.

PROPERTIES OF SEPARATION

Chromatographic separations of compounds depend on the polarity of solvent, solutes, and the stationary phase; solvent flow; solute diffusion; and other factors. Chromatographic separations are carried out by techniques involving a few of the general physical properties of molecules and the molecular interactions within the system. Molecular interactions include weak chemical reactions or bonds and physical interactions or attractions (hydrogen bonding, dispersion, etc). Physical properties of molecules include solubility, adsorption, and volatility.

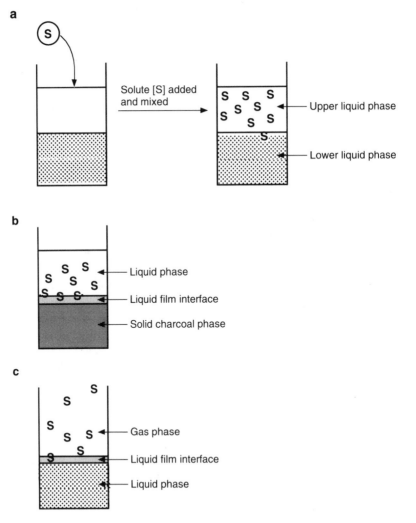

Figure 13-5. Examples of chromatographic separations: (a) Liquid-liquid. Substance (S) is more soluble in the upper phase. (b) Liquid-solid. Substance (S) distributes between liquid and solid. (c) Gas-liquid. Substance (S) distributes between liquid film and gas.

In chromatography, mixtures or substances to be separated are placed in a moving situation where they can exhibit any two of the mentioned physical properties. This may involve using the same property twice, such as solubility in two different liquids, or it may involve two different properties entirely. For example, if a substance is placed in a separatory funnel with two immiscible liquids (chloroform and water) the substance will "distribute" itself or "partition" itself between the two liquids depending on its relative solubility in them (Fig. 13-5a). Thus, an interaction between the solubility properties of the two liquids is used to achieve separation. If a substance is placed in a flask with a liquid and a solid (such as charcoal), the substance will distribute itself between the liquid film and the surface of the solid (Fig. 13-5b). Thus, solubility and adsorption properties are used to achieve separation. And if a volatile substance is dissolved in a nonvolatile liquid, it will distribute or partition itself between the liquid film and the gas in contact with the liquid film (Fig. 13-5c). Thus an interaction between the solubility and volatility properties of the molecule was used to achieve separation.[4] The system used for separation of substances consists of two phases, mobile and stationary, with a substance distributed or partitioned between them.

The differences in physical and chemical properties of the individual components determines their relative affinity for the stationary and mobile phases. Thus, a substance with a relatively high affinity for the stationary phase (as compared to the mobile phase) is more strongly attracted to the stationary phase and moves slowly through the chromatographic system than does a substance with lower affinity. This difference in migration velocity ultimately leads to the physical separation of the components in a sample. The components will migrate through the system at differing rates, thus achieving separation.

Physiochemical Processes of Separation

Physiochemical process refers to the process or mechanism of solute interaction used with the stationary phase to achieve separation, or fixed-phase interactions. *Fixed-phase interactions* are generally classified as four types: adsorption, partition, ion exchange, and size exclusion. Separation is generally based on interactions involving polarity, solubility, ionic charge, and the physical properties of the molecule, including size and shape.

ADSORPTION

Adsorption is a distribution process whereby the solute interacts reversibly with the surface molecules of a finely divided solid. Molecules are usually adsorbed with some degree of spacial orientation to the surface and with only a small part of the molecule (the functional group) actually in contact with the surface. This attraction to the solid stationary phase is based on the degree of polarity of the solute molecules, the solid phase, and the liquid phase. The polar adsorbents interact "attractively" with molecules by forces primarily due to hydrogen bonding. Examples of polar adsorbents include alumina, silica gel (Fig. 13-6), quartz, titanium oxide,

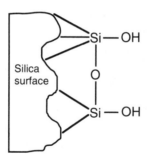

Figure 13-6.   Example of a polar stationary adsorbent: silica gel.

organic ion exchange resins, and cellulose. Nonpolar adsorbents interact primarily by forces due to dispersion. Examples of nonpolar adsorbents are certain charcoals, paraffin, graphite, and some organic resins and plastics.[5]

PARTITION

Partitioning is a process whereby a solute "distributes" or "equilibrates" itself between two immiscible liquid phases depending on its solubility properties. The solubility of molecules is based on solute polarity and the concept of "like dissolves like." Normally, the stationary phase is polar, and the mobile phase is nonpolar (or relatively less polar). This type of system is referred to as a *normal-phase partition.* In a *reverse-phase system,* the stationary phase is nonpolar, and the mobile phase is polar. Reverse-phase partition is useful in separating nonpolar substances that may not be separable by the normal-phase process.[6-7]

ION EXCHANGE

Ion exchange is a process that uses the charge of a molecule to achieve separation. Separation is based on differences in charge (positive or negative) and the magnitude of that charge. The stationary phase is usually an ionized resin with a functional group attached. The functional group's counterion will bind ions of opposite charge reversibly, thereby retarding their elution. The eluent (mobile phase) is usually a buffer of a specific pH and ionic strength. Sample ions "exchange places" with the mobile phase ions on the functional groups of the stationary phase. Ion exchange systems are of two types: *anion exchange* or *cation exchange,* depending on what type of ion exchange is occuring. Like all acids and bases, the exchangers may be strongly ionized or weakly ionized. Strong cation exchangers are usually resins that carry sulfonic acid groups, whereas weak cation exchangers usually carry carboxylic acid groups. Strong anion exchangers are resins that usually carry quaternary ammo-

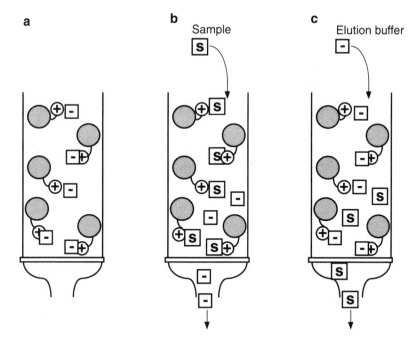

Figure 13-7. Example of an anion exchange system. (a) Ion exchange resin with negatively charged counterion attached to functional group. (b) Sample ion (S) binds to functional group ion by exchanging negative counterion. (c) Elution buffer ion exchanges places for sample ion to be collected as eluate.

nium groups, and weak anion exchangers usually carry amine groups. Figure 13-7 shows an example of an anion exchange system.

SIZE EXCLUSION

Size exclusion is a process of separation that is based on the molecular size of the solute molecule. Molecules of relatively large molecular weights (>2000 g/mol) such as polymers and biomolecules are best suited to this type of separation. Size exclusion is the only noninteractive mechanism of separation. This means that separation is not due to intermolecular forces and interactions. The stationary phase is a porous material of controllable size. Small solute molecules can enter the pores of the stationary phase and will be retained by the stationary phase longer, whereas large solute molecules cannot enter the pores and will be eluted off the column with the mobile phase quickly (Fig. 13-8). Intermediate-size molecules will experience moderate retention. This type of separation process is also referred to as gel filtration, gel permeation, and molecular sieve. Size exclusion chromatography is the preferred term.

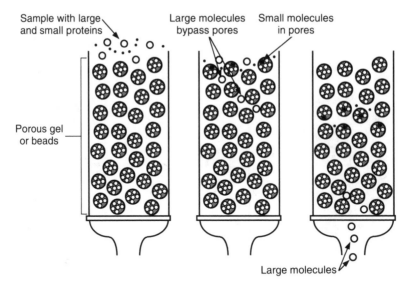

Sample with large and small proteins

Large molecules bypass pores

Small molecules in pores

Porous gel or beads

Large molecules

Figure 13-8.   Example of size exclusion process where large molecules are eluted off the column quickly, whereas the smaller molecules interact with the porous stationary phase and elute later.

PLANAR CHROMATOGRAPHY

Various combinations of mobile and stationary phases are possible, thus leading to the many different branches or types of chromatographic methods known today. Separation of components is achieved by any combination of processes thus far discussed. Basically, chromatographic methods may be divided into two subdivisions: *planar chromatography,* and *column chromatography.* In this chapter we discuss only planar chromatography. Column chromatography is discussed in the following two chapters.

In planar chromatography, there are no physical walls or columns used to retain the phases mechanically. Instead, the limits of the mobile phase are set by its surface tension and viscosity as well as the nature of the stationary phase. Planar chromatography is subdivided into paper chromatography (PC) and thin layer chromatography (TLC) and differs from other chromatographic techniques in the planar arrangement of the stationary phase. Both PC and TLC are closely related in their technical aspects of sample preparation, sample application, development, identification, and quantitation. The two methods differ fundamentally in the composition of the stationary phase.

PAPER CHROMATOGRAPHY

In *paper chromatography,* the stationary phase is simply a type of filter paper. Although ordinary filter paper may be used, special papers are manufactured for PC.

They are highly purified, especially from metal contaminants, and are manufactured under controlled conditions so that properties such as porosity, thickness, and arrangement of cellulose fibers are reproducible from batch to batch. Standard cellulose is most often used (Whatman No. 1 filter paper or its equivalent). Chromatographic paper contains enough water in its natural form to classify PC as a typical partition system, where water is the stationary phase held by adsorption on cellulose molecules, which in turn are kept in a fixed position by the fibrous structure of the paper.[8] The filter paper acts as the solid support for the liquid stationary phase. The forces involved to achieve separation of compounds in PC are derived from the special chemical and structural properties of the paper used and are in part due to partition, adsorption, and ion exchange phenomena. The characteristics of the stationary phase can be changed if the paper is treated with other liquids such as rubber latex, paraffin oil, silicone oil, or petroleum jelly. The paper will be rendered water repellent and will absorb the organic component of the solvent mixture (which then becomes the stationary phase) in preference to the water. Special papers are commercially available that contain adsorbents or ion exchange resins, are specially treated (acetylated), or are made of other fibers such as glass or nylon. The type of paper used for PC systems is usually chosen according to the type of material being separated: whether they are hydrophilic or hydrophobic (lipophilic), neutral or charged. Cellulose is used almost exclusively for separating hydrophilic substances such as amino acids and sugars.

The choice of mobile phase is also determined by the nature of the substances being separated and the stationary phase. The mobile solvent is normally a mixture consisting of one main organic component, water, and various additions such as acids or bases. The organic liquid may or may not be immiscible in water. The water in the mobile phase is somewhat retained by the filter paper so that the stationary phase is considered a water-cellulose complex. A substance in solution will be held more or less strongly in this complex depending on the hydrophilic properties of that substance. Separation is achieved by partitioning with this liquid complex and by adsorption with the paper itself. Examples of common solvent mixtures used for the mobile phase are water and acetonitrile or water, butanol, and acetic acid.[9]

THIN LAYER CHROMATOGRAPHY

In *thin layer chromatography,* the stationary phase is a thin layer of adsorbent material fixed on an inert solid support such as glass, plastic, or aluminum. Commonly used adsorbents include silica gel, alumina, starch, cellulose powder, and their derivatives. Binding agents may be added to the adsorbent to provide better adhesion of the adsorbent layers to the support surface and to stabilize the layers of adsorbent material. Commercially available plates are of high quality and reproducibility. Reproducibility is influenced by the use of uniform-size particles of adsorbent material. As in PC, the choice of the appropriate stationary phase adsorbent and mobile phase depends on the characteristics of the solutes.

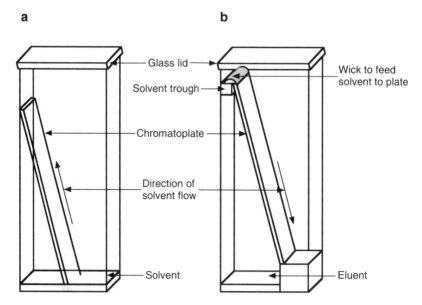

Figure 13-9.   Development methods in PC. (a) Ascending. (b) Descending.

OVERALL PROCESS

The basic system design in planar (PC and TLC) chromatography is quite simple. The filter paper or adsorbent material on a solid support serves as the stationary phase. Separation of components is achieved by movement of the mobile phase over the stationary phase by capillary action or gravity pull depending on whether an ascending or descending system is used. Because reproducibility of chromatograms depends on constancy of temperature and maintenance of saturated atmospheric conditions, separation using this technique often requires an equilibrated, sealed development chamber or tank (Fig. 13-9).

SAMPLE PREPARATION

Some degree of sample preparation is required prior to applying the sample to the stationary phase in PC and TLC. Biological samples commonly used are urine and blood, which may contain certain materials (proteins, lipids, inorganic ions, etc.) in high enough concentration to interfere with the chromatographic procedure. Methods commonly used to rid biological samples of these materials include protein precipitation, extraction, ultrafiltration, and ion exchange techniques. In addition, the analytes being separated may be in such low concentrations in the biological fluid that extraction and concentration techniques are warranted.[10]

STORAGE AND PREPARATION OF STATIONARY PHASE

Because of the nature of the stationary phase, a controlled humidity environment is useful when storing PC and TLC plates prior to use. Prior to sample application, the plates or paper should be activated by drying them in an oven (100°C) for a specific time. Cellulose and silica gel are hydroscopic and readily adsorb water molecules from the atmosphere. The presence of water layers on the surface of the stationary phase affects the interaction of the sample and the mobile phase to its surface and, thus, its separation efficiency.

SAMPLE APPLICATION

Planar chromatography lends itself well to qualitative and quantitative analysis. If qualitative analysis is desired, simply applying an arbitrary amount of sample to the paper or plate is sufficient. But if quantitative analysis is desired, a known amount of sample is applied to the paper or plate using calibrated micropipettes. It is important to apply samples in small spots to minimize diffusion or sample spreading. This is usually accomplished by applying a small amount of sample and drying it quickly with a hair dryer or draft hood. Another small amount of sample may be applied directly on top of the first application. Overapplication of the sample is a common error that causes excess diffusion and band spreading on the chromatogram.

Once the samples have been applied, the system is ready for development by placing the plate or paper into a presaturated chamber. Development of the chromatogram does not begin if the end of the paper or plate is not immersed into the solvent. This allows for a specific equilibration period, during which the paper or adsorbent adsorbs the components of the vapor phase of the chamber and becomes conditioned. This optimizes mobile phase flow over the stationary phase.[11]

DEVELOPMENT OF CHROMATOGRAM

There are several basic methods for development. They can be classified as either one-dimensional or two-dimensional. If the paper or plate is held horizontal and the solvent flows from one end to the other, the term *horizontal chromatography* is used. If the sample is applied to the center of the paper or plate and flows outward, the term *radial chromatography* is used. If the paper or plate is held vertically, the term *ascending* or *descending chromatography* is used, depending on whether the solvent is allowed to flow upward by capillary action or downward by a combination of capillary action and gravity pull (Fig. 13-9).

A more effective separation of substances is sometimes achieved with two-dimensional chromatography. In this system, the sample is applied in a small spot in a lower corner of the chromatographic paper or plate. It is chromatographed in one direction in the first solvent system, and then chromatographed using a second solvent system in a direction perpendicular to the first (Fig. 13-10).

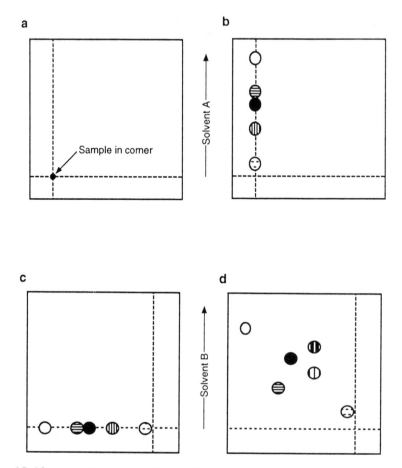

Figure 13-10. Two-dimensional TLC. (a) First development. (b) Results of first separation. (c) Plate rotated 90° for second development. (d) Final chromatogram.

DETECTION AND VISUALIZATION

After chromatographic development, the wet paper or plate is removed from the tank and allowed to dry either at room temperature or in a controlled-temperature environment such as an oven. Visualization of the separated compounds is now possible. This can be accomplished in several ways: direct observation of a naturally colored compound, observation of fluorescence when irradiated with ultraviolet light, radioactive measurement of radioactive compounds, heat charring, or staining the compound by means of a chemical reaction. Specific reagents are available for the detection of certain groups of substances. The detection reagents are usually sprayed on the paper or plate surface in a fine mist to achieve uniform wetting. This is necessary if quantitation of the compound is desired. (Fig. 13-11).

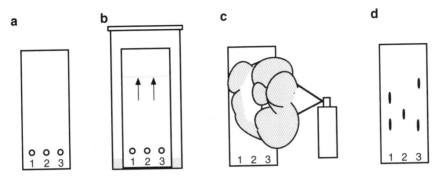

Figure 13-11.   Overall development/visualization process for PC and TLC. (a) Sample application. (b) Development of chromatogram. (c) Visualization with chemical spray. (d) Final chromatogram.

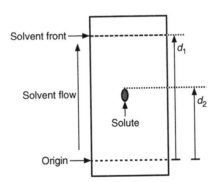

Figure 13-12.   Retention factor (R_f) is a constant used in PC and TLC, reflecting a ratio of distances traveled by the compound and solvent: $R_f = d_2/d_1$.

QUALITATIVE IDENTIFICATION

Once visualization is achieved, qualitative identification of the compound is possible. A compound may be characterized by determination of its retention factor (R_f). A compound's R_f is a constant in a given chromatographic system. It is measured directly on the chromatogram by determining the ratio of the distances traveled by the compound and the solvent[12] (Fig. 13-12). The extent of solute migration both in PC and TLC is commonly described by its R_f value. The retention factor is calculated as follows:

$$R_f = \frac{\text{distance moved by solute}}{\text{distance moved by solvent front}} \qquad \text{(Eq. 13-1)}$$

The R_f of the unknown compound is compared to the R_f of a known compound or standard and is thus identified. The R_f is constant only if measured under strictly constant conditions, specifically temperature, type of paper or adsorbent used, makeup of the solvent system, and amount of sample applied. Qualitative sample identification may also be made by comparison of staining and fluorescence characteristics of the unknown standards.

QUANTITATIVE ANALYSIS

Quantitative analysis of the stained chromatograph is also possible. A certain degree of error is inherent in paper chromatography quantitation because of the nonuniformity of the paper itself. Substances can be quantitatively measured only if a mixture of standards is included on the same paper or plate as the compound of interest. Quantitation can be achieved several ways: by measuring spot size, by use of a densitometer to scan the intensity of the developed spots, by radioactive counting, and by spectrophotometric analysis of eluted compounds. When measuring spot size, an estimate of the quantity of analyte is determined by comparison to a known standard included on the same chromatograph. At best, this is a semiquantitative method. For greater accuracy, the paper or plate can be scanned to obtain relative densities of separated spots by using a densitometer in one of three modes: transmission, reflectance, or fluorescence.

A *densitometer* is a special spectrophotometer (for a review of spectrophotometry, see Chapter 6) that scans the chromatogram and measures the transmission of monochromatic light through the separated components. This simple photometer is composed of a light source (usually tungsten if measuring in the visible wavelength range); a filter or grating for isolating wavelength; a means of scanning the plate (either by physically moving the plate over the stationary light source and detector or by moving the light beam and detector across a stationary plate; and a photodetector (Fig. 13-13). A densitometer usually has several variable slits through which the optical system focuses the beam. The size of the slit width is selected to give optimum absorption as well as optimum separation of the fractions. The signal output of the chromatogram as seen on a strip chart recorder will appear as peaks with areas proportional to the density of the spots scanned (Fig. 13-14). The areas of the unknown peaks can be compared to the areas of the standard peaks to determine the amount of unknown present in the original mixture. Many times, the absorbance of each unknown as compared to the total absorbance of all peaks is calculated and the results are reported as relative percentages.

If the sample is radioactively tagged, radioactivity may be counted by using a radioactive scanning device or more accurately using a scintillation counter. Quantitation may also be accomplished by spectrophotometric analysis of eluted components from the chromatogram. Again, known standards must be included on the same chromatogram as the unknown for accurate quantitation.

APPLICATION

Paper chromatography is not used much today because TLC is usually better. Generally, paper is used to separate and identify amino acids and simple sugars that

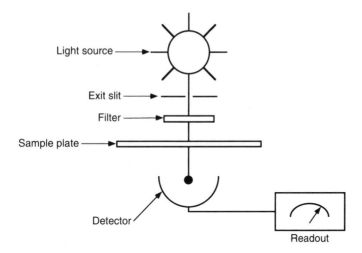

Figure 13-13. Densitometer.

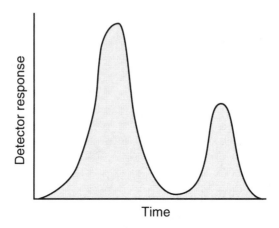

Figure 13-14. Chromatogram of separated compounds from a strip chart recorder.

have elevated concentrations in some inborn errors of metabolism. PC is also used in toxicology screening. Thin layer chromatography is used in amino acid screening, toxicology screening, and to identify pulmonary surfactants in amniotic fluid. Paper chromatography and TLC techniques can be used analytically as well as for preparative work.

ADVANTAGES

The main advantage of TLC is its speed and simplicity. The planar arrangement of PC and TLC has several advantages over column techniques, such as simplicity, flexibility, two-dimensional development, and applicability of specific or selective chemical detection methods directly to the chromatogram. The major disadvantages are that automation is difficult and, more important, the sensitivity and accuracy of the quantitative analysis are lower than for other methods such as column chromatography.

Maintenance and Quality Assurance

Precision of the measurement depends on preparing reproducible chromatograms. This is accomplished by using high-quality adsorbents of uniform particle size and applying small samples to the plate. Better resolution of compounds will result from careful application of sample and use of a uniform adsorbent.

Quality assurance of any chromatographic procedure includes running appropriate standards and controls with each run. Control values should be within established limits (usually 95% confidence) before accepting the chromatograph as valid. If quantitation of a chromatogram is accomplished using a densitometer, the densitometer must be checked as well. A neutral density standard with several bands of specific quantitative value (relative % density) should be checked and recorded daily. The linearity of the instrument should also be verified and recorded weekly. A standard strip range (e.g., 0.100 to 3.000 absorbance units) is often used to verify that the peak area recorded is linear to the density or amount of the spot on the densitometer scan. Further information pertaining to quality assurance of a photometer can be found in Chapter 6.

Summary

Chromatography is a technique used to separate and analyze components of a mixture. The separation process depends on the compound's interactions between the stationary and mobile phases. Interactions basically classified as: (1) adsorption, where separation is based on the polarity of the molecule; (2) partition, where separation is based on the relative solubility of the molecule; (3) ion exchange, where separation is based on the relative charge on the molecule; and (4) size exclusion, where separation is based on the size and shape of the molecule.

Paper chromatography and TLC differ from other chromatographic techniques because of the planar nature of their stationary phase. The type of stationary phase and mobile phase to be used in a chromatographic separation depends on the nature of the substances being separated.

The overall process of planar chromatography is basically quite simple. Planar chromatography is versatile because the stationary and mobile phase combination, and the choice of chromatographic development and detection technique, may be chosen to best isolate and identify a compound of interest.

Questions and Problems

1. The tendency of a molecule to attach itself to a finely divided solid is referred to as (a) partition; (b) adsorption; (c) ionic interaction; (d) elution.

2. Size exclusion chromatography separates solutes in a sample based on the (a) solubility of the solutes; (b) molecular size and shape; (c) sign and magnitude of the ionic charge; (d) adsorption ability of the solutes.
3. Which of the following chromatography systems is characterized by a stationary phase of Whatman filter paper and a moving phase of liquid? (a) thin layer; (b) ion exchange; (c) paper; (d) size exclusion.
4. Construct a block diagram of a densitometer.
5. Reproducibility of thin layer chromatograms is ensured by which of the following: (a) application of small sample spots; (b) uniform porosity and size of adsorbent material; (c) constancy of temperature and maintenance of saturated atmospheric conditions; (d) all of the above.

References

1. Bobbitt JM, Schwarting AE, Gritter RJ. Introduction to chromatography. New York: Reinhold Science Studies, Reinhold Book Corp., 1968:1-65.
2. Bruno TJ. Chromatographic and electrophoretic methods. Englewood Cliffs, NJ: Prentice-Hall, 1991:1-16.
3. Miller JM. Chromatography: Concepts and contrasts. A Wiley-Interscience Publication. New York: John Wiley & Sons, 1988:40-64.
4. Bobbit JM. Schwarting AE, Gritter RJ. Introduction to chromatography. New York: Reinhold Science Studies, Reinhold Book Corp., 1968:1.
5. Mikes O, Chalmers RA. Fundamental types of chromatography. In: Mikes O, ed. Laboratory handbook of chromatographic methods. New York: Van Nostrand Reinhold, 1966:23-4, 189.
6. Bobbitt JM, Schwarting AE, Gritter RJ. Introduction to chromatography. New York: Reinhold Science Studies, Reinhold Book Corp., 1968:30.
7. Mikes O, Chalmers RA. Fundamental types of chromatography. In: Mikes O, ed. Laboratory handbook of chromatographic methods. New York: Van Nostrand Reinhold, 1966:23-4.
8. Braithwaite A, Smith FJ. Chromatographic methods, 4th ed. New York: Chapman and Hall, 1985:50.
9. Miller JM. Chromatography: Concepts and contrasts. New York: John Wiley & Sons, 1988:239-42.
10. Snyder LR. Theory of chromatography. In: Heftmann E, ed. Chromatography, 5th ed. Fundamentals and applications of chromatography and related differential migration methods, part A: Fundamentals and techniques. Journal of Chromatography Library, vol. 51A. New York: Elsevier Scientific Publishing, 1992:A1-A68.
11. Bobbitt JM, Schwarting AE, Gritter RJ. Introduction to chromatography. New York: Reinhold Science Studies, Reinhold Book Corp., 1968:59-60.
12. Nyiredy S. Planar chromatography. In: Heftmann E. Chromatography, 5th ed. Fundamentals and applications of chromatography and related differential migration methods, part A: Fundamentals and techniques. Journal of Chromatography Library, Vol. 51A. New York: Elsevier Scientific Publishing, 1992:A109-A150.

Suggested Readings

Heftmann E, ed. Chromatography, 5th ed. Fundamentals and applications of chromatographic and electrophoretic methods, part I: Fundamentals and techniques. Journal of Chromatography Library, Vol. 51A. New York: Elsevier Scientific Publishing, 1992.

Jönsson JA. Common concepts of chromatography. In: Jönsson JA, ed. Chromatographic theory and basic principles. Chromatographic Science Series, vol. 38. New York: Marcel Dekker, 1987.

Touchstone JC, Sherma J, eds. Techniques and applications of thin layer chromatography. New York: John Wiley & Sons, 1985.

14

LIQUID CHROMATOGRAPHY

Peggy L. Bottjen

Objectives

After completing this chapter, the reader will be able to:

1. Describe how separation occurs in each of the following methods:
   A. Partition
   B. Adsorption
   C. Ion-exchange
   D. Size-exclusion
2. Explain why filtration and degassing are important during preparation and storage of the mobile phase.
3. Discuss various liquid chromatography (LC) pump designs and their uses.
4. State which LC column is the most widely used.
5. Discuss the detectors available for LC and an advantage/disadvantage to each.
6. Establish and follow a maintenance program for an LC system.

Definitions

Gradient Elution: Separation with changing flow rate, column temperature, or mobile phase polarity.

High Pressure Liquid Chromatography (HPLC): Separation on columns with small (3–10 μm) particles, in fairly short times (typically <1 hour), and at pressures up to 6000 psi.

Internal Standard: A compound similar to the analyte that is added to all standards, controls, and unknowns in equal concentration. Its ratio to the analyte will compensate for extraction, injection volume, and other variation.

Isocratic Elution: Separation with constant flow rate, column temperature, or mobile phase polarity.

Normal Phase: A chromatographic method that uses a stationary phase (column) that is more polar than mobile phase.

Peak Height: Measurement from baseline to tip of peak, used to quantitate the analyte.

Resolution: Degree of separation of two adjacent peaks.

Retention Time: Time elapsed from injection to maximum peak detection.

Reverse Phase: A chromatographic method that uses a stationary phase (column) that is less polar than the mobile phase.

Introduction

Liquid chromatography (LC) is a multifaceted chromatographic technique for the separation, detection, and quantitation of a wide variety of analytes. It employs a liquid mobile phase and a coated, solid stationary phase to separate such analytes as drugs, amino acids, vitamins, sugars, and proteins. In this chapter we examine the principles, instrumentation, and maintenance of LC systems.

Principles

Liquid chromatography is a process in which a mixture of analytes is separated by passing through a column. The mixture is injected into a flowing stream of mobile phase where it is distributed between the mobile phase and a stationary phase present in the column. Repeated sorption/desorption of the analytes occurs during movement along the stationary phase and results in separation due to differences in the distribution constants of the individual analytes.

Separation of a mixture of analytes on a LC column is depicted in Figure 14-1. Step (a) shows a mixture of three analytes, A, B, and C, injected in a tight band at the head of the column. As mobile phase continues to flow, the analyte C is not retained as much as A and B as it move along the column, so separation begins as in step (b).

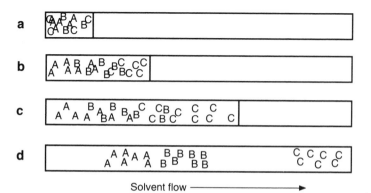

Figure 14-1.   Separation of a mixture on an LC column. (a) Analytes A, B, and C are injected at front of column. (b) Separation takes place as solvent flows through the column. (c) Further separation takes place. (d) Analytes A, B, and C are separated.

Step (c) shows a further separation, and by step (d) the analytes are essentially separated from each other. A strip-chart recording of these analytes as they flow through a detector is shown in Figure 14-2. Analyte C is retained the least by the column and is the first peak detected. Analyte B is retained longer than C but less than A, so it is the next peak, followed by A, which is retained the longest. Each analyte then has a unique retention time (a, b, c) that can be measured from injection to maximum peak detection.[1]

As seen in Figure 14-1, the analytes each interacted differently with the column and were retained on the column for different periods of time. This interaction with the column occurs by one of four separate mechanisms, depending on the mobile phase and column chosen. The four basic methods of LC separation are partition, adsorption, ion exchange, and size exclusion chromatography.

Partition, or *liquid-liquid chromatography,* is the most commonly used in LC. It uses a liquid stationary phase with a polarity different from that of the mobile phase. Solute molecules tend to stay in the phase with a similar polarity. If the mobile phase is very polar, then the most polar analytes will flow swiftly through with the mobile phase while the less polar analytes will be retained by the column longer, and thus separation occurs.

In *normal phase partition chromatography* the stationary phase in the analytical column is usually a polar compound such as silica (SI), diol (2OH), aminopropyl (NH2), or cyanopropyl (CN) bonded to silica gel. The mobile phase is a more nonpolar liquid such as chloroform, hexane, or isopropanol. *Reverse phase partition chromatography* is the opposite of normal phase. It uses a nonpolar stationary phase such as octadecyl (C18), octyl (C8), phenyl (PN), or cyano (CN) bonded to silica gel. The mobile phase is an aqueous buffer combined with solvents such as methanol or acetonitrile. *Ion-pairing* is a technique that uses ionic analytes that are not normally

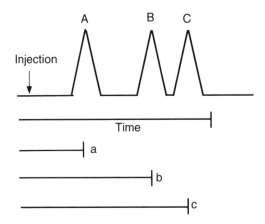

Figure 14-2. Chromatogram of separation of analytes A, B, and C. Analyte C from Figure 14-1 was the least retained by the column, so it elutes first, followed by B, then A. The retention time of analytes A, B, and C from injection to maximum peak detection are represented as a, b, and c.

separated by reverse phase chromatography and adds a counterion that binds to form a more neutral pair. This pairing of ions can then be separated by reverse phase chromatography.

Adsorption, or *liquid-solid chromatography,* involves a porous, solid stationary phase such as silica gel or alumina with a relatively nonpolar mobile phase such as chloroform, hexane, or isopropanol. Although not widely used, this method of separation may be useful for mixtures whose analytes vary widely in polarity such as lipids or fat-soluble vitamins.

Ion-exchange chromatography involves a stationary phase made up of an ion-exchange resin that has charged functional groups that bind ions of the opposite charge. The mobile phase is an aqueous solution buffered to a pH that permits the exchange resin and the analyte to have opposite charges. A counterion is present in the mobile phase and competes with the analyte for a spot on the resin. Either anion- or cation-exchange resins may be used. Figure 14-3 is a diagram of the process with a cation-exchange resin used to quantitate amino acids. Lithium ion (Li^+) is used as the counterion. During retention (a), the low concentration of Li^+ ion in the mobile phase allows the amino acids to be retained on the column. As the Li^+ ion concentration is increased (b), it exchanges with the amino acids on the resin with subsequent elution of the amino acids.

Size-exclusion, or *gel-filtration chromatography,* involves separation of analytes by their molecular size. A packing material such as silica gel, cross-linked dextran, or vinyl polymer that contains many pores and channels serves as the stationary phase. As the analyte mixture passes through the packing, smaller molecules are trapped in the pores while the larger molecules pass through more quickly, thus achieving

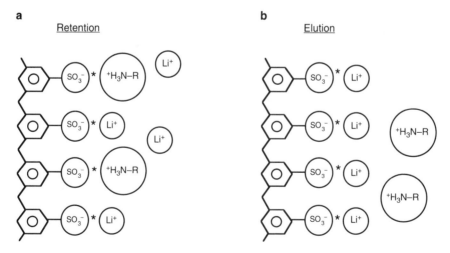

Figure 14-3. Cation exchange of amino acids. (a) Retention of amino acids. The low concentration of Li^+ ions in the mobile phase allows amino acids to react with column resin. (b) Eolution of amino acids. The increased Li^+ ion concentration causes amino acids and Li^+ ions to exchange places so amino acids are eluted from column.

separation by size. An important application of size-exclusion chromatography is removal of salts from protein-containing fluids.[2]

Component Parts

A liquid chromatography system is made up of six basic components as depicted in Figure 14-4. These components can be separate pieces of equipment from one or more manufacturers or may be combined into one piece of instrumentation such as a dedicated amino acid analyzer.

MOBILE PHASE RESERVOIR

The mobile phase and reservoir may be one bottle or several bottles if a gradient pump is used. The bottle must be clean and of sufficient strength to withstand vacuum pressure. The line going into the reservoir should have a 2-micron filter attached to prevent particles from entering the LC system. The mobile phase should be made with high-purity water and chemicals. Most manufacturers offer "HPLC" grade solvent and water for LC mobile phases. Filtration of the mobile phase with a 0.45-micron filter is recommended to remove any particles that would clog the system.

Degassing or removal of dissolved air in the mobile phase is very important to minimize noise in the detector baseline and bubble problems in the pump. Mobile phase degassing may be accomplished by vacuum, sonication, heating, or helium sparging applied to the reservoir. Helium sparging is most commonly used. In this technique helium is gently bubbled through the mobile phase to remove the dissolved air. Another effective technique that is frequently used is simultaneous vacuum application and sonication. Heating effectively degasses mobile phases but is not very convenient.[3]

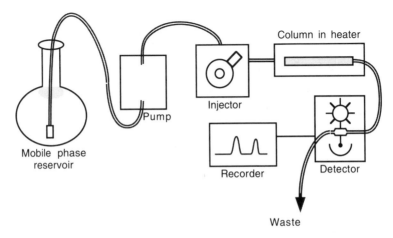

Figure 14-4.   Components of a liquid chromatography system.

Table 14-1
Gradient Program Example

Time(min)	%A Solvent	%B Solvent	Flow (mL/min)
0.0	95	5	1.0
4.0	80	20	1.0
10.0	50	50	1.0
15.0	0	100	1.0
17.0	0	100	1.5
20.0	95	5	1.5
24.0	95	5	1.0

PUMPS

A liquid chromatography pump is the heart of the LC system. The pump draws the mobile phase from the reservoir and forces it through the rest of the system. One mobile phase may be used and pumped at a constant flow rate, called isocratic elution, or several solvents can be used to make a gradient elution. Table 14-1 is an example of a gradient elution program using two different solvents and changing flow rates.

Several different types of pumps may be used including reciprocating-piston, syringe, tandem-piston, and piston-diaphragm pumps. *Reciprocating single-, double-, or triple-piston pumps* are used most commonly. Single-piston pumps deliver the mobile phase in a series of rapid pulses as depicted in Figure 14-5a. Usually, they need to have a pulse dampener attached to smooth out the flow, but that increases the back pressure in the system. Double-piston pumps are an improvement over the single-piston because as one piston is delivering the mobile phase, the other is refilling (Fig. 14-5b). Triple-piston pumps use three pump heads, offset to deliver and refill with mobile phase at different times to further reduce pulses in the flow rate (Fig 14-5c).

Modern *syringe pumps* use a single syringe compartment with plunger to push mobile phase througout the system. This configuration gives smooth, pulse-free flow. The limitation is that flow is interrupted while the syringe is refilling, so elution of the analytes must be completed within the volume of mobile phase contained in the syringe.

Tandem-piston, or *two-stage pumps,* use two pistons, but one delivers mobile phase at twice the rate of the other. As the faster pump delivers it also refills the first pump's chamber with mobile phase. This design is intended to smooth out pulses in the flow and is about as effective as the reciprocating double-piston pump.

Piston-diaphragm pumps have a diaphragm that separate the mobile phase from the pump. The piston pumps oil against the diaphragm, which then pushes the mobile phase through the system. The mobile phase does not come in contact with the piston, so no piston seals are needed.

All of the described pumps can be used in the isocratic mode for LC methods. To

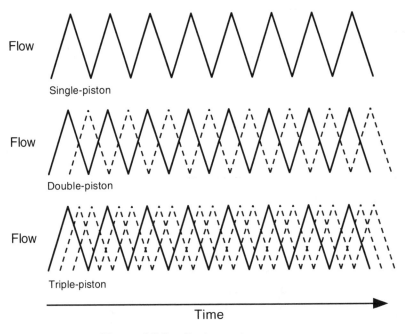

Figure 14-5. Reciprocating pumps.

do gradient elution, the pump must have a mixing device, either low pressure or high pressure. Low-pressure gradient systems mix the solvents needed before entry into the pump, and high-pressure gradient systems mix solvents after they have gone through the pump but before the mobile phase gets to the column.[4]

INJECTORS

The next component in a LC system is an injector (Fig. 14-4). Introduction of the sample mixture into the stream of mobile phase is accomplished through a sample injection valve. This valve can be a manual injector or an automatic injector such as an autosampler.

A *manual injector* has two positions, load and inject. In the load position the valve sends the flowing mobile phase straight through the valve, bypassing the sample loop. Sample can then be injected by a syringe into the sample loop without being carried away immediately by the mobile phase. When the valve is manually turned to the inject position, the mobile phase is rerouted through the sample loop and the sample mixture is then pushed into the stream and on to the column.

An *autosampler,* or *auto-injecter,* employs the same type of valve as the manual injector except that the sample loop is automatically filled between injections. A needle- or syringe-type apparatus withdraws sample from a vial and injects it into the sample loop. The valve automatically changes from the load position to the inject position by air pressure or electricity. The autosampler allows the LC

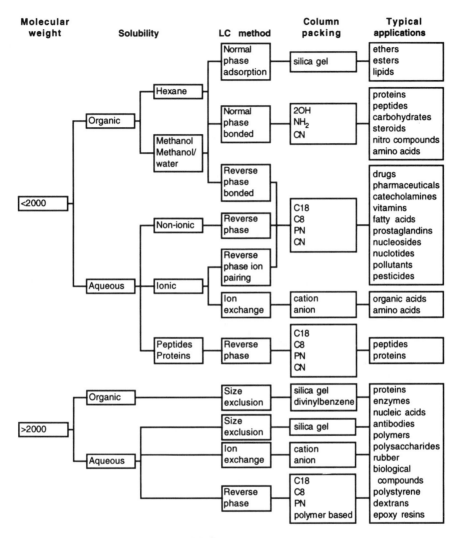

Figure 14-6. Column selection.

system operator to "walk-away" from the system, because sample injection is automatic.

COLUMNS

After injection, the sample encounters the *analytical column* where separation takes place (Fig. 14-4). A particular column is chosen based on the mixture that needs to be separated. Figure 14-6 is a flow diagram for selecting a column. First, the molecular weight of the analyte should be calculated. Then its solubility in water, hexane, and methanol is evaluated. Once these are known, then the LC method is determined and a column packing can be chosen. Each packing listed is manufactured by several different companies, and may differ slightly in selectivity for certain analytes. Also included in Figure 14-6 is a list of typical applications for the columns listed. Keep in mind that the reverse phase, C18 column is the most universally used column in LC chromatography.[5]

Small inner-diameter, microbore columns (1-2 mm) are relatively new and are used for *microbore LC*. They offer increased sensitivity, reduced solvent consumption, and reduced sample requirements.[6] Their disadvantage is that an LC system must be dedicated to that method. Microbore LC needs a syringe (pulseless) pump, small volume injectors, and detectors with low-volume flow cells.

Columns are relatively expensive, so they should be protected by a guard column placed between the injector and the column. The guard column is packed with the same material as the column and serves to collect particles and contaminants that would damage the analytical column. Guard column packing can be purchased loose and packed by the user or is available as a cartridge that can be discarded after use.

Some applications require that the column be at a temperature other than ambient or room temperature. Heating may be as simple as submersing the column in a temperature-controlled water bath or surrounding the column in a water jacket attached to a cold or warm water supply. More sophisticated heaters are available, such as forced air ovens or solid block heaters, with temperature controllers that more accurately regulate the temperature.

The most efficient separations are achieved when the entire system is plumbed with the proper tubing and fittings. Connections between components should be made with low-volume fittings especially made for LC work. Tubing is generally of two types, either stainless steel or polymeric such as Teflon or PEEK (poly-ether-ether-ketone). Tubing lengths should be as short as possible and the inner diameter small, generally 0.010 in.[3]

DETECTORS

In general, LC detectors are similar to other laboratory detectors described in this book, but they have flow cells instead cuvettes. Table 14-2 lists common detectors and their advantages/disadvantages.

Absorbance detectors, which measure absorbed light in the visible or UV regions of the spectrum, are probably the most used in LC. The detector responds to those analytes that absorb light at the selected wavelength. Absorbance detector types include: (1) Fixed wavelength absorbance detectors operate with monochromatic light given off by a specific lamp such as a low-pressure mercury arc discharge lamp at 254 nm. (2) Variable wavelength detectors operate with a broad spectrum light source (usually a deuterium lamp). A diffraction grating or prism monochromater is used to select a wavelength of light that passes through the flow cell to a single diode. (3) The diode array detector uses a deuterium lamp to pass light of all wavelengths through the flow cell. A monochromater splits the light into component wavelengths, which passes through the sample and strikes an array of diodes.

Table 14-2
Liquid Chromatographic Detectors

Detectors	Advantages	Disadvantages
UV/VIS fixed wavelength	Inexpensive Sensitive	Nonspecific
UV/VIS variable wavelength	Versatile	Less sensitive
UV/VIS diode array	Specific	Expensive
Fluorescence	Very sensitive Specific	Not all compounds fluoresce Instrument instability
Refractive index	Detects all compounds	Poor sensitivity
Electrochemical	Very sensitive Specific	High purity mobile phase free of O_2 and metal ions Frequent calibration

Fluorescence detectors measure light at a specific wavelength emitted from an analyte after it has been excited by light of a lower wavelength. (For principles of fluorometry, see Chapter 9). The intensity of the light emitted and detected by the photomultiplier tube is proportional to the concentration of the analyte. Fluorescence detection is very sensitive and selective, but not all compounds fluoresce, making its use somewhat limited.

Refractive index (RI) detectors measure the refractive index of an analyte as it flows through the cell. These detectors respond to all compounds, which makes the method nonspecific but useful when absorbance or fluorescence do not work. Its sensitivity is lower than other types of detectors.

Electrochemical detectors measure current caused by an electrochemical reaction (oxidation or reduction) that takes place at the surface of an electrode. As solute concentration increases, so does the current detected. These detectors are very specific and sensitive but must be calibrated often and demand high-purity mobile phases.[7]

DATA RECORDERS

The electronic signal generated by an LC detector is sent to a recording device that transforms the signal into an interpretable report for the user. *Strip-chart recorders* are the simplest data-gathering devices for an LC system. They convert the analog signal from the detector into a mechanically drawn picture or chromatogram of the analytes detected (Fig. 14-7). *Integrators* convert detector signals to chromatograms just as recorders do but are also able to do calculations of the peak height, peak area, and analyte concentration.

Computer data systems have been developed to act as recorders and integrators, as well as to store chromatogram information electronically. The data can be used, stored, or manipulated the next day or the next year. One step more advanced are *system controllers* that not only gather and manipulate the data from the detector but also control the pump, autoinjector, column heater, and detector. These

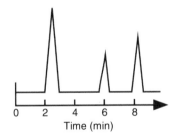

Figure 14-7.   Chromatograph as displayed by a strip-chart recorder.

system controllers enable LC operators to leave the system unattended as it is running.

SYSTEMS

Generally LC system are a series of modular components from one or several different manufacturers that are put together in a configuration necessary for the desired separation. As separation needs change, the components can be swapped around or replaced. However, there are some integrated systems built for a specific purpose—the component parts are not modular. The Beckman Amino Acid Analyzer model 6300 or 7300 (Beckman Instruments, Inc., Palo Alto, CA 94304) is a good example of an LC system in which all the component parts have been assembled in one instrument for a specific purpose—analyzing amino acids. The mobile phases, pumps, injector, column, detector, recorder, and system controller work as one unit. Additional data management is achieved with System Gold™ specialized software.

Bio-Rad's REMEDI™ Drug Analyzer (Bio-Rad Laboratories, Inc., Hercules, CA 94547) is another example of an LC system that is designed for a specific function. It has all the usual LC components but also can extract drugs from urine or blood using sample clean-up cartridges placed before the analytical column. In addition, the computer stores a library of UV scans to which unknowns are compared for identification.

The miniaturization of component parts enables manufacture of integrated LC systems that are not restricted to a single type of analysis. The Waters™ LC Module I (Millipore Corp., Waters Chromatography Div., Milford, MA 01757) is an example of a complete LC system with UV detection that requires just $17'' \times 20''$ of counter space, considerably less than a traditional modular LC system.

ADVANTAGES/DISADVANTAGES

One of the major advantages of LC is that most interferences can be eliminated either through the extraction process or by proper selection of the analytical column. If an interference is seen in the chromatogram, the mobile phase can usually be changed to separate the interferant from the analyte of interest. Thus, complex mixtures can be separated.

Table 14-3
Liquid Chromatography System Maintenance

Component	Activity	Frequency	Reference
Mobile phase	Filter and degas	Daily	Ref. 1, p. 140
Reservoir	Clean or replace	Monthly	Ref. 1, p. 155
Inlet-frit	Replace	As needed	Ref. 1, p. 158
Pump	Measure flow rate	Daily	Instrument manual
	Change seals	3-6 months	Instrument manual
	Clean check values	As needed	Instrument manual
Injector	Change manual injector seals	As needed	Instrument manual
	Prime autosampler lines and syringe	Daily	Instrument manual
Column	Record back pressure	Daily	Instrument manual
	Change in-line filter	50-100 injections	Instrument manual
	Change guard column	50-100 injections	Instrument manual
	Check column performance	3-6 months	Ref. 1, p. 298
	Check method linearity	6 months	Procedure manual
Detectors	Change lamp	As recommended	Instrument manual
	Clean flow cell	As needed	Ref. 1, p. 352
Recorder and integrators	Replace paper and pens	As needed	Instrument manual
Data system	Backup and store files	Weekly	Data system manual
LC system	Flush with water, then organic solvent	Daily	Instrument manual
	Clean air-intake filters	Monthly	Instrument manual
	Other	As recommended	Instrument manual

A disadvantage of LC compared to most laboratory analyses is that a sample extraction of some type is almost always needed to clean up the sample before injection on the system. Because LC is complex, method development and trouble-shooting of procedures are time-consuming and often tedious.

Maintenance and Quality Assurance

Most components of LC systems do not need large amounts of maintenance, but there are a few tasks that should be done regularly.[8] The manufacturer's maintenance guidelines for the component parts should be followed. General maintenance guide-lines are outlined in Table 14-3. The most important thing to remember is that a very clean mobile phase and sample reduce system maintenance.

Controls and standards should be run with each sample or group of samples.

Summary

Liquid chromatography is a chromatographic technique for the separation, detection, and quantitation of a wide variety of analytes. Four basic LC methods of separation are partition, adsorption, ion-exchange, and size exclusion. Reverse-phase partition chromatography is the most commonly used method. The components of the LC system include a mobile phase reservoir, pump, injector, column and heater, detector, and data recorder. Systems may be made up of modular components or an integrated instrument. Liquid chromatography can separate complex mixtures with few interferences, but method development can be difficult and labor-intensive. Instrument maintenance is necessary but not extensive.

Questions and Problems

1. Draw an LC system, and briefly describe the function of each component part.
2. List and describe the four basic methods of LC separation. Which is the most commonly used in LC?
3. Describe the differences in the flow of a liquid mobile phase produced by single-, double-, or triple-piston reciprocating pumps.
4. Which type of LC detector is the most versatile?
5. When developing an LC method for the detection of phenobarbital (an antiepileptic drug), your laboratory has available a cation exchange column, a C18 reverse phase column, and a silica gel column. Which would be the most logical choice with which to begin your method development?

References

1. Snyder LR, Kirkland JJ. Introduction to modern liquid chromatography. New York: John Wiley & Sons, 1979:17-24.
2. Burtis CA, Bowers LD, Chattoraj SC, Ullman MD. Chromatography. In: Tietz NW, ed. Fundamentals of clinical chemistry, 3rd ed. Philadelphia: WB Saunders, 1987:105-24.
3. Dolan JW, Snyder LR. Troubleshooting LC systems. Clifton, NJ: Humana Press, 1989:139-64, 201-34.
4. Parris NA. Instrumental liquid chromatography, 2nd ed. Journal of Chromatography Library, Vol. 27. New York: Elsevier Science Publishing, 1984:61-74.
5. Poole CF, Schuette SA. Contemporary practice of chromatography. New York: Elsevier Science Publishing, 1984:215-32.
6. Wong SHY. Supercritical fluid chromatography and microbore liquid chromatography for drug analysis. Clin Chem 1991, 37:1210-5.
7. Scott RPW. Liquid chromatography detectors, 2nd ed. Journal of Chromatography Library, Vol. 33. New York: Elsevier Science Publishing, 1986:89-151.
8. College of American Pathologists. Laboratory instrument manual: Evaluation, verification, and maintenance, 4th ed.: College of American Pathologists, Chicago, IL 1989:73-74.

Suggested Readings

Bowers LD. Liquid chromatography. In: Kaplan LA, Pesce AJ. Clinical chemistry: Theory, analysis, and correlation. St. Louis: CV Mosby, 1989:94-109.
Brown PR. High performance liquid chromatography: Past developments, present states, and future trends. Anal Chem 1990, 62:998-1008A.
Hanai T. Liquid chromatography in biomedical analysis. New York: Elsevier Science Publishing, 1991.

15

GAS CHROMATOGRAPHY

David S. Hage

Objectives

After completing this chapter, the reader will be able to:

1. Define gas chromatography and describe its basic principles.
2. Describe the different types of carrier gases and stationary phases used in gas chromatography (GC).
3. List the instrumental components of a gas chromatographic system.
4. Describe the operation and use of common gas chromatographic detectors.
5. Discuss the routine maintenance and quality control of a gas chromatographic system.

Definitions

Acylation: Conversion of a compound into an acetate derivative for injection on to a GC system.

Adjusted Retention Time or Adjusted Retention Volume (t_r' or V_r'): A measure of compound retention calculated by subtracting the system void time or volume (t_m or V_m) from the compound's retention time or volume (t_r or V_r).

Alkylation: A derivatization method in which an alkyl group is added to some active functional group on the solute.

Bonded-Phase Gas Chromatography: A technique in GC that uses a stationary phase that is chemically bonded to the support material.

Carrier Gas: A term used to describe the mobile phase in GC.

Chromatogram: A plot of detector response versus elution time or volume on a chromatographic system.

Chromatography: A separation technique based on the different interactions of sample compounds with two phases, a mobile phase and a stationary phase, as the compounds travel through a supporting medium.

Electron Capture Detector (ECD):   A radiation-based GC detector selective for compounds containing electronegative elements.

Flame Ionization Detector (FID):   A GC detector based on the ability of compounds to produce ions when burned in a flame.

Gas Chromatography (GC):   A chromatographic technique in which the mobile phase is a gas.

Gas Chromatography/Mass Spectrometry (GC/MS):   An analytical method that uses GC for compound separation and mass spectrometry for compound detection.

Gas-Liquid Chromatography (GLC):   A GC technique that uses a liquid stationary phase coated on to a solid support.

Gas-Solid Chromatography (GSC):   A GC technique that uses the same solid material as both the support and stationary phase.

Headspace Analysis: An injection technique based on the presence of volatile solutes in the vapor phase above a liquid sample.

Height Equivalent of a Theoretical Plate (H or HETP):   The length of a column needed to generate one theoretical plate.

Inlet Splitter: Device used to apply only a portion of an injected sample onto a GC column.

Isothermal Elution: Elution of compounds on a chromatographic system at a constant temperature.

Kovat's Retention Index: A measure of retention determined by comparing the adjusted retention time of the solute of interest to the adjusted retention times of *n*-alkanes analyzed under the same chromatographic conditions.

Mobile Phase: The solvent used to elute sample components from a chromatographic column.

Nitrogen-Phosphorus Detector (NPD):   A GC detector based on the ability of compounds to produce ions when burned in the presence of an alkali metal vapor.

Number of Theoretical Plates (N):   A measure of the efficiency or width of sample peaks on a chromatographic system.

Porous Layer Open Tubular Column (PLOT):   Capillary column coated with a thin layer of a glass powder or a microcrystalline material, followed by a film of liquid stationary phase.

Retention Time or Retention Volume (t_r or V_r):   The time or elution volume required for a retained compound to elute from a chromatographic system.

Silica Capillary Column: Capillary column with silica stationary phase chemically bonded to the walls of the capillary.

Silylation: A derivatization method in which hydrogens on a compound are replaced with alkylsilyl groups.

Single-Ion Monitoring (SIM):   A detection mode in GC/MS in which only a few ions characteristic of the compound(s) of interest are monitored.

Splitless Injection: Sample injection method in which solute is applied in a large volume of a volatile solvent in order to help to decrease the initial width of the sample peak on the chromatographic system.

Stationary Phase: A chemical layer that is coated or covalently attached to the support material in a column.

Support-Coated Open Tubular Column (SCOT):   A capillary column coated with a thin layer of a particulate support, followed by a thin film of a liquid stationary phase.

Temperature Programming: An elution technique in which the temperature of the chromatographic system is varied with time.

Thermal Conductivity Detector: A GC detector based on the ability of solutes in the carrier gas to conduct heat away from a hot wire.

Total Ion Current (TIC):   A GC/MS detection mode in which all ions produced from eluting compounds are monitored.

Void Time or Void Volume (t_m or V_m):   The time or volume it takes a nonretained compound to elute from a chromatographic system.

Wall-Coated Open Tubular Column (WCOT):   Capillary column using a thin film of a liquid stationary phase coated directly on the walls of the column.

Introduction

Gas chromatography (GC) has long been a popular method for separating and analyzing compounds. The popularity of this technique comes from its high resolving power and low limits of detection, as well as its speed, accuracy, and reproducibility. Gas chromatography is used if the compounds to be separated are either naturally volatile or can be easily converted into a volatile form. This makes it especially useful in the determination of small organic molecules, including drugs, amino acids, and numerous other biologically active compounds. Common clinical applications include therapeutic drug monitoring, detection of drugs of abuse, emergency room testing, and amino acid analysis.

In this chapter I will begin with a short description of the theory behind GC, discuss what factors affect its ability to separate compounds, and offer a detailed look at instrumentation used in GC and common techniques used in GC sample analysis. I will then present some guidelines for the maintenance and quality control of GC systems.

Principles

Gas chromatography may be defined as a chromatographic method based on the use of a mobile phase that is a gas. Like any other type of chromatography, the separation of compounds by GC is based on the different interactions of sample compounds with two phases, a mobile phase and a stationary phase, as the compounds travel through a supporting medium. The mobile phase refers to the solvent (a gas in the case of GC) that is continuously applied to a column. The stationary phase refers to a solvent or chemical layer that is coated or attached to a solid support in the column.

As sample components travel through a GC column, they interact with the mobile phase and stationary phase to different degrees. Those interacting strongly with the stationary phase spend a longer time in the column and elute later than weakly interacting components. This results in the separation of sample components as they pass through the column. A plot of the amount of each component eluting off the column with time (or mobile phase volume) is referred to as a *chromatogram*. An example of a typical GC chromatogram is shown in Figure 15-1.

As with any chromatographic system, the ability of GC to separate two compounds depends on two factors: the difference in the retention of the two compounds,

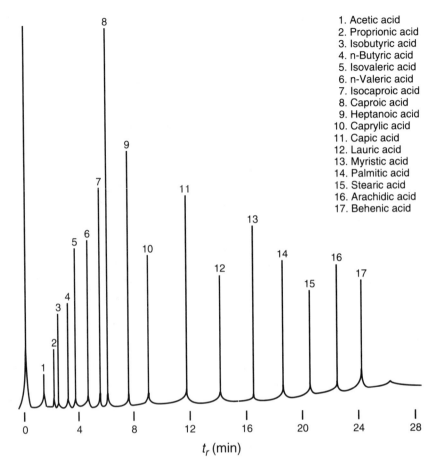

Figure 15-1. Typical gas chromatogram. *(Restek Corporation, 110 Benner Circle, Bellefonte, PA 16823. Reproduced with permission.)*

and the width of their peaks, or the efficiency of the system. As already discussed, the retention of a compound depends on how it interacts with the stationary phase and mobile phase present in the system. This can be described by using the *retention time* (t_r) or *retention volume* (V_r) of a compound. If the system's *void time* (t_m) or *void volume* (V_m) is known (i.e., the elution time or elution volume of a nonretained solute), then the *adjusted retention time* (t_r') or *adjusted retention volume* (V_r') of a compound can also be used in describing retention, where

$$t_r' = t_r - t_m \qquad\qquad\qquad \text{(Eq. 15-1)}$$

$$V_r' = V_r - V_m \qquad\qquad\qquad \text{(Eq. 15-2)}$$

Any of these retention parameters can be used in solute identification, because the values of t_r and V_r (or t_r' and V_r') are characteristic for a compound under a given set of chromatographic conditions. The identity of an unknown compound injected on to a GC system can often be determined by comparing the retention parameters for the unknown to those determined for reference compounds. Another measure of retention commonly used in GC is the Kovat's retention index (I). The value of I for a compound is determined by comparing the compound's adjusted retention time to the adjusted retention times of n-alkanes injected on to the same column and under identical conditions. The value of I for the compound of interest is then calculated as follows:

$$I = 100\,n + 100\,[\log t_{r'(X)} - \log t_{r'(n)}]/[\log t_{r'(n+1)} - \log t_{r'(n)}] \qquad \text{(Eq. 15-3)}$$

where

$t_{r'(X)}$ = adjusted retention time of the compound of interest
n = carbon number of the n-alkane eluting just prior to compound X
$t_{r'(n)}$ = adjusted retention time of the n-alkane eluting just prior to compound X
$t_{r'(n+1)}$ = adjusted retention time of the n-alkane that elutes just after compound X

One advantage of using the Kovat's retention index over other measures of retention, such as t_r and V_r, is that the value of I shows less variation with temperature. The Kovat's retention index also provides a measure of compound polarity that is useful in stationary phase selection.

The efficiency of a chromatographic system is determined by the stationary and mobile phases used in a separation, as well as the type of support in the column, the flow rate of the mobile phase, and many other factors. To compare the efficiencies of different chromatographic systems, one measure that may be used is the number of theoretical plates (N), where

$$N = 16\,(t_r/W_b)^2 \qquad \text{(Eq. 15-4)}$$

where

t_r = retention time of a compound
W_b = baseline width of the compound's peak.

The larger the value of N is for a column, the greater the column's separating power or efficiency. To compare columns of different lengths, another measure of efficiency that is used is the height equivalent of a theoretical plate (H or HETP):

$$H = L/N \qquad \text{(Eq. 15-5)}$$

where

L = length of the column
N = number of theoretical plates

Note that H is simply a measure of the distance along the column that is needed to generate one theoretical plate. Thus, the smaller the value of H is, the better the separating power or efficiency of the column.

Mobile and Stationary Phases

Gas chromatography differs from other chromatographic techniques in that its mobile phase, a gas, plays little or no role in determining a compound's retention on the GC system. Retention is instead determined mostly by a compound's volatility and the degree to which it interacts with the stationary phase. This results from the fact that the gaseous mobile phase has a much lower density and chance for interacting with the compound than the solid or liquid that makes up the stationary phase. Because the main purpose of the gas in GC simply is to move solutes along the column, the mobile phase in this technique is often simply referred to as the carrier gas. Examples of common carrier gases used in GC are hydrogen, helium, nitrogen, and argon.

Although the carrier gas does not greatly affect solute retention, the choice of which gas to use is important in other ways. Factors that need to be considered in choosing a carrier gas include: (1) efficiency of the chromatographic system, (2) stability of the column and compounds to be studied, (3) type of detector being used, and (4) possible risks or hazards involved in using the gas. Efficiency is affected by the carrier gas through changes it creates in a compound's rate of diffusion into the stationary phase. Low-molecular-weight gases, such as helium or hydrogen, produce much larger rates of compound diffusion than heavier gases, such as nitrogen or argon. This is important because faster diffusion produces narrower peaks and allows faster separations.

Column or compound stability can be important when using a carrier gas such as hydrogen, which can react with sample components or with the stationary phase. Detector performance must also be considered in carrier gas selection. For example, a thermal conductivity detector requires the use of hydrogen or helium, carrier gases that have thermal conductivities very different from those of most sample components. Hazards associated with the carrier gas are important to consider when working with hydrogen, which is potentially explosive and requires special precautions in its use.

The stationary phase in GC is important because it is the main factor in determining the selectivity and retention of compounds. There are three types of stationary phases used in GC: solid adsorbents, liquids coated on solid supports, and bonded-phase supports.

If solid adsorbents are used, the separation method is referred to as *gas-solid chromatography (GSC)*. In this technique, the same material acts as both the stationary phase and support material. Examples of supports used in GSC include alumina, silica, molecular sieves, and active carbon. Although GSC was the first type of gas chromatography developed, it is currently not as widely used as other GC methods. One reason for this is the strong retention that GSC columns have for most solutes. Catalytic changes in sample components can also occur on GSC supports. In addition, GSC supports tend to have a range of chemical and physical environments present on their surfaces, often giving rise to nonsymmetrical peaks and variable retention times. Advantages of GSC include its long column lifetimes and its ability to retain and separate some compounds, such as geometrical isomers or permanent gases, that are not easily resolved by other chromatographic methods.

Gas-liquid chromatography (GLC) is a GC technique in which the stationary phase is a liquid coated on a solid support. Liquids used for GLC can be based on polymers, hydrocarbons, fluorocarbons, and even molten salts or liquid crystals. These liquids are typically coated onto supports prepared from diatomaceous earth, such as Chromosorb P or Chromosorb W. Over 400 liquid stationary phases are available for use in GC, but only about 6 to 12 are needed for most applications. Liquid stationary phases recommended[1,2] for use in GLC cover a wide range of

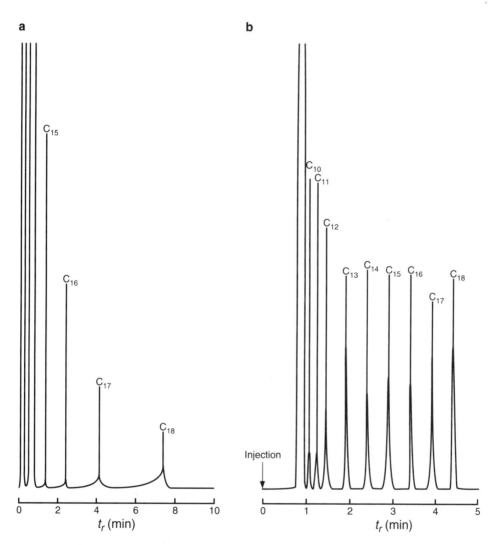

Figure 15-2.   Comparison of C_{10} to C_{18} *n*-alkanes determined by (a) isothermal elution and (b) temperature programming. *(Nygren S. Fester GC analyses performed by flow programming in short capillary columns. J Hiph Resolut Chromatogr 1979, 2:319-23. Reproduced with permission.)*

polarities. Because polar compounds will be most strongly retained on a polar material and nonpolar compounds will be most strongly retained on a nonpolar material, proper selection of the stationary phase is an important factor in controlling the retention and selectivity of compounds on a GLC column.

One problem with using a liquid stationary phase in GC is that the liquid may slowly be lost from the column with time. This is particularly a problem if high temperatures are being used in the GC system. Such loss of the stationary phase is undesirable because it contributes to the background signal of the detector and changes the characteristics of the column with time. One way this loss can be avoided is to use stationary phases that are covalently attached to the support. The use of covalently linked stationary phases in GC is known as a *bonded-phase gas chromatography*. Advantages of using bonded-phase supports are that they are more stable than liquid stationary phases and allow for faster, more efficient separations. As with liquid stationary phases, many bonded phases are available, but only a few are required for most separations.

Besides changing the stationary phase used in the GC system, retention of compounds can also be adjusted by changing the temperature of the column. This affects the volatility of the compounds and the degree to which they interact with the stationary phase. If a constant temperature is used in a GC separation, the technique is referred to as an *isothermal method*. If the temperature is varied with the time, the technique is called *temperature programming*. Temperature programming is commonly used in GC for samples containing a large number of different components. By proper selection of the starting temperature and the way in which the temperature is changed during the run, good resolution of both weakly and strongly retained compounds can be achieved in a minimum amount of time. An example of the use of temperature programming in GC is given in Figure 15-2.

Instrumentation

A schematic diagram of a typical GC system is illustrated in Figure 15-3. An example of a commercial GC system[3] is shown in Figure 15-4. The basic design of a GC system consists of five main components: a mobile phase source, an injector, a column, a detector, and a computer or recorder for data acquisition.

MOBILE PHASE SOURCE

The mobile phase source in a GC system is usually a standard gas cylinder with a two-stage regulator for pressure control. By regulating the pressure of the released gas, the flow rate of the gas through the column is also controlled. The flow rate of the carrier gas can be measured by using either bubble or thermal mass flow meters. The carrier gas used in GC should be of high purity (i.e., >99.995% pure) or should be purified prior to use. Impurities can be removed by passing the gas through a series of traps for water, oxygen, or organic matter. Particulate matter may be removed by

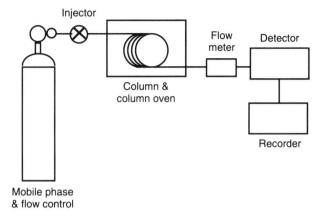

Figure 15-3.   Typical GC system.

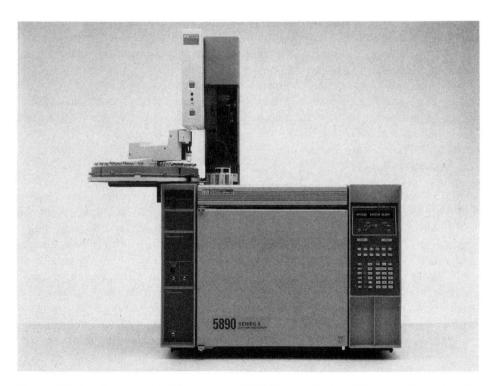

Figure 15-4.   Commercial GC system. *(© 1992 Hewlett-Packard Company. Reproduced with permission.)*

fritted filters. Removal of such impurities is needed to avoid contamination of the chromatographic system, giving rise to a loss in sensitivity and resolution.

In some cases it is necessary to use special control devices to maintain constant flow of the carrier gas as the temperature or pressure of the system is varied. This is particularly important in systems where capillary columns or temperature programming[4] are being used. Good flow rate and pressure control are also important in obtaining highly reproducible column efficiencies and resolutions. This is best done by regulating pressure and flow rate at both the inlet and outlet of the column.

INJECTION METHODS AND DERIVATIZATION TECHNIQUES

Either manual methods or autoinjectors can be used to inject compounds on to a GC system. For naturally volatile compounds, direct injection onto the GC system is often possible. For gaseous solutes, this is done by using a gas-tight sampling valve and syringe. The valve usually has two positions, one for loading sample into the loop, and one for placing the contents of the loop into the carrier gas stream.

Volatile liquids or solids can be applied directly to the GC system as long as they are dissolved in a solvent that does not overlap with their peaks or contain nonvolatile material that will deposit in the injector or column. If a packed column is being used, such compounds are injected by using a microsyringe placed into a heated injection port. As the compounds are injected into the port, they are quickly volatilized and taken by the carrier gas to the column.

For thermally unstable compounds, a heated injection port can be a problem in that it may cause decomposition of the sample. For these types of compounds, direct injection of the sample on to the column is sometimes used. This allows for a lower injection temperature.

Headspace Analysis

Headspace analysis is an injection technique used for compounds that are naturally volatile but as present in a solution that also contains nonvolatile or interfering components. This method is based on the fact that volatile solutes in solution will also be present in the vapor phase immediately above the solution. By sampling this vapor phase, known as the headspace, volatile solutes can be collected and injected without interference from less volatile sample components. Headspace analysis can be performed in one of two ways: the static method, and the dynamic method. In the *static method,* the sample solution is placed in a closed container, and solute is allowed to distribute between the liquid and vapor phases at a constant temperature. After equilibrium has been reached, a sample of the vapor phase is taken and injected on to the GC system. One problem with this method is that good control of the temperature and volume of sample withdrawn are needed for reproducible results. In addition, compounds with only modest volatilities may be difficult to detect by this approach. An alternative technique is the *dynamic method,* in which an inert gas is continually passed over or through the liquid sample. This gas carries with it any volatile compounds. This gas is then passed through a cold trap or solid adsorbent that collects and concentrates the volatile solutes. After collection, the solutes are then removed from the trap and applied to the column. Although this technique requires more time and effort than the static method, it is also more reproducible and allows better detection of compounds with relatively low volatilities.

Derivatization

For many compounds, the molecule of interest may not be volatile enough for any of these injection techniques to be used. One approach that is used in this case is to derivatize the compound into a more volatile form. *Derivatization* can be used not only to increase the volatility of a compound but also to increase its thermal stability, its response on the detector, and its separation from other sample components. Most derivatization reactions used in GC can be classified into one of three groups: (1) silylation, (2) alkylation, and (3) acylation. Almost all such reactions are designed to be performed with minimal amounts of sample or reagents (i.e., 0.1-2.0 mL) and are typically carried out at room temperature. Most of these reactions can be performed using kits that are commercially available.

Silylation is probably the most common of these derivatization techniques. It involves replacing hydrogens on a solute (e.g., R-OH, R-CO$_2$H, R-NH$_2$, etc.) with alkylsilyl groups, such as $-SiMe_3$. The result is that the compound is converted into a less polar, more volatile, and more thermally stable form. The most common reagent used in silylation is trimethylchlorosilane (TMS). However, a number of other silylation reagents can also be used.

The second type of derivatization, *alkylation,* involves the addition of an alkyl group to some active functional group on the solute. A common example is the esterification of a carboxylic acid, forming a volatile methyl ester. It is commonly performed by using borontrifluoride in methanol as the reagent.

The third technique, *acylation,* involves the conversion of a solute into an acetate derivative. It is often used to improve the volatility of alcohols, phenols, and amine-containing compounds or to increase their response on an electron-capture detector. Trifluoroacetic anhydride (TFAA) is one common reagent used for acylation. Other reagents used for this are the N-fluoroacylimidazoles. The latter group of reagents is used for compounds containing hydroxy groups, secondary amines, or tertiary amines in their structure.

Inlet Splitters and Splitless Injectors

Beside compound volatility, another factor that must be considered in choosing an injection technique for a GC system is whether a packed column or capillary column is being used. This is important because capillary columns are much more efficient than packed GC columns, which also makes them more susceptible to peak broadening due to large injector volumes. To overcome this problem, several special injection techniques have been developed for use with capillary columns. Two common approaches are to use inlet splitters and splitless, or direct, injection. In both cases the aim is to apply a narrow plug of sample to the column without causing excessive broadening of the resulting peaks in the chromatogram.

Inlet splitters are used if the compounds of interest are reasonably volatile, thermally stable, and make up between 0.001 and 10% of the sample composition. In this method, the sample is placed into the injection port and vaporized. As the sample leaves the injection port, only a small portion is applied to the column while the remainder goes to waste. To minimize the time that the sample spends in the injector, a high carrier gas flow rate and high injector temperature are used. The main difficulty with inlet splitters is that solutes with different volatilities may not be divided between the column and waste streams in the same ratio. This can cause variability in the recovery of these compounds and can affect their final quantitation.

In *splitless injection* the sample is injected with a large volume of a volatile solvent. As this combination is applied to the column, the volatile solvent travels ahead of compounds in the sample. This forms a thick layer of liquid around the support material at the top of the column and greatly increases retention of the sample components as they reach that region. The result is that a narrow sample plug forms at the top of the column, helping to decrease the initial width of the sample peak on the chromatographic system.

COLUMNS

In a GC system the column is usually enclosed in an oven that precisely and accurately controls its temperature. The oven is well insulated and is equipped with fans to produce a uniform temperature. Most GC ovens allow control over a wide range of temperature (e.g., -50 to $450°C$) and can be programmed for a variety of temperature changes during a run. Typical temperature changes performed with these ovens involve linear gradients of 0 to $30°C/min$.

The column used in GC can be either a packed column or a capillary column. *Packed columns* are usually 1 to 2 m long, a few millimeters in diameter, and filled with support particles coated with the desired stationary phase. *Capillary,* or *open-tubular, columns* range from 10 to 30 m in length, have inner diameters of 0.1 to 0.5 mm, and have stationary phase located only on or near their interior surface. Capillary columns generally have higher efficiencies and better limits of detection than packed columns, making them better for analytical applications. However, packed columns have a larger sample capacity and require less care and training in their use.

For capillary columns, there are several ways in which the stationary phase can be coated on the column's interior surface. In wall-coated open tubular columns (WCOT), a thin film of a liquid stationary phase is coated directly on the walls of the column. These columns are typically very efficient but have a small sample capacity due to their low surface area. In support-coated open tubular columns (SCOT), the column is coated with a thin layer of a particulate support, such as diatomaceous earth. A thin film of a liquid stationary phase is then coated on this layer of support material. This gives SCOT columns a larger surface area and thicker layer of stationary phase than WCOT columns. The result is a less efficient system but also one with a larger sample capacity. Porous layer open tubular columns (PLOT) are similar to SCOT columns but use a thin layer of a glass powder or a microcrystalline material on the walls of the column rather than a particulate support. Their behavior is the same as SCOT columns. Silica capillary columns consist of a stationary phase chemically bonded to the walls of the capillary. They are highly efficient and stable but do have a limited sample capacity. This type of column is becoming increasingly popular in clinical methods based on GC.

DETECTORS

After the column, the next important component of the GC system is the detector. There are many types of detectors available for GC, but only a few are commonly used. Examples of the more common GC detectors include (1) the thermal conductivity detector, (2) the flame ionization detector, (3) the nitrogen-phosphorus detector, (4) the electron capture detector, and (5) detectors based on mass spectrometry.

Thermal Conductivity Detectors

The *thermal conductivity detector,* also known as a *katherometer,* or *hot-wire, detector,* was the first universal detector developed for GC. It measures a bulk property of the carrier gas, namely, its ability to conduct heat away from a hot wire. This ability changes as solutes elute from the column, allowing the solutes to be detected.

To detect the thermal conductivity of the carrier gas, an electronic circuit known as a Wheatstone bridge (explained in Chapter 1) is used. This circuit (Fig. 15-5) consists of four resistors, arranged in a parallel circuit with two resistors in each arm. When the resistors in the circuit are properly balanced, the potential measured by the

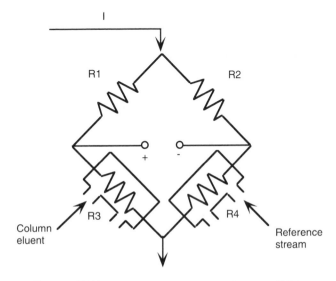

Figure 15-5.   Thermal conductivity detector (TCD).

electrometer at the center is equal to zero. If the resistance of one of the arms changes, a nonzero potential is produced. This circuit is used in a thermal conductivity detector by placing one of the resistors in contact with carrier gas leaving the column (i.e., column effluent). A second resistor is usually placed in a reference stream containing only pure carrier gas. As current is passed through the circuit, the wires in the resistors are heated. For the resistors in contact with the carrier gas, some of this heat is removed. The extent of the heat removal depends on the carrier gas's thermal conductivity. As compounds elute from the column, thermal conductivity in the carrier gas changes. This changes the amount of heat removed from the corresponding resistor and the resistor's temperature. As the resistor heats or cools, its resistance changes. The result is that the Wheatstone bridge is no longer balanced and a voltage difference is produced that can be measured.

In order for a thermal conductivity detector to respond to a compound, it is necessary that the carrier gas have a thermal conductivity different from that of the compounds to be detected. Hydrogen and helium are the carrier gases with thermal conductivities most different from those of common inorganic and organic compounds, but hydrogen is not usually used with thermal conductivity detectors because it can react with metal oxides present on the resistors. Thus, helium is the carrier gas of choice for this type of detector.

The main advantage of the thermal conductivity detector is that it is applicable to the detection of almost any compound. It is also nondestructive, making it useful for preparative scale work. The fact that it is nondestructive means that it can also be used in combination with other types of GC detectors. Some disadvantages of a thermal conductivity detector are that it responds to impurities in the carrier gas and is highly sensitive to changes in flow rate. Another disadvantage is its limit of detection, which is approximately 10^{-6} to 10^{-8} g of solute/mL carrier gas. This level is 10^3 to 10^7 times higher than can be measured by other types of GC detectors.

Flame Ionization Detectors

The *flame ionization detector (FID)* is perhaps the most common type of GC detector. It is also a "universal" detector because it is capable of measuring the presence of almost any organic substance and many inorganic compounds. An FID detects compounds by measuring their ability to produce ions when burned in a flame. A diagram of a typical FID is shown in Figure 15-6. In an FID, the flame is usually formed by burning the compounds in the carrier gas with a mixture of hydrogen and air. Ions produced by the flame are collected by an electrode surrounding the flame. As ions are produced, they create a current, allowing the eluting compound to be detected.

One advantage of an FID is that it will detect essentially any organic compound, yet will not respond to many common carrier gases or impurities, such as water, ammonia, nitrogen, helium, hydrogen, and carbon dioxide. The limit of detection of an FID for organic compounds is also quite good, being approximately 10^{-13} g of carbon/sec. This is approximately 100 to 1000-fold lower than the limits of detection that can be obtained with a TCD.

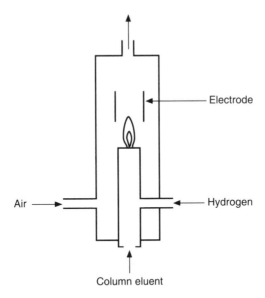

Figure 15-6.   Flame ionization detector (FID).

Nitrogen-Phosphorus Detectors

A more selective type of GC detector is the *nitrogen-phosphorus detector (NPD),* also known as an *alkali flame ionization detector* or a *thermionic detector.* As its name implies, the NPD is used mainly in the determination of nitrogen- or phosphorus-containing compounds. In principle, the NPD is similar to an FID in that both are based on the measurement of ions produced by compounds burning in a flame. The main difference is that the flame used in an NPD contains a small amount of vapor from an alkali metal, such as rubidium, that greatly enhances the formation of ions from nitrogen- and phosphorus-containing compounds.

The ability of an NPD to preferentially detect compounds containing nitrogen or phosphorus makes it especially useful in the detection of organophosphate pesticides and in the determination of amine-containing drugs. Like an FID, the NPD does not detect many common carrier gases or impurities. The NPD differs from an FID in that it is more sensitive when detecting nitrogen- and phosphorus-containing compounds. It does have some response to organic compounds, but at a level typically less than that seen in an FID. Beside nitrogen and phosphorus, an NPD also has an improved response versus an FID for the detection of compounds containing sulfur, halogens, and arsenic.

Electron Capture Detectors

The *electron capture detector (ECD)* is another type of selective detector used in GC. An ECD (Fig. 15-7) is a radiation-based detector that is selective for compounds

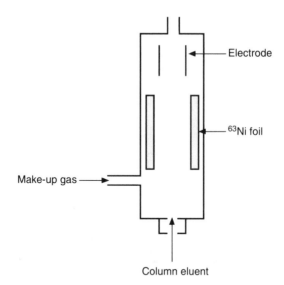

Figure 15-7.   Electron capture detector (ECD).

containing electronegative elements, such as halogen atoms. It detects compounds based on the capture of electrons by electronegative atoms in the molecule. The electrons to be captured are produced by a radioactive source, such as ^{3}H or ^{63}Ni. Both of these radiation sources emit beta-particles (i.e., high-energy electrons) as part of their natural decay process. As these high-energy electrons are released, they collide with the carrier gas, usually argon or nitrogen. This produces a large number of secondary, or thermal, electrons containing lower amounts of energy. In the absence of compounds eluting from the column, a steady stream of secondary electrons is produced that goes to a collector electrode and produces a current. When a compound containing electronegative atoms elutes from the column, the compound's atoms capture some of the secondary electrons and reduce the current produced at the collector electrode. This decrease in current allows the compound to be detected.

The design of an ECD consists of a radiation source and a collector electrode. The carrier gas used must be one that is easily ionized, such as argon or nitrogen. This is needed for the production of secondary electrons in the detector. A trace amount of methane is also usually included in the carrier gas to maintain the production of secondary electrons and to create a stable detector response.

An ECD can be used to detect most compounds containing electronegative atoms, such as halogen-, nitro-, and sulfur-containing compounds. It can also be used to detect polynuclear aromatic compounds, anhydrides, and conjugated carbonyl compounds. The ECD is widely used for the determination of chlorinated pesticides, polynuclear aromatic carcinogens, and organometallic compounds.

Mass Spectrometers

One additional type of detector commonly used in GC is the *mass spectrometer.* The resulting combination of GC and mass spectrometry, known as GC/MS, is a powerful tool for both quantitating and identifying compounds in complex samples. This technique is presently the technique of choice for many analytical applications. It is especially useful in screening for drugs in urine or serum, as well as in identifying the presence of a wide range of other components in biological fluids. The basis of mass spectrometry (MS) is discussed in detail in the following chapter.

RECORDERS

The last component of a typical GC system is the data-recording system, which can range from a simple strip-chart recorder to a dedicated computer. Its purpose is to acquire and store data obtained from the GC detector. For many types of detectors, such as a thermal conductivity detector or an FID, a simple strip-chart recorder or integrator is adequate for most analytical applications. Most detector manufacturers have computers and software available for processing data from their equipment. Beside data management and analysis, computer systems for GC are also increasingly being used in compound identification and in maintaining records for quality control of the GC system.

Maintenance and Quality Assurance

The reliable performance of any analytical method requires the establishment of a preventive maintenance and quality control program. The exact maintenance required by a GC system depends on its individual components; however, there are several guidelines that apply to most systems. For example, one item that frequently needs periodic care is the carrier gas supply and gas flow system. In order to obtain reproducible system behavior, it is necessary to verify that these components are free of leaks and contaminants. We have already discussed techniques for reducing carrier gas contaminants. Leaks in a GC system can be detected by pressurizing the suspected components, capping off the components, turning off the gas supply, and looking for a decrease in pressure with time. The exact location of a leak can be determined by using a leak detection fluid.

The injection port may require routine cleaning and replacement of parts. One item that needs frequent replacement is the septum. A leaky septum will give rise to low column flow rates, producing longer apparent retention times and/or decreased detector response. The lifetime of a septum will be determined by the number of injections made on the system and the quality of the injection needle. A smooth, sharp needle with no burrs or rough edges is best for obtaining long septum lifetimes. Regular replacement of septa is recommended. Daily replacement may be required if large number of samples are injected.

New columns or columns that have been stored for extended periods often have volatile contaminants present that have been adsorbed from the air or that remain from previous injections. It is recommended that these columns be conditioned prior to routine use to remove such contaminants. The specific procedure to use in column conditioning will depend on the column type. The manufacturer will typically provide detailed instructions for this process. The conditioning process usually involves first turning off the detector and its support gases and connecting the column to the carrier gas inlet flow stream, while leaving the outlet end disconnected from the detector. Disconnecting the column from the detector avoids contamination of the detector by adsorbed components leaving the column during the conditioning. A He or N_2 carrier gas is next applied to the column at a stable flow rate. The column is initially held at 100°C for an hour and is then slowly heated until a temperature about 30°C below its maximum operating temperature is reached. The column is kept at this temperature for 8 to 12 hours and then allowed to cool. After the conditioning process, the column can either be capped and stored or connected to the rest of the GC system for use in routine analysis.

Once a column is in use, two items that should be routinely monitored are the column's efficiency and retention. Both of these parameters can be examined by periodically making injections of a standard test solution on to the system and recording the retention time (t_r) or Kovat's retention index (I) for each test solute. The peak widths can be used to determine the efficiency of the system (i.e., N or H). The test solution for this monitoring may contain common analytes determined by the laboratory or a test mixture suggested by the column manufacturer. Many column manufacturers use a test mixture developed by the Grob team[5] or a mixture outlined in Rotzsche[6] for this type of evaluation.

The GC detector also requires routine maintenance for optimum performance. Most GC detectors will need periodic cleaning to remove accumulated particulate matter, such as silica or soot. If not removed, these deposits can lead to decreased detector sensitivity and increased detector noise. Flame ionization and nitrogen-phosphorus detectors can be cleaned by partially disassembling the detector cell and wiping with a swab dipped in an appropriate solvent. Cleaning of an ECD or TCD is sometimes done by "backing out" adsorbed impurities. This process is performed by placing an empty column into system, establishing a normal flow of gas through the detector, and raising the detector temperature to 350 to 400°C for an extended period of time. The exact conditions to use can be obtained from the detector's manufacturer.

Items that need periodic replacement on GC detectors include the resistor filaments in a TCD or parts of the gas flow valves in an FID or NPD. If an ECD is found to be defective, the entire detector cell should be exchanged for a new assembly to avoid contamination from the radioactive source. An ECD should also be monitored for radioactive leaks at least once every 6 months by using a wipe test. More frequent testing for leaks may be required with heavy detector use.

Summary

Gas chromatography remains one of the most common and popular analytical methods available for sample separation and analysis. In this chapter we examined some of the basic principles behind the operation of GC and have discussed various carrier gases and stationary phases used in this technique. Types of GC described included gas-solid chromatography, gas-liquid chromatography, and bonded-phase GC. We also discussed the use of packed and capillary columns. Instrumental components for GC systems include the carrier gas sources, injectors, column ovens, recorders, and various detectors. Together, these components allow GC to be used for a variety of different types of samples with fast and sensitive detection. This is particularly true for naturally volatile compounds. For compounds that are less volatile, this chapter presented a number of different approaches that can be used for sample injection or derivatization. Means were also described for assessing the efficiency and retention of GC systems. Implementing these procedures allows for effective quality control of a GC analysis. The overall result is a powerful and reliable analytical technique.

Questions and Problems

1. Describe what is meant by the terms *gas-liquid chromatography* and *bonded-phase gas chromatography.* How do these techniques compare?
2. What are the differences between a packed GC column and a capillary GC column?
3. Which GC detectors can be used to monitor the following compounds: (a) A series of acidic drugs containing only C, H, and O in their structure? (b) A chlorinated organic pesticide? (c) A drug containing an amine (H_2N-) group in its structure?
4. Describe how each of the following GC detectors works: (a) ECD. (b) TCD. (c) FID.
5. Compare and contrast each of the following injection techniques: (a) Direct injection. (b) Headspace analysis. (c) Splitless injection.
6. The following data were obtained for a series of compounds injected on to a GLC system. Air, which is not retained by the system, elutes at 1.00 min. Calculate the adjusted retention times and Kovat's retention indexes for solutes A and B.

Compound	Retention Time (min)
n-Alkanes	
Ethane ($n = 2$)	3.51
Propane ($n = 3$)	4.98
Butane ($n = 4$)	7.30
Pentane ($n = 5$)	11.00
Hexane ($n = 6$)	16.85
Other Compounds	
Solute A	6.50
Solute B	10.35

References

1. Hawkes S, Grossman D, Hartkopf A, Isenhour T, Leary J, Parcher J. Preferred stationary liquids for gas chromatography. J Chromatogr Sci 1975, 13:115-7.

2. Rotzsche H. Stationary phases in gas chromatography. Journal of Chromatography Library, vol. 48. New York: Elsevier Science Publishing, 1991:302-51.

3. Hewlett Packard. Reference manual: 5890A gas chromatograph. Avondale, PA: Hewlett Packard, 1984: chaps. 12, 18.

4. Nygren S. Faster GC analyses performed by flow programming in short capillary columns. J High Resolut Chromatogr 1979, 2:319-23.

5. Grob K Jr, Grob G, Grob K. Comprehensive, standardized quality test for glass capillary columns. J. Chromatogr 1978, 156:1-20.

6. Rotzsche H. Stationary phases in gas chromatography. Journal of Chromatography Library, vol. 48. New York: Elsevier Science Publishing, 1991:74.

Suggested Readings

Grob RL, Modern practice of gas chromatography, 2nd ed. New York: John Wiley & Sons, 1985.

Guiochon G. Quantitative gas chromatography. Journal of Chromatography Library, vol. 42. New York: Elsevier Science Publishing, 1988.

Jennings W. Analytical gas chromatography. Orlando, FL: Academic Press, 1987.

Lee ML, Yang F, Bartle F. Open tubular gas chromatography. New York: John Wiley & Sons, 1984.

Willet J. Gas chromatography. New York: John Wiley & Sons, 1987.

16

MASS SPECTROMETRY

James H. Nichols

Objectives

After completing this chapter, the reader will be able to:

1. Describe mass spectroscopy.
2. List the components of a mass spectrometer.
3. Understand how mass spectra are affected by instrumentation and methodology.
4. Know common clinical applications of mass spectrometry.
5. Interpret simple mass spectra.
6. Describe how the three types of gas separators work.
7. Understand four ionization techniques suitable for gas phase specimens.
8. Understand two desorptive ionization techniques for liquid or solid phase specimens.
9. Describe magnetic sector, quadrupole, and time-of-flight mass analyzers.
10. List the three common mass spectrometry detectors: photographic emulsions, Faraday cups, and electron multipliers.
11. List the advantages of sending digitized mass spectrometer detector signals to a dedicated computer.
12. Describe calibration and quality assurance procedures for mass spectrometry.
13. Recognize common problems and interferences encountered in mass spectrometry.
14. Understand basic technical literature on mass spectrometry.

Definitions

Abundance: A measure of the quantity of ions present at a given mass/charge ratio. Abundance can be presented as an absolute value, an ion intensity, or as a percentage of the total ion yield.

Base Peak: The most abundant ion in the mass spectrum.

Derivative: The result of chemical modification, derivatization, with an agent that changes a physical property of a molecule before injection on a gas or liquid chromatograph. The most common derivatives increase the volatility of compounds to improve gas chromatography resolution.

Desorptive Ionization: Production of ions from the surface of a liquid or solid by bombardment with high-energy particles or photons.

Fragmentation: The process where unstable high mass ions break apart to form more stable, lower-mass ions (fragments).

Ion Intensity: The abundance of an ion presented as a percentage of the base peak abundance.

Ion Source: The component of the mass spectrometer where ions are formed from molecules introduced into the instrument.

Ion Yield: The total amount of all ions detected in a spectrum, obtained by summing the individual abundances of each ion.

Mass Analyzer: The component of the mass spectrometer where ions are physically separated based on differences in mass.

Parent (Molecular) Ion: The ion corresponding to the nominal molecular weight of the analyte and attached derivative, without fragmentation.

Resolution: The ability to discriminate between two different masses, whether at unit difference or fractions of an amu. In chromatography, the ability to discriminate between two peaks, a measure of peak separation.

Select Ion Monitoring (SIM): Spectra representing only a few chosen ions and their abundance. The process of monitoring only preselected ions of a given mass rather than an entire spectrum of ion masses.

Total Ion Chromatogram (TIC): Spectra representing all resolvable ions and their abundance detected over a range of masses.

Introduction

Mass spectrometry is an analytical technique to determine mass and structural information about a molecule. In the mass spectrometer, energy is transferred to a molecule, resulting in ionization. Excess energy causes the newly formed ion to rearrange and "fragment" into more stable configurations. The resulting ions are separated by mass to generate a pattern or spectrum that is characteristic of the parent molecule. In theory, each spectrum is a molecular "fingerprint" that can be used to identify the compound. This process can be visualized in Figure 16-1.

The components of the mass spectrometer are an ionizing chamber or source, a mass analyzer, a detector, and a recorder or computer. The ionizing chamber creates ions from sample molecules. Several methods are used to generate ions: electrical and chemical for gas phase analytes, and desorptive techniques for solid and liquid phase analytes. Because each method of ion generation is different, the appearance of the final spectra depends on the mechanism of ionization and how much energy is transferred to produce ionization. Most mass spectrometers separate positive ions, though some configurations are designed for negative ion generation. Positive ion separation is considerably more common in the clinical laboratory and will be a focus of this chapter.

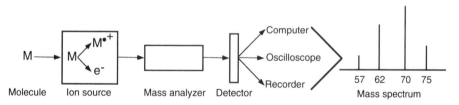

Figure 16-1. Mass spectrometer demonstrating the principal components: ion source where ions are generated, the mass analyzer where ions are separated by mass, a detector and a data-recording/storage device.

Once formed, positive ions are electrically focused and accelerated into a mass analyzer, whereas negative ions are deflected into an anion trap. In the mass analyzer, the velocities and paths of the positive ions are related to their mass and charge. Compounds with larger mass (greater molecular weight) will travel more slowly and be deflected less by an imposed magnetic or electrical field than compounds of lower mass. The mass analyzer can select ions of discrete mass for detection based on their mass/charge ratio. Once an ion reaches the detector, a signal is produced and recorded. The analog signal can be monitored directly by an oscilloscope or converted to a digital signal for storage and analysis by computer. Although instruments differ in the manner of ion generation and mass analysis, these components are common to all mass spectrometers.

Mass spectrometry is a powerful tool for both the qualitative and quantitative analyses of molecules in the nanomolar concentration range. In conjunction with gas and liquid chromatography, mass spectrometry provides convincing proof of peak purity and identification that is independent of shape and retention time. Clinical laboratory applications of mass spectrometry include identification and quantitation of drugs (prescription, over-the-counter, and "recreational"), study of metabolism and pharmacokinetics of drugs, detection of environmental toxicants such as pesticides, and detection of hormones, cytokines, or other naturally occurring compounds.

Principles

THE MASS SPECTRUM

The *mass spectrum* is a total ion summation at each resolvable mass over a given range. Figure 16-2 presents the total ion spectrum obtained from 2 μg of L-ephedrine derivatized with *N*-trifluoroacetyl-L-propyl chloride (TPC). The *x* axis represents the mass/charge ratio, m/z. Because most chemicals encountered in the clinical laboratory will generate ions with a +1 charge, m/z is equivalent to the molecular weight of the ion in atomic mass units (amu). Most mass spectrometers can scan an m/z of 0 to 1000, but resolution and ion yield are severely compromised at higher masses. The scale of the *y* axis on the left side of the spectrum represents ion abundance. The height of each line of the spectrum corresponds to the total number of ions with a specific mass. In Figure 16-2, the m/z 166 ion is the base peak, as it is the most abundant ion, with an abundance of 1.85×10^6. Abundance is the magnitude of the detection signal at any given mass. An alternative presentation of abundance, the ion intensity, sets the height of the most abundant ion at 100% and expresses the quantity of all other ions as a percentage of this ion. In Figure 16-2, the *y* axis on the right side of the spectrum represents intensity (I) as a percentage of the *m/z* 166 ion. A third method of presenting abundance involves summing all the ions in the spectrum and reporting the amount of each ion mass as a percentage of the total detectable ions. This value is termed the ion yield, $\Sigma_{50}^{\%}$. The subscript number indicates the low end of the range for summation. The high end of the range is the largest ion on the spectrum. On the far right in Figure 16-2, the ion signals are summed from *m/z* 50 to 438, and *m/z* 166 is 30% of the total ion abundance. Looking at the *m/z* 251 ion, one can see that this ion has an absolute abundance of 0.25×10^6, which is 15% as frequent as the *m/z* 166 ion and is 5% of the total detectable signal from *m/z* 50 to 438, $\Sigma_{50}^{\%}$. All three methods of presenting abundance are found in mass spectrometry literature. The manner of presentation is more a matter of preference than an absolute rule.

Several hundred spectra may be collected over a period of several minutes at each analysis. An individual spectrum, as in Figure 16-2, displays only a single scan from all of those collected. If the spectra were collected from a pure analyte at an equal ion concentration, they would all be identical, and any single scan would be representative of the entire population. This ideal is rarely achieved, because pure specimens are seldom analyzed in the clinical laboratory. Instead, purification is

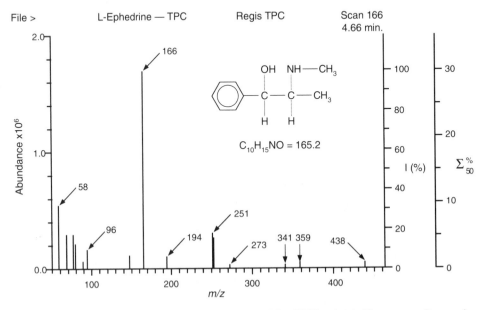

Figure 16-2. Total ion mass spectrum of L-ephedrine-TPC, s (−) (trifluoroacetyl) propyl chloride, derivative.

achieved by connecting mass spectrometers directly to the effluent from gas or liquid chromatography columns. The mass spectrometer then becomes the detector for the chromatography system. By combining high-resolution chromatography with mass spectrometry, individual components of a complex sample mixture can be separated and mass-analyzed. Hundreds of scans can be collected over the entire elution period, but only a few of them actually contain information pertaining to a single analyte.

Computer ion selection can assist in determining which scans contain relevant information. Figure 16-3a shows the total ion chromatogram (TIC) obtained by separating 2 μg of phentermine derivatized with TPC on a gas chromatography (GC) column and monitoring the mass spectra of the eluent. The lower x axis scale represents time from injection in minutes, which is equivalent to number of mass scans shown on the upper x axis scale (i.e., 250 scans were collected in 6 minutes). Abundance is indicated on the y axis. Peaks on the TIC represent increases in the magnitude of all ions at the detector, indicating elution of an unresolved peak of two or more compounds. If the operator knows that the analyte of interest (e.g., phentermine) contains mass ions at m/z 91, 194, and 251, the computer can be used to select and display only those ions (Fig. 16-3b). Peaks on the selected ion chromatogram (select ion monitoring, SIM) indicate the individual scans, from the hundreds collected, that should be examined for this analyte (scan numbers 97 to 102). Figure 16-3c shows scan number 101, which contains the spectrum matching the TPC derivative of phentermine. Thus, phentermine has been positively identified in the 3.62-minute retention time peak, and no other peaks need to be examined for this analyte. A patient sample can produce hundreds of eluate peaks on a chromatogram. The selection of single ions from a total ion chromatogram is especially useful in finding specific analytes within overlapping or unresolved peaks.

This example demonstrates the power of mass spectrometry. Individual mass spectra give detailed information about the masses of ions reaching the detector at a given time. For a purified but unknown substance, mass spectrometry allows identification and quantitation. Mass spectrometry also allows identification and quantitation of a mixture containing a known substance. Mass spectrometry has advantages over other detection methods: it works with almost all compounds, and each compound produces a unique mass spectrum.

INTERPRETATION OF MASS SPECTRA

Mass spectra contain structural information in addition to the mass data about a particular molecule. Energy imparted to a molecule at the source produces ionization. Excess energy, beyond that required for ionization, creates an unstable, high-energy ion. This unstable ion undergoes rearrangement and fragmentation. The result is two smaller "fragment" ions. These ions can undergo further fragmentation. The masses and abundances of parent fragment ions are recorded in the mass spectrum.

The mass spectrum of caffeine obtained by electron impact ionization is displayed in Figure 16-4a. The first step in interpreting a mass spectrum is to identify the parent or molecular ion (M^+). The mass of M^+ equals the sum of the nominal atomic weights for the atoms comprising the parent molecule, because the most abundant

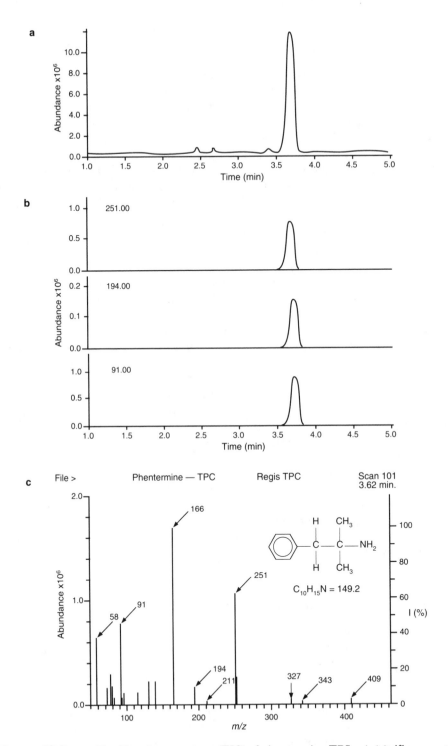

Figure 16-3. (a) Total ion chromatogram (TIC) of phentermine-TPS, s (−) (trifluoroacetyl) propyl chloride, derivative. (b) Selected ion monitoring (SIM) of phentermine-TPC at m/z 251, 194, and 91 ions. (c) Total ion mass spectrum of phentermine-TPC derivative.

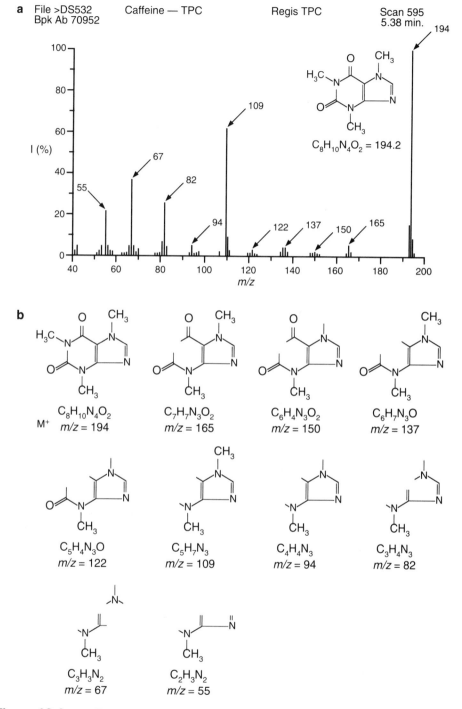

Figure 16-4. (a) Total ion mass spectrum of caffeine in methanol. Percentage ion intensity is shown on *y* axis. (b) Electron impact (EI) fragmentation pattern of caffeine collected at 70 eV. Molecular diagram represents only one way that caffeine could fragment resulting in a particular *m/z* value. There may be other possibilities for some ions.

isotopes in all naturally occurring elements have the lowest atomic mass. Thus, carbon = 12 (not 12.011), nitrogen = 14 (not 14.0067), and oxygen = 16 (not 15.9994), because the most abundant isotopes of these atoms are ^{12}C, ^{14}N and ^{16}O. Therefore, caffeine's M^+ mass is 194 amu [4×14 (N) = 56, 8×12 (C) = 96, 2×16 (O) = 32, and 10 $\times 1$ (H) = 10; 56 + 96 + 32 + 10 = 194]. The m/z value of caffeine's parent ion is 194, which is also the highest mass and the most abundant ion in this example. The highest m/z and most abundant ions are not always the parent ion, especially in electron impact mass spectrometry (see Electron Impact Ionization subsection). Note the two less abundant ions at m/z 195 and 196. These are due to the presence of natural isotopes: ^{13}C, ^{15}N, ^{17}O, and ^{18}O in a small proportion of caffeine molecules. Most mass spectra demonstrate stable isotope lines in proportion to the percentage of isotope commonly found in nature.

Besides the parent ion at m/z 194, the mass spectrum of caffeine contains other ions at lower m/z. These ions are fragments of the parent ion. The m/z 109 ion fragment is more abundant and therefore more stable than the m/z 67, 82, or 55 ions. In turn, these fragment ions are considerably more stable than those with still lower abundances.

The exact mechanism of fragmentation depends on the molecule and the mode of ionization. A complete discussion of this topic is beyond the scope of this text. The composition of a fragmentation ion can usually be deduced from its m/z value and knowledge of the parent ion's structure. In the caffeine example, the difference between m/z 194 and 165 is 29 amu. The only way to remove 29 mass units from caffeine is loss of a •NCH_3 group (14 + 12 + 3 = 29). To know which of caffeine's three •NCH_3 groups are lost, each group would have to be labeled with a stable isotope such as deuterium. This may not be necessary, because examination of the fragmentation patterns at lower m/z values may provide additional information on the nature of the m/z 165 ion. The loss of 28 units (•C=O) or 15 units (•CH_3) can also be seen during caffeine fragmentation. The configuration of each fragment ion is given in Figure 16-4b. As an exercise, the reader should perform the analysis and determine how the actual weights are calculated. Precise rules for rearrangement, fragmentation, and determination of the number and types of atoms in a parent ion from m/z values alone can be found in the Suggested Readings section.

Instrumentation

The component parts of a mass spectrometer are the gas separator, ion source, mass analyzer, detector, and recorder. Mixtures are usually separated by GC or high-performance liquid chromatography (HPLC) before introduction into the mass spectrometer (see Chapters 14 and 15). A separator is required when effluent from a noncapillary GC column is to be analyzed by mass spectrometry.

GAS SEPARATOR

Three types of gas separators are used to concentrate samples and decrease the flow of carrier gas into the ion source of the mass spectrometer: membrane, fritted glass, and jet (Fig. 16-5).[1,2]

Membrane Separator

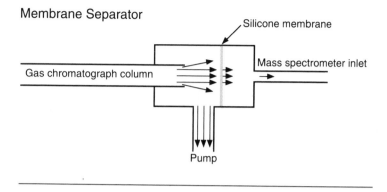

Fritted Glass Separator

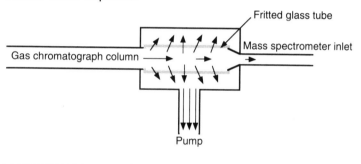

Jet Separator

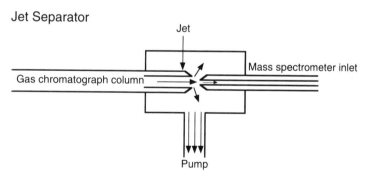

Figure 16-5. Three gas separators for use in GC/MS instruments.

Membrane Separator

This separator employs a silicone rubber membrane across the separator chamber. Organic analyte molecules are more soluble in silicone rubber than typical carrier gases. They dissolve in the membrane and are drawn out by the vacuum produced in the ion source. Carrier gas (and some analyte) molecules are removed from the GC side of the membrane by a pump.

Fritted Glass Separator

This separator takes advantage of the ease with which small gas molecules pass through a tube made of fritted glass. Large analyte molecules are retained within the fritted glass tube in the separator chamber. A high-efficiency pump removes most of the carrier gas from the effluent stream; only a low-pressure stream with a high proportion of analyte molecules reaches the ion source.

Jet Separator

Effluent gas from the GC column is directed through a narrow jet. Gas velocity increases and pressure decreases as the tube diameter narrows (Bernoulli's law). Once gas passes the jet, pressure drops rapidly. Small carrier gas molecules move away from the central gas stream much faster than larger analyte molecules. A narrow opening aligned with the center of the jet nozzle allows only gas molecules that remain in the central gas stream to pass through to the ion source. A high-efficiency pump removes carrier gas from the separator chamber.

ION SOURCE

Electron Impact Ionization

In *electron impact (EI) ionization* analyte molecules and carrier gas from a gas chromatography column are directed into a beam of electrons (Fig. 16-6). Collisions with electrons generate both positive and negative ions. Positive ions are collected and focused by a series of exit plates with negative potentials. These plates align and focus the positive ions into a single beam directed into the mass analyzer. Negative ions and uncharged molecules that avoided collisions are drawn away by the anion trap and vacuum system. The ion source produces a collimated beam of positive ions from the effluent of a GC system.

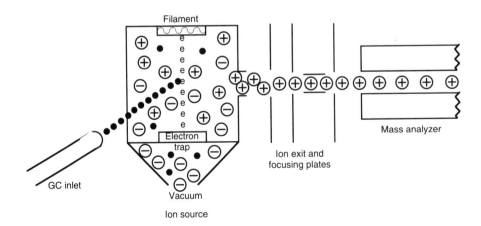

Figure 16-6. Electron impact ion source. Molecules enter with the GC column effluent and collide with a stream of electrons, resulting in ionization. Positive ions are collected and focused into the mass analyzer.

The electron beam is critical in EI mass spectrometry. Electrons are produced by electrically heating a rhenium filament. The emitted electrons are attracted by the positive potential of an electron trap. When equilibrium is attained, a steady stream of electrons flows from the heated filament to the electron trap. A small magnetic field forces the electrons to travel in a helical path. This longer helical path increases the probability of collision with a molecule. Column carrier gas containing analyte molecules enters perpendicular to the electron stream.

Factors relating to ion production can be monitored. These include the current in the rhenium filament, the total emission of electrons, and the electron trap current. Total emission is always greater than the trap current, because some electrons collide with gas molecules and do not enter the trap. The difference between trap current and total emission is directly proportional to the number of collisions.

The energy of the electron beam is directly related to the potential difference in electron volts (eV) between the filament and the trap. Ion production increases as the electron beam energy increases. The increase in ion production is nonlinear and follows a sigmoidal curve when plotted against potential difference. Few ions are produced at potentials less than 5 eV. The production of ions increases dramatically at 10 to 30 eV and approaches a maximum at electron beam energies greater than 50 eV. Most reference spectra are collected at an electron beam energy of 70 eV, because fluctuations in the electron beam at this energy level will have little effect on the production of ions.

Mass spectra from EI ionization contain numerous fragment ions. Parent molecular ions, if present at all, have a relatively low abundance. Instead, many fragmentation ions are produced because of the excess energy absorbed during the collisions. Figure 16-7 compares cocaine mass spectra from EI ionization to those produced by other modes of ionization. Cocaine demonstrates a parent ion of minimal abundance at m/z 303, with fragmentation ions at 182 and 82 due to the loss of $[\cdot OCOC_6H_5]$ and $[\cdot COOCH_3 + \cdot CHCH_2CH_2 + \cdot OCOC_6H_5]$, respectively (Fig. 16-7a). Parent ions are usually identified by using a low-potential (10-15 eV) electron beam. The lower energy decreases ion yield but also limits fragmentation, allowing the detection of M^+.

Although the identity of the parent ion may be more difficult to determine from EI spectra, the fragmentation ions provide more detailed structural information than do other forms of ionization. The number and abundance of fragmentation ions in EI ionization enhance the specificity of the spectra and decrease the probability of two different compounds having fragments with identical masses and similar abundances. This makes EI ionization especially useful in the clinical laboratory as a method for confirming the identity of unknown compounds.

The sensitivity (ability to detect low analyte concentrations) of EI ionization can be enhanced by maximizing either the flow of electrons or the number of analyte molecules in the source. Sensitivity increases with increasing trap current, dimensions of electron beam, and sample pressure. As the trap current increases, more electrons flow between the filament and the trap, increasing the probability of collisions with analyte. However, the strength of the target current is limited by heat generation of the filament. Large target currents burn out the filament faster. The

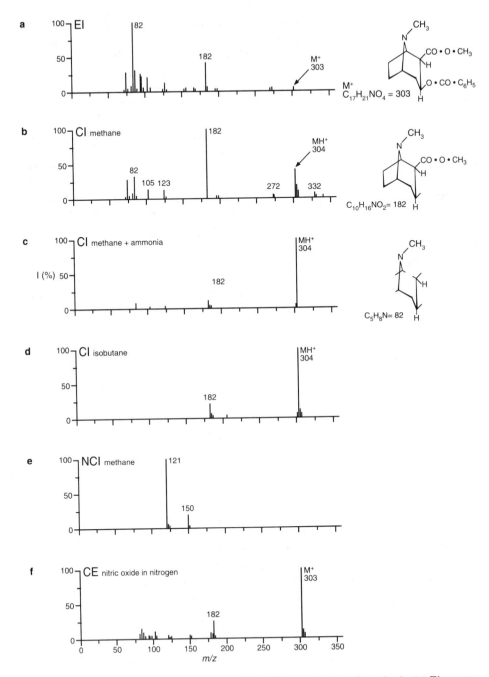

Figure 16-7. Spectra of cocaine obtained by different ionization methods. (a) Electron impact ionization. (b-d) Chemical ionization with different reagent gases. (e) Negative chemical ionization. (f) Charge exchange ionization.

maximum dimension of the electron beam is limited by the design of the ion source. The pressure of the carrier gas is restricted to 10^{-6} to 10^{-4} torr (atmospheric pressure is about 760 torr). Pressures less than 10^{-6} torr allow most analyte molecules to pass through the electron beam without collision. Pressures greater than 10^{-4} torr cause frequent collisions between analyte molecules and carrier gas molecules before entering the electron beam or between analyte ions and carrier gas ions after leaving the electron beam. In either case, the collisions produce directional changes in analyte molecules, resulting in fewer analyte ions entering the mass analyzer. Mass analysis thus requires strong vacuum conditions for optimal sensitivity. The rate of effluent gas influx is limited by the efficiency of the vacuum pump in the ion source. With most single-pump systems, a flow rate of 1 cm³/min from a capillary GC column can be accommodated. Larger-diameter columns run at higher flow rates, typically around 20 cm³/min, and require a stream splitter. The splitter allows only a fraction of the effluent gas to enter the ion source. Dual differential or molecular turbo pumping systems, with their higher pumping speeds and efficiencies, can handle higher flow rates. However, only 10 to 20% of the effluent gas from an open tubular packed column can be used with even the most efficient pumping system. This restriction on sample flow limits the sensitivity of mass spectrometry.

Chemical Ionization

Chemical ionization (CI) is milder than EI ionization and achieves ionization without a transfer of excess energy. A reagent gas (methane, ammonia, hydrogen, isobutane, etc.) is introduced at a pressure of approximately 1 torr into an ionization chamber similar to that of an EI ionization source. The filament voltage is increased to allow electron penetration into the reagent gas. Reagent gas molecules collide with high-energy electrons to produce reagent ions. Reagent ions then collide with analyte molecules with resultant ionization. Filament voltage is monitored in CI rather than trap current, because few electrons penetrate the reagent gas and enter the trap. Electron ionization of analyte molecules does not occur even though a beam of high-energy electrons is present because of the large excess of reagent gas in the center of the source. Maintenance of strong vacuum is more difficult than in EI ionization because of the addition of reagent gas. At least two high-efficiency pumps need to be connected directly to the source to achieve pressures of 10^{-6} torr.

The reagent gas ions produced by collision with the electron beam contain a reactive hydrogen group, XH^+. Collisions of these reagent ions with analyte molecules result in the formation of adduct ions in addition to fragmentation ions. The parent ion predominates in CI in the form of $(M^+ + 1)$ because of protonation by reagent ions. The CI spectra of cocaine (Fig. 16-7b) shows the parent ion at m/z 304 [303 + 1 (H^+)].

Although CI produces higher yields of parent ion, fragmentation is not prohibited, and many reagent gases induce fragmentation of particular analytes. The CI mass spectra depend on the proton affinity of the reagent gas and the difference in proton affinities between the reagent gas and the analyte. Reagent proton affinity is increased from methane to ammonia to isobutane. In the cocaine example, decreased fragmentation and adduct formation (methane can produce a 332 amu $\cdot CH_2CH_2^+$ adduct) occur as reagent gas proton affinity increases (Fig. 16-7b-d).

Negative ions can also be induced by *negative chemical ionization (NCI)*. Its mass separation method is similar to CI's, except that the ion extraction and focusing plates are positively charged to select negative analyte ions. Negative ion generation is due to resonance capture from low-energy electrons (approximately 0.1 eV) and is virtually undetectable at normal EI and CI energies of 70 eV or more. Negative chemical ionization recently gained popularity after reports of enhanced sensitivity compared to positive CI and EI. However, spectra are less predictable with this newer technique. Note the lack of a parent ion in the NCI spectra of cocaine (Fig. 16-7e).

Charge Exchange

Charge exchange (CE) ionization is identical to CI but uses reagent gases without donatable protons (helium, argon, nitrogen, carbon dioxide, xenon, etc.). Because there are no hydrogen atoms to exchange in the reagent gas, the predominant ion in CE spectra is the parent ion. The CE spectrum of cocaine is shown in Figure 16-7f.

Field Ionization

Field ionization (FI) is similar to EI ionization, but it uses a strong electrical field to produce ionization. Analyte molecules entering the field are stripped of an electron. There is little transfer of excess energy and little fragmentation. It has a lower ion yield, and it is 10 to 100 times less sensitive than EI ionization mass spectometry.

Desorptive Ionization

Up to this point the discussion of ionization has been limited to gas phase analytes. However, there are numerous mechanisms for producing ions from solid and liquid phase molecules. The simplest is to atomize, heat, and volatilize the effluent from an HPLC column. Then, any of the ionization techniques we discussed may be used. Of course, this technique requires volatile analytes in a volatile solvent and cannot be used with nonvolatile solvents or samples or with analytes that break down when heated.

Desorptive ionization techniques do not require a volatile sample. Therefore, fragile compounds that would be destroyed by derivatization or heating and nonvolatile compounds can be analyzed. Liquid and solid phase ionizations are diagrammed in Figure 16-8. Analyte diffusion in liquid samples is decreased by the addition of glycerol. High-energy particles (ions, atoms, fission fragments, etc.) are focused on the specimen. They collide at the surface layer of the sample and form ions. Many of the ions are propelled from the sample by the force of the impact. In fact, most of the excess energy (beyond that needed for sample ionization) is lost as kinetic energy. The spectra obtained using desorptive techniques contain adducts resulting from the addition of H^+, Na^+, K^+, and other cations used as buffering salts in the specimen. Parent molecular ions and fragmentation ions are rare. Another problem with desorptive ionization is the large background signal produced by ionization of solvent

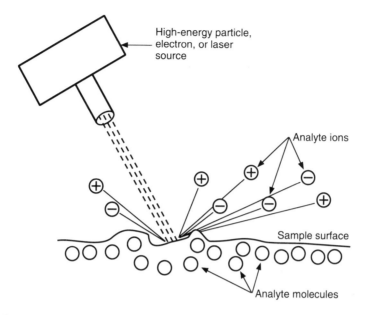

Figure 16-8. Desorptive ionization. A beam of high-energy particles, electrons, or photons is directed at the surface of a solid or liquid sample. Sample molecules struck by the beam are ionized and ejected.

and glycerol. The magnitude of the background signal depends on the striking angle of high-energy particles and the concentration of solvent at the sample surface. There is no easy way to subtract the background signals from the analyte spectra.

There are several desorptive ionization techniques. *Fast atom bombardment (FAB)* uses a stream of high-energy xenon, argon, or other gas that does not contain hydrogen atoms. This is the most popular desorptive ionization technique in clinical laboratories. *Field desorption* uses a beam of high-energy electrons. *Laser desorption* uses photons to generate ions. *Massive particle bombardment (MPB)* bombards a sample with particles accelerated from a ^{252}Cf source. This technique has been employed to ionize large molecules, such as proteins, in the range of 10,000 to 20,000 daltons. Because of the low yield of high-mass analyte ions, scanning times of several hours to days are required to collect enough data for accurate integration.

High-performance liquid chromatography/mass spectrometry systems using desorptive ionization techniques deposit droplets of column effluent on a conveyor belt leading into the ion source. Usually, the droplets are heated and vaporized before ionization. However, it is difficult to rapidly vaporize aqueous eluents before ionization. Most successful applications of this system use reverse-phase HPLC with more volatile organic solvents. Sample carryover can occur with belt systems because of the difficulty of continuously cleaning the belt during a run. Despite these problems, HPLC/MS is gaining popularity.

MASS ANALYZER

There are several configurations and technologies to separate ions in a collimated beam by mass. These include magnetic sector, quadrupole, and time-of-flight mass analyzers. We present the magnetic sector first, for historical reasons, but it is usually employed in research laboratories rather than clinical laboratories. Quadrupole and time-of-flight mass analyzers are the most common types in clinical laboratories.

Magnetic Sector Mass Analyzers

The *magnetic sector mass analyzer* deflects the ion beam by using a perpendicular magnetic field (Fig. 16-9). Ions generated in the source are focused and accelerated into a magnetic field.[3] The amount of ion deflection is based on the strength of the imposed field and the weight and charge of the ion. For ions of equal charge (usually 1 unit), the greater momentum of heavy ions makes them less susceptible to deflection than are light ions. Greater field strength is required to deflect heavier ions to the detector.

Single m/z values can be focused on to a stationary detection slit by either adjusting the magnetic field strength or the accelerating voltage. The relationship is described mathematically in Equation 16-1.

$$m/z = r^2 B^2 / 2V \qquad \text{(Eq. 16-1)}$$

where

r = radius of the flight path (m)
B = magnetic field strength (gauss)
V = potential (V)

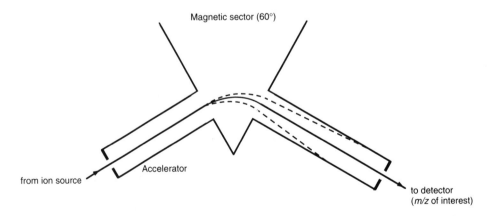

Figure 16-9. A 60° magnetic sector mass analyzer. A focused collimated beam of ions is deflected by a perpendicular magnetic field. The magnitude of the field is varied to direct individual m/z to the stationary detection slit.

For a magnetic sector mass analyzer of fixed radius, only one ion will reach the detector for any given combination of magnetic field strength and accelerating voltage. Varying the acceleration voltage while keeping magnetic field strength constant is only practical over a tenfold range of m/z values. Acceleration affects the quality of the ion focus and the ultimate abundance of ions reaching the detector. Too great a change from the optimum setting decreases the sensitivity of the system. Therefore, to detect ions of different mass/charge ratios, most magnetic sector instruments vary the strength of the magnetic field while holding acceleration potential to a constant optimal value.

Sensitivity is also affected by the scanning speed. Scanning speed is the rate of change of magnetic field strength. A faster scan allows fewer ions of given m/z value to reach the detector. The magnetic field strength cannot be instantaneously altered. This resistance of the field to change keeps scanning speeds to 0.1 s per decade (50 to 500 amu) or less. Scanning at the maximum speed still yields a resolving power of 10^4 (0.1 amu over a 1000-amu range), making the magnetic sector mass spectrometer extremely sensitive for exacting research applications.

The magnetic sector instrument shown in Figure 16-9 is a single-focusing device. Double-focusing instruments use two sectors to separate ions. These instruments are accurate to six significant figures. In single-focusing magnetic sector instruments, the ions in any given flight path have a distribution of kinetic energies centered around the mean kinetic energy. These nonuniform energies limit resolution, because ions of a given mass with differing kinetic energy will diffuse away from a theoretically focused path and blur the separation between individual mass units during their flight to the detector. Double-focusing instruments eliminate this problem by separating ions based on mass and energy. An electric sector separates ions by their kinetic energies. Only a narrow range of isokinetic ions is allowed to enter the magnetic field sector. Resolution is greatly enhanced in these instruments.

Quadrupole Mass Analyzers

The *quadrupole mass analyzer* actually acts like a mass filter rather than a mass separator.[4] Ions from the source are accelerated between four parallel ceramic electrodes (Fig. 16-10).[3] Direct current (dc) and radio frequency (RF) voltages are applied to the quadrupole. Ions oscillate because of the effects of the constant (dc) and alternating (RF) electric fields. Resonant ions complete their path and arrive at the detector, while all other ions collide with the mass analyzer. Ions lighter than the resonant ions collide with the quadrupole because the alternating RF field induces ever-widening oscillations. Ions heavier than the resonant ions gradually drift toward a charged quadrupole electrode because they are relatively unaffected by the alternating RF field. Only ions with a selected m/z value achieve uniform oscillatory motion and reach the detector. A complete mass spectrum is scanned by varying the voltage that produces both the dc and RF fields. Changing the field strength allows ions with different m/z values to reach the detector. For all ions, the most stable path from the source to the detector occurs at a single dc/RF ratio. Therefore, the electronics is designed so that altering the voltage keeps the dc/RF ratio constant.

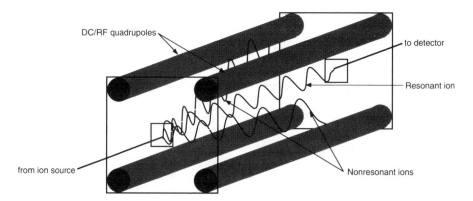

Figure 16-10.   Quadrupole mass analyzer. Four ceramic rods conduct direct current and oscillating radio frequency waves that stabilize the flight paths of selected m/z value ions. Only the stabilized ions reach the detector. Other ions are lost by collision with the quadrupole rods.

Quadrupole mass analyzers have several advantages over magnetic sector instruments: (1) Complete scans can be conducted in tenths of a second. Therefore, quadrupole mass analyzers are good for selected ion monitoring. However, as with magnetic sectors, their sensitivity is decreased at high scan speeds. (2) Quadrupole instruments can be operated at pressures an order of magnitude higher than for magnetic sectors. This allows the application of more sample without significant loss of sensitivity. (3) Because quadrupole instruments do not have a magnet, they are considerably smaller and lighter than magnetic sector instruments.

The major disadvantage of quadrupole mass analyzers is low resolution (about 1 amu over a 1000-amu range). Because unit resolution is adequate for most confirmation procedures, quadrupole instruments are common in clinical laboratories.

Time-of-Flight Mass Analyzers

Time-of-flight instruments measure the time required for an ion to travel from the source to the detector. There are two modes of operation, pulsed and continuous. In the *pulsed mode,* an electron beam or laser pulse produces a microsecond burst of ions that are accelerated into the mass analyzer. In the time-of-flight analyzer, ions travel at speeds based on the momentum gained during acceleration. As mentioned in the section on mass sectors, heavier ions have greater momentum than lighter ions and will therefore travel more slowly. Separation occurs in a region that is shielded from external fields, allowing the ions to travel straight paths dependent only on mass. Ions of a particular m/z value are detected by monitoring a selected period of time after ionization. Scanning is performed by detecting ions in successive nanosecond time periods. The time-of-flight instrument is ideally suited for selected ion monitoring. Spectra from time-of-flight mass analyzers have a greater abundance of parent ions because low-source temperatures for ion production (100–150°C) are used.

In the *continuous mode,* ions are produced over 50- to 100-microsecond periods and are collected in potential wells. These ions are released in a single brief burst (a packet) for simultaneous release into the mass analyzer. The accumulation of ions in the continuous mode can increase the sensitivity by over tenfold, but it can also decrease resolution if the ion packet is not properly focused.

Resolution in time-of-flight instruments is determined by the accelerating voltage, the spatial distribution of ions, and the length of the separating region. Because ion packets are neither infinitesimally small nor monoenergetic, instrument resolution is limited by the broadening that occurs during separation. Ultimate resolution depends on the speed at which a packet of ions can be detected. Current technology allows successive m/z readings every few nanoseconds—an entire spectra is scanned in 0.1 millisecond. Therefore, time-of-flight instruments can be used to study rapid gas phase kinetic reactions.

DETECTOR

Three detection methods are employed in mass spectrometry: photographic emulsions, Faraday cups, and electron multipliers.

Photographic Emulsions

A *photographic emulsion detector* is the simplest type of detector and is mostly used with magnetic sector mass analyzers. An entire spectrum can be collected at one time. Photographic emulsions are sensitized by ions just as they are to photons or radioactive particles. Each m/z value will appear as a discrete line on the emulsion. The spectrum will consist of a series of parallel lines. Sensitivity and resolution are related to grain size and homogeneity of the emulsion and to image widening due to scatter in the emulsion. Developed emulsions can be scanned by densitometers or comparators to measure the abundance of each ion. Disadvantages of this type of detection are the time for analysis (emulsions must be developed and scanned), nonlinear response to ions, and the restriction to mass analyzers that can focus the entire dispersed ion beam on a plane.

Faraday Cups

A *Faraday cup* is an insulated metal cup connected to a ground through a very large load resistor. When positive ions strike the Faraday cup, they pick up electrons from the metal. This results in a minute current (10^{-17} to 10^{-19} A). This current produces a voltage drop across the resistor between the cup and ground. This voltage is amplified and measured by a solid-state electrometer with field effect transistor input. Faraday cup detectors have a quick response time and good sensitivity.

Electron Multipliers

Electron multipliers are sensitive devices that can detect a single ion. They are analogous to photomultiplier tubes (Fig. 16-11). Ions strike a cathode that emits secondary electrons. These electrons accelerate to the first dynode and release an even greater number of electrons. Cascade amplification occurs with each successive

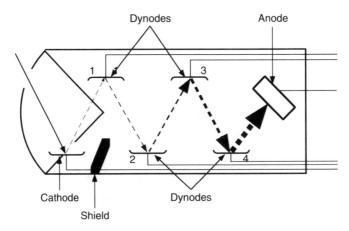

Figure 16-11. Electron multiplier detector.

dynode. A 10- to 12-dynode electron multiplier produces a signal amplification of 10^5 to 10^6. Electrons from the final dynode are collected by the anode. The current produced by the electrons is amplified and measured. Electron multipliers have excellent response time and superb sensitivity.

RECORDER

Developed Photographic Emulsion

A *developed photographic emulsion* can be inspected for ion locations and abundances. Visual inspection is only semiquantitative. Accurate quantitation is achieved by densitometric scanning.

Recording Oscillograph

The signal from the detector is sent to the *oscillograph* that records signal strength versus time on a strip chart. Oscillographs are simple, reliable, and inexpensive. The recorded spectra require manual interpretation: each m/z value must be identified on the spectrum, and the amplitudes need to be converted into some measure of abundance.

Microcomputer

Most mass spectrometer detectors in clinical laboratories are connected to a dedicated *microcomputer*. Signals from the detector are digitized and stored in computer memory. Spectra can be displayed on a monitor or printed. Computer software aids in data analysis. The more prominent m/z values are identified, and relative abundances are calculated. The computer can display graphs of total signal versus time (to identify retention times for GC or HPLC peaks) or the mass spectrum at a given time.

Many mass spectrometry computers also have a stored database of spectra for thousands of compounds. Computer software can identify unknown compounds using algorithms that match the relative abundance of the unknown's m/z values with those of compounds stored in the database. If no match is found, the computer will list the chemicals most similar to the unknown compound.

Maintenance and Quality Assurance

The quality of mass spectrometer operation is most commonly assessed by examining the ion yield of a known chemical each day of operation. Consistent abundance of parent and fragmentation ions with constant ion ratios is an excellent indication that mass spectrometer reproducibility and accuracy are acceptable. Decreased ion yields are an early indicator of mechanical failure or suboptimal running conditions.

TUNING THE MASS SPECTROMETER

Before this quality control check, the mass spectrometer should be "tuned." Tuning is performed to calibrate the accuracy of ions' m/z values and to maximize relative abundance throughout the scanning range. Perfluorinated compounds are commonly used for tuning. These compounds have well-characterized spectra in the 50- to 650-amu mass range. Tuning can be performed manually or automatically, using an internal supply of calibrator connected to the ion source by a special valve. Instruments with this capability do not have to run special injections to calibrate, and one needs to refill the calibrator supply only about once a year. During tuning, the voltages applied to the ion focusing plates at the source exit are adjusted to maximize the relative abundance of detected ions and to ensure that these ions coincide with the exact known ion masses of the calibration compound.

Even with perfectly tuned mass spectrometers, interlaboratory differences in absolute abundances of identical compounds are unavoidable. Tuning emphasizes certain regions of the spectrum, depending on the preference of the operator. In addition, different types of mass analyzers give dissimilar results. Quadrupole instruments, for example, tend to have lower yields for heavier ions. On these instruments it is acceptable to set relative abundance of a low-mass ion to 100% and detect only 1 to 2% of an ion around m/z 500. However, for heavy ion sensitivity, the ion exit plate voltages can be adjusted to improve the yields of heavier ions while diminishing yields at lower masses. Comparisons of unknowns or standards to published or commercial reference standards rarely result in perfect matches because of differences in instrumentation and tuning among laboratories. Better matches with reference spectra occur when library reference spectra are from the same instrument with similar tuning and ionization conditions. The best matches will occur when the reference spectrum is collected from a sample extracted, chromatographed, and mass-analyzed in a manner identical to the patient specimen.

OVERCOMING NONLINEARITY DUE TO ADSORPTION

Nonspecific adsorption and sample matrix differences present other difficulties. Nonspecific adsorption to column active sites or to exposed metal in the mass spectrometer can produce nonlinear response curves. This is because a greater percentage of compound adsorbs at lower concentrations than at higher concentrations. Nonlinearity can be overcome by spiking the sample with a large amount of a deuterated internal standard. The deuterated compound saturates all adsorption sites, preventing adsorption of the compound of interest. Unfortunately, most deuterated standards contain a small percentage (<1-2%) of unlabeled standard. Thus, the assay becomes a standard addition one and cannot reliably quantitate the compound of interest if its concentration is less than 1% of that in the internal standard.

CONTAMINANTS, INTERFERANTS, AND MATRIX EFFECTS

Contaminants can affect ion abundance and decrease sensitivity by increasing background noise for ions in certain regions of the chromatogram. Vacuum-pump oil can contaminate the ion source if vaporized into the mass spectrometer. Loss of stationary phase solvent from a gas-liquid chromatography column (column bleed) can increase baselines near the end of a GC run, because the stationary phase solvent is volatile at high temperatures. This problem can be minimized by keeping column temperatures below 325°C or by switching to chemically bonded stationary phases, in which the stationary phase is covalently bound to the column matrix.

Plasticizers and phthalates (used to catalyze the polymerization of plastics in solvent bottles, tubes, and seals) can appear in trace quantities in patient samples or solvents during extraction. In addition, mobile phase gas tanks, if completely emptied, can contaminate GC columns and the mass spectrometer with organic chemicals often found at the bottom of the tanks. These interferants can be avoided by using GC/MS-grade reagents and high-purity gases; switching to brands of storage vials, syringes, and processing tubes that exhibit less leaching of plasticizers; and using a gas purification system.

If low levels of interferants cannot be eliminated, spectra can be corrected by performing baseline subtractions. This works well in total ion monitoring (TIM) applications. However, baseline subtraction is not as reliable in select ion monitoring (SIM) applications. In SIM the entire instrument is dedicated to monitoring a few chosen ions. The spectra are not truly representative of the entire chromatograph, and the presence of interferants may be missed. If interferants decrease the sensitivity of selected ions, a problem is usually noted. However, a new contaminant might be undetected until enough of it adsorbs to the column to grossly affect instrument performance. Contaminants may falsely elevate the abundance of an ion. This produces inconsistencies in the abundance ratios of two or three ions in a given compound. Monitoring several ion ratios for compounds undergoing SIM analysis is recommended to detect such contaminants.

MAINTAINING SEPARATION COLUMN AND ION SOURCE INTEGRITY

Samples containing particulate matter and unextracted or crudely extracted samples can clog inlet valves and injection syringes. This may decrease the abundance of later samples. Certain compounds in samples can bind to the separation column or can coat exposed surfaces in the ion source. This may create new active sites that interfere with later analyses. Frequent injection of samples derivatized with different compounds can result in damage to exposed metals if the derivatizing agents interact to produce corrosive products. All of these problems can be prevented by injecting only clean, nonparticulate sample extracts on to the instrument, by using quality solvents and derivatizing compounds, and by avoiding the frequent injection of samples prepared with different derivatizing reagents and solvents. Periodic inspection and cleaning of instrument parts will reduce the frequency of these problems.

Summary

Mass spectrometry is an analytical technique to determine mass and structural information about a molecule and to identify and quantify compounds.

Mass spectrometers have four components: an ion source, a mass analyzer, a detector, and a recording device. Gas chromatography instruments also have a gas separator.

Ions are generated in the ion source by collisions with electrons (EI) or activated gas molecules (CI). Ions can also be produced by electrically stripping an electron from the analyte (FI). Desorptive ionization processes are employed with nonvolatile compounds. Ions are produced by bombarding the surface of the specimen with atoms, electrons, or photons.

Ions are resolved by m/z value in the mass analyzer. Magnetic sector mass analyzers deflect the flight path of a collimated ion beam and relate mass to distance of deflection. Quadrupole mass analyzers stabilize the flight path of specific ions using dc and oscillating rf fields. Time-of-flight mass analyzers relate ion masses to the time required for ions to reach the detector.

Detectors include photographic emulsions, Faraday cups, and electron multipliers. The latter two detectors are connected to recorders. The older recording oscillographs have largely been displaced by computerized recorders.

The mass spectrum is a total accumulation of the amount and mass of ions reaching the detector at any given time. The mass spectrum allows determination of the parent molecular ion and provides structural information about the analyte.

Mass spectrometers require daily tuning and quality assurance. Problems are avoided by proper specimen processing, use of high-purity chemicals and carrier gases, and periodic cleaning and inspection.

Questions and Problems

1. List the component parts of a mass spectrometer and describe their functions.
2. Describe the differences in mass spectra obtained using EI ionization versus CI.
3. Determine the fragmentation patterns of ephedrine-TPC (Fig. 16-2) and phentermine-TPC (Fig. 16-3) for the ions at m/z 251, 194, and 166.
4. Isotope lines that add 1 or 2 amu to parent and fragmentation ions are generally detected in mass spectra due to the natural occurrence of stable isotopes. Given the following abundance of isotopes in the environment, calculate the expected abundances of the $(M^+ + 1)$ and $(M^+ + 2)$ lines for the spectrum of nonderivatized caffeine. Do they agree with the amounts shown in Figure 16-4a? $^{13}C = 1.1\%$; $^{15}N = 0.37\%$; $^{17}O = 0.4\%$; $^{18}O = 0.2\%$; $^{2}H = 0.015\%$.
5. There is considerable interest in GC/MS confirmation assays to identify the source of morphine positive urine drug screens. Both street heroin and poppy seeds, obtained in baked food products, can be metabolized to morphine, giving positive urine results and posing a legal problem for prosecution cases. Heroin, however, is first metabolized to 6-monoacetylmorphine (MAM) and then to morphine, whereas poppy seed ingestion does not result in MAM production. Given the structure of these opiates (Fig. 16-12a), (a) Determine which of the reagents in Figure 16-12b would be the most appropriate derivatization agent for the separation of these compounds based on mass alone. Why? (b) You decide to derivatize these compounds with N-methyl-bistrifluoroacetamide (MBTFA) and obtain m/z 477, 380, and 364 ions for morphine; m/z 423, 380, 364, and 267 for MAM; and m/z 369 and 310 for heroin. Indicate possible fragmentation patterns

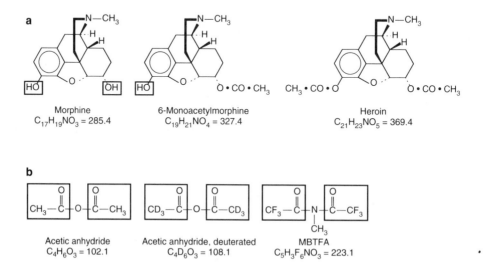

Figure 16-12. (a) Chemical structures of morphine-related opiates. The shaded hydroxy-groups are susceptible to acetylation. (b) Chemical structures of three common derivatizing agents. The shaded groups are transferred to analyte molecules during derivatization.

generating these ions. (c) Which compounds would be most appropriate to use as internal standards?

6. Draw schematics of magnetic sector and quadrupole mass analyzers that illustrate their components and operating principles.

7. List the advantages of using computers to record mass spectrometry data.

References

1. Andresen BD, Wise BL. Mass spectrometry. In: Tietz NW, ed. Textbook of clinical chemistry. Philadelphia: WB Saunders, 1986:204-05.

2. Poklis A. Gas chromatography. In: Kaplan LA, Pesce AJ. Clinical chemistry: Theory, analysis, and correlation, 2nd ed. St. Louis: CV Mosby, 1989:123-05.

3. Willard HH, Merritt LL Jr, Dean JA, Settle FA Jr. Instrumental methods of analysis, 7th ed. Belmont, CA: Wadsworth Publishing, 1988, 476-77.

4. Skoog DA, Leary JJ. Principles of instrumental analysis, 4th ed. Fort Worth: Saunders College Publishing, 1992:429-32.

Suggested Readings

Gudzinowicz BJ, Gudzinowicz MJ, Martin HF. Fundamentals of integrated GC-MS (in three parts). Chromatographic Science Series, vol. 7. New York: Marcel Dekker, 1977.

Lawson AM. Mass spectrometry. Hawthorne, NY: Walter de Gruyter & Co., 1989.

McLafferty FW. Interpretation of mass spectra, 2nd ed. Reading, MA: WA Benjamin, 1973.

Watson JT. Introduction to mass spectrometry, 2nd ed. New York: Raven Press, 1985.

Yinon J. Forensic mass spectrometry. Boca Raton, FL: CRC Press, 1987.

17

FLOW CYTOMETRY

Michaeleen M. Collins
Samuel J. Pirruccello

Objectives

After completing this chapter, the reader will be able to:

1. Explain the basic principles of flow cytometry.
2. Describe the workings of flow cells.
3. Explain the relationship between sample flow rate and analysis resolution and sensitivity.
4. List the advantages and disadvantages of jet-in-air and closed quartz flow cells.
5. List the advantages and disadvantages of arc lamp and laser light sources.
6. Describe how an argon laser works.
7. List the types of measurements available with flow cytometers, and describe their uses.
8. Describe the following optical components of a flow cytometer: lenses, dichroic filters, and dielectric mirrors.
9. Explain when logarithmic signal amplification is necessary.
10. Interpret single-parameter histograms and dual-parameter contour plots of mixed cell populations.
11. Describe maintenance and quality assurance procedures for flow cytometry.

Definitions

Arc Lamp: A light source containing mercury or xenon gas under high pressure. When stimulated by an electrical discharge between closely spaced electrodes, the gas emits a continuous spectrum of light from about 200 nm into the infrared.

Coherent Light: Light in which all the waves are in phase and parallel.

Dichroic Filter or Mirror: Filter coated with a substance that reflects light above or below a certain wavelength and transmits other wavelengths. Dichroic filters are usually placed at a 45° angle to the incident light beam.

Dielectric Mirror: A device composed of alternating thin layers of high and low refractive index glass. A portion of light is reflected each time the beam reaches a high refractive index layer. Wavelengths that are multiples of four times the layer thickness undergo constructive interference with reflection. All other wavelengths undergo destructive interference.

Fluorochrome: A fluorescent pigment.

Forward Angle Light Scatter: Light scatter in nearly the same direction as the incident beam. The intensity of forward light scatter is directly related to the size of the particle.

Frequency Distribution Plot: A plot of counts or frequency (*y* axis) versus numeric or category group (*x* axis) (also known as a histogram). In flow cytometry the *x* axis is usually a channel defined by a range of light scattering or fluorescence intensities.

Gating: Selection of specific ranges of signal intensities from forward angle light scatter, 90° light scatter, or a fluorochrome's fluorescence. Multiple gating or backgating involves selecting two or more parameters for analysis. This allows mixtures of particles or cells to be resolved into discrete groups such as lymphocytes, monocytes, and granulocytes.

Hydrodynamic Focusing: Use of pressures and tube diameters to alter position, diameter, and flow rate of the sample stream.

Hydrodynamics: The relationship between motion and forces affecting motion in fluids.

Laminar Flow: Nonturbulent flow of fluid in layers near a boundary. In flow cytometry the boundaries are between sample and sheath fluids and between sheath fluid and air or the flow cell walls.

LASER: Light Amplification by Stimulated Emission of Radiation. A device that uses oscillations of atoms or molecules between energy levels for generating coherent electromagnetic radiation.

Resolution: In flow cytometry, the ability to separate signals from individual particles or cells.

Sensitivity: The ability to differentiate between low-intensity sample signals and background noise.

Sheath fluid: Pressurized fluid that surrounds the sample stream in the flow cell and chamber.

Introduction

Flow cytometers are laser- or arc lamp-based instruments capable of discrete analysis of single particles in suspension as they pass through an aperture at high velocity. Particles may be whole cells, cellular components such as nuclei, latex beads, or any other particle suited for specific analysis. Cytometry allows for the measurement of multiple properties of a single cell or particle and allows measurements to be made rapidly on thousands of cells from heterogeneous mixtures. The measured parameters in flow cytometry include light scatter, which yields structural information about the particles analyzed, and fluorescence emission from dyes that are bound to specific molecular structures of the cell such as nuclei, chromosomes, cytoplasm, organelles, or membranes. These measurements are performed by illuminating the cells or particles with light at the specific absorption wavelength of the dyes used as detector molecules.

Flow cytometers employ a multiplicity of technologies, including lasers, hydrodynamics, optics, and computers. Flow cytometers analyze cells with a high degree of specificity, and some instruments can also physically sort cells based on defined parameters. In this chapter we will focus on the basic operation of flow cytometers. A more in-depth discussion of fluorescence is given in Chapter 9. Detailed information on laser technology, optics, and electronics is given in *Flow Cytometry and Sorting.*[1]

Principles and Component Parts

A flow cytometer is composed of a flow cell with inlets for sample and sheath fluids, a flow chamber in which sample passes through one or more high-intensity light beams, a laser or arc lamp light source, optics for focusing and selecting light, filters and mirrors, multiple detectors, and a computer for signal processing and recording output. Some flow cytometers also have a cell-sorting device.

FLOW CELL

Discrete analysis can occur only if the sample in suspension is appropriately presented to the detection area.[2] All flow cytometers use some type of *flow cell* with hydrodynamic focusing to present the particles to the laser beam. This hydrodynamic focusing makes use of laminar flow (Fig. 17-1). First, water or saline from a pressurized container is introduced into the flow cell (sheath fluid). Then, the sample fluid is injected into the center of the sheath fluid. The sample containing the cells or particles is then hydrodynamically confined to the center of the sheath stream.

The diameter of the sample stream determines the resolution of analysis. Better resolution is achieved with smaller-diameter streams that decrease the likelihood of more than one cell at a time encountering the laser beam.

Speed of sample delivery changes the sensitivity of analysis. A slower-moving stream allows each particle to spend more time within the light beam. This increases light scatter and fluorescence from each particle, resulting in stronger signals reaching the detectors.

The sheath pressure, sample pressure, and sample delivery rate control the velocity and diameter of the sample stream. Cytometers employ either a differential pressure system or a volumetric injection system to control these variables. In the differential pressure system, the sample tube and the sheath tank are at different pressures. The magnitude of the pressure difference between the two fluids determines the sample flow rate (Fig. 17-2). The primary advantage of differential pressure systems is their ability to precisely control sample delivery. A disadvantage of these systems is their inability to determine the number of cells or particles per unit volume of sample.

In the volumetric injection system a fixed volume of sample is aspirated and delivered by syringe. Sample volume and injection rate are selected by the operator. Therefore, the number of cells per unit sample volume can be calculated from the number of cells recorded per unit of time. Sample velocity is controlled by the sheath

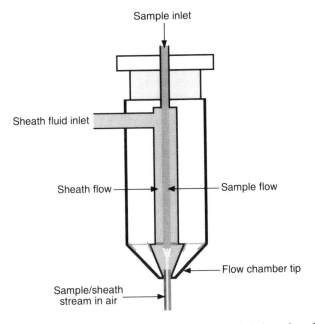

Figure 17-1. Flow cell with a jet-in-air type chamber. Sample is introduced under pressure in the sample inlet. The sample stream is later contained within the sheath fluid (also under pressure). These streams are focused at the flow cell tip. The sheath fluid functions as a cuvette.

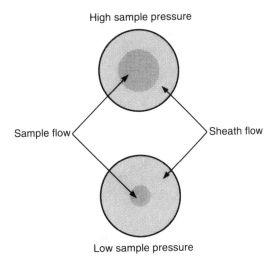

Figure 17-2. Changes in sample stream diameter with changes in sample fluid pressure.

pressure, and sample stream diameter is controlled by both the sheath pressure and the volumetric sample delivery rate. Increasing the sheath pressure while keeping the sample delivery rate constant increases sample stream velocity and decreases sample stream diameter. This improves resolution but decreases sensitivity. Increasing the sample delivery rate while keeping the sheath pressure constant increases sample stream diameter but does not affect its velocity. This increases the analysis rate at the expense of resolution. Care must be taken to flush between samples when this injection system is employed to avoid carryover from cells remaining in the syringe or tubing.

FLOW CHAMBERS

Flow chambers direct the specimen through the light beam. The two types of flow chambers are jet-in-air and closed quartz flow cells. In *jet-in-air flow chambers,* the sample stream is focused in the flow cell and intersects the laser beam immediately upon emerging from the orifice of a conical nozzle. The nozzle diameter is usually 70 to 100 μm, but larger nozzles may be used for analysis of large diameter particles such as plant cells.

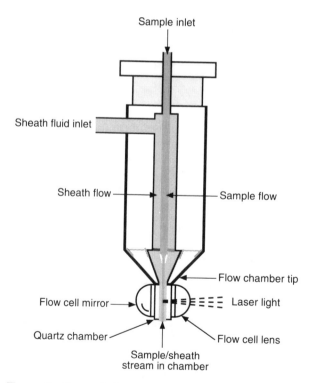

Figure 17-3. Flow cell with a sealed quartz chamber. Sheath and sample streams are directed through the quartz chamber. The optical properties are improved, and flow velocities can be lower than with a jet-in-air chamber.

Quartz flow cell chamber tips are also available on some instruments to improve sensing. The sample is illuminated and sensed through the quartz flow cell rather than in air (Fig. 17-3). In the closed chamber, the flow cell orifice leads to a tube that facilitates better sensitivity than jet-in-air flow chambers. To maintain laminar flow in air, stream velocity cannot be reduced below certain limits because of air friction. (For a 100-μm orifice the minimum velocity is about 3 m/sec.)[1] Velocity in a closed flow chamber is limited only by the diameter of the flow cell channel. Therefore, much lower sample stream velocities are practical. The closed chamber also avoids the intense reflection and scattering of excitation light that occurs at the air-stream interface.

LIGHT SOURCE

Numerous light sources have been employed in flow cytometry. These include argon, krypton, helium, and neon ion and dye lasers. The most common excitation light sources for clinical laboratory instruments are air-cooled argon ion lasers and mercury arc lamps. The original flow cytometers, which were actually spectropho- tometers modified to perform analysis on continuously flowing cells in suspension, used arc lamps for illumination. Some models currently use mercury arc lamps, but lasers now predominate as excitation light sources. This preference for lasers is based on the spectral characteristics and power profile of the emitted light, the types of dyes (i.e., absorption profiles) available, and the relative ease of focusing laser light over arc lamp light.

Arc Lamps

Several types of *arc lamps* are available, but the 100-watt mercury short arc lamp is best suited for use in flow cytometry. Brightness or radiance of the light source is a critical consideration for fluorescence excitation. This relates to the ability to focus the excitation light at the area of particle analysis while maintaining a constant power profile across the diameter of the sample stream. The mercury short arc lamp has the highest radiance of available arc lamps.

Mercury arc lamps produce several emission lines. The strongest emission is at 365 nm. Hence, the most appropriate fluorochromes for use with mercury arc lamps are dyes that have absorption maxima in the near ultraviolet range. A weaker mercury emission line at 436 nm (blue light) can be used for excitation of dyes such as fluorescein (450 nm absorption maximum) or acridine orange (500 nm absorption maximum). However, when both dyes are used in combination, excitation with single laser line at 488 nm is more efficient.

Two major drawbacks of arc lamp sources are the requirements for focusing optics and for a monochromator. Multiple lenses (condenser, relay, and objective), diaphragms (aperture and field), and filters (heat, red, and excitation) make arc lamp systems much more difficult to maintain. A third drawback is the difficulty of maintaining a constant power output from the arc lamp. Power fluctuations of the excitation light produce large variances in the measurement of individual particles with the same brightness.

Lasers

Lasers have the distinct advantage of being tunable to specific emission lines so that emitted light is of a single selected wavelength. Lasers are therefore superior to standard arc lamps and filters when discrete excitation wavelengths are required for analysis.

In most clinical laboratory flow cytometers, the lasing material is the inert gas argon. An electric current excites orbiting electrons of the argon ions to one or more higher energy states in the gas plasma tube of the laser (Fig. 17-4). These excited electrons then fall back to their ground state, and energy is released as a photon of light. (This is the same principle as the hollow cathode lamp described in Chapter 7.) Mirrors at both ends of the plasma tube reflect emitted light back into the argon plasma tube so it can stimulate other ions to emit photons of light of the same wavelength and direction as the incident photons. A dielectric mirror on the emission end of the plasma tube allows a small amount of light to be emitted to form the laser

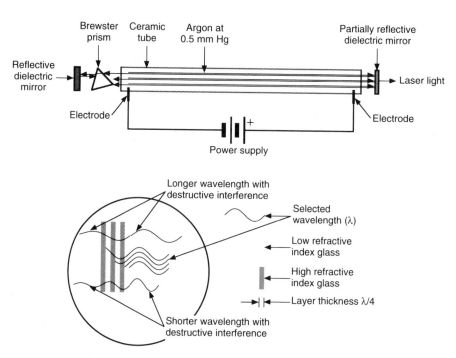

Figure 17-4. Argon laser. Electric current is generated within a ceramic tube containing argon gas at low pressure. Collision of an electron with an argon atom produces a positively charged argon ion and a second electron. Collision between an argon ion and an electron kicks an electron from the 3p orbital to the 4p orbital. This excited state is unstable, and the electron drops to the 4s orbital with the emission of a photon. Emitted light passes through the clear glass ends of the tube and reaches a dielectric mirror. A selected wavelength undergoes constructive interference when reflected. Other wavelengths undergo destructive interference or pass through the dielectric mirror (see inset). Wavelength selection is controlled by the Brewster prism and by the thickness of the layers in the dielectric mirrors. The dielectric mirror at the output end of the laser lets approximately 1% of laser light through.

beam. The remainder of the light is reflected back into the plasma tube to maintain stimulated emission. A prism between the laser tube and the rear mirror diffracts wavelengths of light at different angles. Changing the angle of the rear mirror changes the laser's wavelength. Unwanted emission wavelengths are reflected away from the rear aperture of the plasma tube. A second dichroic mirror in the path of the laser beam reflects a portion of the beam to a photodiode. The photodiode is directly coupled to the electrical input driving the laser and continuously adjusts the current across the plasma tube to maintain constant laser light intensity. The emitted light beam is thus monochromatic, coherent, and of fixed intensity. The argon ion laser is tuned to its major emission line at 488 nm for most clinical laboratory applications.

Laser light sources do have a few drawbacks. High electrical current is required to excite the argon ions in large plasma tubes. The plasma tubes give off large amounts of heat. Early flow cytometers use lasers with high-power outputs (3–5 watts maximum) that require circulating water to cool the lasers and transformers. Approximately 2 gallons of water per minute are required to cool a standard 5-watt laser. Newer instruments use air-cooled 400-mW lasers that operate on standard 120-V alternating current. The decrease in sensitivity resulting from illuminating particles at lower beam strengths is offset by the addition of a small parabolic mirror on the closed flow cell. The parabolic mirror captures scattered and fluorescent light and refocuses it into the detectors.

OPTICS FOR FOCUSING AND SHAPING THE LASER BEAM

Single-cell analysis requires that the laser beam be tightly focused to prevent illuminating more than one cell at a time. In addition, the power profile of the beam across the sample stream should vary by no more than 2 to 5%, so that cells positioned anywhere in the stream will receive the same amount of excitation light. Many flow cytometers use two *crossed cylindrical lenses* to focus the laser beam (Fig. 17-5). The

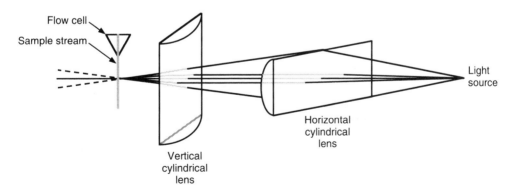

Figure 17-5. Crossed cylindrical lenses used to focus laser light on the flow cytometer sample stream. The horizontal lens decreases the vertical dispersion of the light. The vertical lens decreases the horizontal dispersion. The net result in a small ellipse of light focused on the sample stream.

horizontal lens reduces the height of the beam. The vertical lens reduces the width of the beam. Used together, the crossed lenses focus the laser beam to a horizontal ellipse. A Gaussian distribution of light intensity is produced across the focused beam, with maximum intensity at the center of the ellipse.

Forward Angle Light Scatter Detection

When particles in the sample stream encounter the laser beam, several events occur. First, each particle scatters some of the laser light. Although light is scattered in all directions when a particle is entirely within the laser beam, the intensity of light scatter is not symmetrical (see Chapter 8 and Fig. 8-4). The amount of light scattered along the forward axis or at narrow angles to the axis of the laser beam is roughly proportional to the size of the particle or cell. This *forward angle light scatter* is used to measure cell size. The light scatter detector located at a forward direction from the laser beam is commonly a solid-state silicon photodiode. The photodiode produces current when exposed to light, and this current is transformed to a voltage pulse proportional to the total amount of light collected (integrated pulse). The amount of light is usually high, so neutral density filters are used to reduce the intensity. An absorber bar in front of the photodiode prevents the incident laser beam and stray light from striking the detector.

Fluorescence and 90° Light Scatter Detection

Perpendicular to the laser beam and the sample stream is a lens that collects 90° light scatter and fluorescence. Light scattered at a 90° angle (orthogonally) has been shown to relate to the internal structure or granularity of the cell.[3] For example, smooth small lymphocytes exhibit little forward angle or 90° light scattering. Larger, granular neutrophils exhibit much higher forward angle and 90° light scattering. Monocytes exhibit intermediate forward and 90° light scattering. On the flow cytometer, these three cell types can be distinguished by their light scatter properties alone without adding additional reagents (Fig. 17-6).

As cells or particles pass through the laser beam, fluorescent dyes bound to the cell or incorporated into the particle are excited. The fluorochromes absorb the incident laser light and reemit light of a lower energy and longer wavelength. Emitted light is collected by the optics located 90° to the laser beam. A barrier filter blocks out laser excitation light and stray light. Dichroic filters are then used to select the specific wavelengths of fluorescence to be measured. The typical argon laser light emission at 488 nm is in the excitation spectrum for commonly used fluorochromes such as fluoroescein isothiocyanate (FITC), phycoerythrin, and propidium iodide. These fluorochromes are ideal for clinical flow cytometry because they have overlapping absorption spectra, allowing excitation by a single laser line. The fluorescent emission wavelengths for these three dyes are dissimilar, allowing adequate separation with filters. The emission signals from each fluorochrome are quantitated by separate detectors with the appropriate dichroic filters. Several characteristics of the cell can be measured simultaneously by using two or three dyes in combination. This is termed *multicolor analysis.* Fluorochrome dyes can bind to different cell compo-

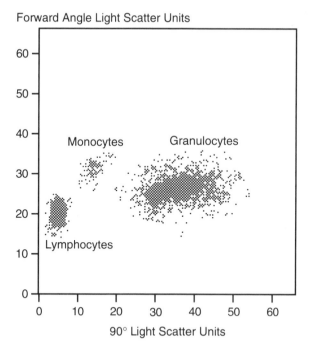

Figure 17-6. Plot of forward angle versus $90°$ light scattering intensities for leukocytes. Lymphocytes, monocytes, and granulocytes are easily resolved without staining. Forward angle light scattering relates mostly to particle size. Monocytes and granulocytes give similar responses. $90°$ light scattering relates mostly to particle granularity. Granulocytes exhibit strong $90°$ light scattering.

nents: cell membranes, cytoplasm, organelles, nuclei, or chromosomes. Fluorochrome-tagged antibodies can bind specific receptors, proteins, or nucleic acids.

FILTERS AND MIRRORS

Dielectric mirrors are mirrors that allow some light to pass through the mirror while reflecting the remaining light. Dielectric mirrors are used to reflect light of specified wavelengths while allowing light of different wavelengths to pass (see inset in Fig. 17-4). They function like multilayer interference filters (see Fig. 6-6). *Dichroic filters* are used to spectrally separate the emitted fluorescent light and to reflect the specific emission from a given dye to the appropriate detector.

One of the most basic systems, for example, uses a 500-nm wavelength dichroic filter to reflect $90°$ light scatter (488 nm) into the first detector while allowing only wavelengths of light longer than 500 nm to pass through. Additional dichroic filters can be used to divert two or more longer wavelengths of fluorescent light to an array of detectors located below the $90°$ scatter detector.

DETECTORS

Photomultiplier tubes are used to measure $90°$ light scatter and fluorescence. Photomultiplier tubes are shown and described in Chapter 6 (see Fig. 6-12).

SIGNAL PROCESSING

The analog signals generated through conversion of light photons to electrical impulses may be processed in several ways. All the signals generated by any one particle while in the laser beam can be summed to give the total light scatter or fluorescence emitted by that particle. This integrated signal equals the area under the curve of the electrical pulse.

The peak height of the electrical pulse can also be measured. The peak height is proportional to the maximum light scatter or fluorescence signal generated by the particle while it passes through the laser beam.

Detector signals can undergo linear or logarithmic amplification. Linear amplification is used when the cell-to-cell differences in light scatter or fluorescence emission are small. Logarithmic amplification is used when cell-to-cell differences in light scatter and especially fluorescence emission are very large (orders of magnitude). Three and four decade logarithmic amplifications are common on most clinical flow cytometers.

Analog signals produced in the detectors are converted to digital signals by using analog-to-digital converters. Each pulse is measured and converted to a relative number proportional to the light intensity from the particle. Instruments may use low-resolution signal collection with 256 channels or higher-resolution collection with 1000 or more channels. Each channel represents a fluorescence intensity value that may be collected as a linear or log data set for each sample analyzed.

Fluorescence Compensation

In many dual-color immunofluorescence applications in which two dyes are excited by a single wavelength of light, the emission spectra of the two dyes may overlap. The high- or low-energy emission signal from one fluorochrome may therefore be measured by the detector set up to measure the second fluorochrome. This results from the inability of the dichroic filters to separate the entire emission spectrum from both dyes. *Fluorescence compensation* is an electronic correction where a portion of the signal from each of the channels is subtracted.[4] The percentage of fluorescence compensation required for a particular dye combination is determined by the percentage of spectral emission overlap and the dichroic filters and mirrors used.

DATA ANALYSIS

Data may be measured as a single-parameter frequency distribution or histogram where the magnitude of the measured parameter (e.g., fluorescence or light scatter) is graphed on the x axis and the frequency or number of cells analyzed is plotted on the y axis (Fig. 17-7).

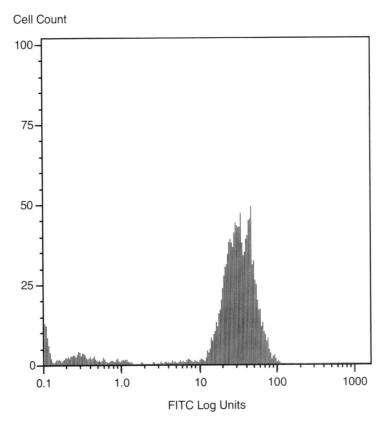

Cell Count

Figure 17-7. Single-parameter histogram of FITC fluorescence. The *y* axis is the number of cells. Each line on the histogram represents a channel of the fluorescence detector. This histogram shows two populations. About 25% of cells have FITC fluorescence intensities between 0.1 and 1.0. About 70% of cells have intensities between 10 and 100.

Two-parameter histograms plot two measurement parameters as defined by the operator. One commonly used two-parameter histogram plots forward angle light scatter on the *x* or *y* axis and 90° light scatter on the other axis. The result is a scattergram that reflects the cell populations within a given mixture, as forward angle light scatter represents cell size and 90° light scatter represents granularity (Fig. 17-6). Another commonly used two-parameter histogram plots red fluorescence (phyco-erythrin) against green fluorescence (FITC) (Fig. 17-8). Monoclonal antibodies to cell surface antigens conjugated with these dyes may be used to enumerate specific cell populations within a heterogeneous sample such as peripheral blood or bone marrow. For two-color fluorescence histograms, cell number or frequency is generally plotted as a density or contour map. Two-color analysis therefore allows one to calculate the frequencies of four or more discrete populations of cells depending on the cell mixture and the antibodies used.

Phycoerythrin Log Units

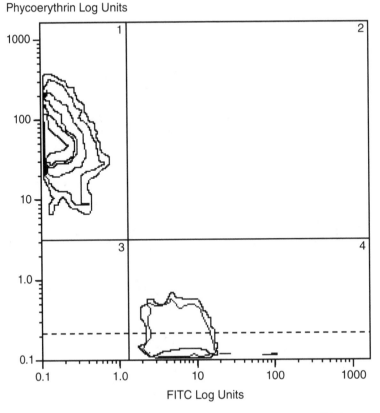

Figure 17-8.   Dual-parameter contour plot of phycoerythrin versus FITC fluorescence intensities. Each contour line represents a specified number of particles. For example, the horizontal dashed line indicates that the number of cells with about 0.25 phycoerythrin and 2.5 FITC fluorescence units is the same as the number of cells with 0.25 phycoerythrin and 20 FITC fluorescence units. This dual parameter contour plot shows two distinct populations of cells. They can easily by resolved with two cutoffs: FITC at 1.5 and phycoerythrin at 3.0 fluorescence units. This yields four zones, with the cells of interest being in zone 1 or zone 4.

Unless the operator specifies otherwise, the flow cytometer will present data measurements on all particles as they pass through the laser beam. Analysis of discrete populations is accomplished through electronic gating where a cell must exhibit appropriate magnitude of particular parameters to be included in the analysis. These parameters may be either light scatter characteristics, fluorescence characteristics, or some combination of both. Gates are defined by delineating specific channels on the *x* and *y* axes to encompass the region of interest for analysis. Two or more gates may be used to define and measure discrete cell populations. This multiple gating or backgating as it is commonly called, allows the flow cytometer operator to answer very specific questions about the properties of a given cell population.

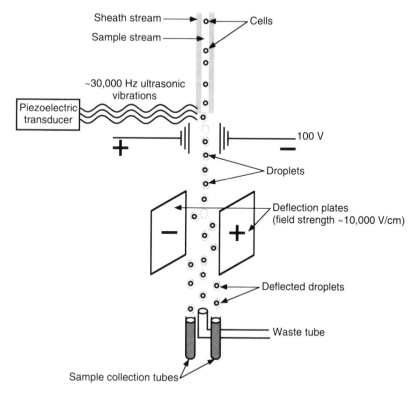

Figure 17-9. Flow cytometer cell sorter. After passing through the flow chamber and detection system, the streams are subjected to ultrasonic radiation from a piezoelectric transducer. This disperses the streams into fine droplets. If conditions are right, no droplet will contain more than one particle. Selected droplets are given a pulse of a positive or negative charge before reaching the deflector plates. Uncharged droplets pass straight through to the waste tube. Charged droplets move toward one plate or the other. The deflected droplets are collected into two containers.

Listmode is a computer list of every cell analyzed with the channel values for each measured parameter. Most flow cytometers can store this list of data in the computer. The operator can convert the list data to histogram form, adjust the gates, and recompile the data list. Listmode analysis is particularly useful for complicated analysis protocols of heterogeneous populations or when a sample contains rare events. Parameter selections and gates may be changed for a run, and the run can then be repeated using only a small amount of sample.

CELL SORTING

Cell sorting is possible because computers can analyze detector signals in less than a millisecond. Cells meeting preselected criteria can be sorted into collection tubes (Fig. 17-9).[5] Sheath fluid is directed away from the cell sorter. The sample stream passes into the sorter. First, ultrasonic waves disrupt the sample stream and produce fine droplets at the sound wave frequency (30,000 Hz in Fig. 17-9). Flow rate and sample dilution are adjusted so that each droplet contains only one cell. A droplet with a cell of interest is subjected to a positive or a negative potential (100 V) that gives the cell a temporary surface charge. Charged cells are deflected by the deflection plates into sample collection tubes. Uncharged cells pass straight through. The collected cells may be a single cell type or a few cell types with some common characteristics. The sorting process can be repeated to yield smaller volumes of single cell types.

Maintenance and Quality Assurance

Flow cytometers are precision instruments that must be scrupulously maintained for optimum functioning. All optical surfaces must be kept clean and free of abrasions. This is especially true in the flow chamber, where buildup of proteins and cellular debris must be prevented. The high-pressure hydrodynamics of flow cytometry requires smooth, clean surfaces. Contamination of walls or nozzle tips will produce turbulence and disrupt stream flow.

Periodic assessments of optical alignment, detector response to fluorescence, and linearity of response are necessary. In addition, the light source and monochromators need periodic inspection and evaluation (as for spectrophotometers). Finally, control materials are analyzed at regular intervals.

VERIFICATION OF OPTICAL ALIGNMENT

A solution of fluorospheres (uniform plastic particles incorporating a fluorescent dye) must be sampled each day of operation to verify alignment of the flow cytometer optics and sample stream. Alignment is adjusted to achieve maximum signal intensity and minimum signal variability. These parameters are monitored by recording the mean channel number of fluorescence and light scattering and the coefficient of variation (CV) of the peaks. All parameters that will be used to analyze test specimens must be monitored (e.g., forward and 90° light scattering, red and green fluorescence).

STANDARDIZATION OF FLUORESCENCE INTENSITY

Reference fluorospheres with stable fluorescence intensity similar to that of antibody-stained lymphocytes are used to optimize fluorescence amplification or gain settings. Ideally, settings are chosen so that peak fluorescence is near the midpoint of the intensity scale. All fluorosphere results should be less than the highest channel of the histogram. Amplification should be adjusted with unstained lymphocytes. Their signal should be greater than the lowest channel. Fluorospheres are monitored at least daily to ensure that changes in the level of antigen expression (antibody fluorescence) on a patient's cells are biological rather than analytical.

DETERMINATION OF LOGARITHMIC AMPLIFIER LINEARITY

Reference particles of specific fluorescent intensities are available for determining instrument linearity. These should be used periodically (monthly) to ensure that the low-intensity and high-intensity signals are amplified at the same ratio.

VERIFICATION OF REAGENT QUALITY AND PROCEDURAL STEPS

Commercially prepared control cells are available to monitor reagents and procedures. These controls are handled and assayed in the same way as patient samples. Selection of the appropriate controls depends on the use of the flow cytometer and will not be fully discussed here. Examples include isotypic controls for immunophenotyping applications and gating controls for cellular applications.

Summary

Flow cytometry is a powerful technique for analysis of fluid suspensions of cells and particles. A flow cytometer consists of a flow cell for injecting and hydrodynamically focusing a sample stream, a flow chamber that functions as cuvette, a powerful light source such as an argon laser, optics for focusing and selecting light, photomultiplier tube detectors, a signal processor, and a computer for data analysis and reporting. Multiple parameters—forward angle and 90° light scatter and fluorescence of at least two fluorochromes—can be evaluated simultaneously. This enables classification and enumeration of cells in blood, bone marrow, and tissue suspensions. Some flow cytometers also can sort cells based on predefined parameters.

Questions and Problems

1. You switch from a jet-in-air to a closed quartz flow chamber. Sample stream velocity is reduced by a factor of 4. What are the effects on analysis?
2. List the advantages of a laser light source over an arc lamp.
3. How is light produced in an argon laser?
4. List the measurement parameters available for flow cytometry and their uses.
5. Sketch a dielectric mirror and describe how it works.
6. In the histogram shown in Figure 17-7, what three FITC fluorescence intensities had cell counts of approximately 12?
7. What can be achieved by analyzing solutions containing fluorospheres of uniform size with stable fluorescence?

References

1. Steen HB. Characteristics of flow cytometers. In: Melamed MR, Lindmo T, Mendelson ML, eds. Flow cytometry and sorting, 2nd ed. New York: Wiley-Liss, 1990:2-25.

2. Wood JCS. Clinical flow cytometry instrumentation. In: Bauer KD, Duque RE, Shankey TV, eds. Clinical flow cytometry: Principles and application. Baltimore: Williams and Wilkins, 1993:71-92.

3. Salzman GC, Crowell JM, Martin JC, Trujillo TT, Romero A, Mullaney PF, LaBauve PM. Cell classification by laser light scattering: Identification and separation of unstained leukocytes. Acta Cytol (Praha) 1975, 19:374-77.

4. Loken MR, Parks DR, Herzenberg LA. Two-color immunofluorescence using a fluorescence-activated cell sorter. J Histochem Cytochem 1977, 25:899-907.

5. Salzman GC. Flow cytometry: The user of lasers for rapid analysis and separation of single biological cells. In: Goldman L, ed. The biomedical laser, New York: Springer-Verlag, 1981:33-53.

Suggested Readings

Dorros G. Understanding lasers. Mount Kisco, NY: Futura Publishing, 1991.
Keren DF, ed. Flow cytometry in clinical diagnosis. Chicago: ASCP Press, 1989.
Shapiro HM. Practical flow cytometry, 2nd ed. New York: Alan R. Liss, 1988.

18

AUTOMATED CHEMISTRY ANALYZERS

Gregory A. Tetrault
Catherine Leiendecker-Foster
John H. Eckfeldt
Ronald D. Feld
Jimmie K. Noffsinger

Objectives

After completing this chapter, the reader will be able to:

1. Define automation, and list commonly automated testing steps.
2. Classify automated chemistry analyzers.
3. Define and compare unidirectional and bidirectional interfaces.
4. Describe how sampling and testing throughput affect turnaround time.
5. Explain how centrifugal analyzers operate.
6. Describe four sequential multiple analyte analyzers.
7. Describe four simultaneous multiple analyte analyzers.
8. Describe Kodak Ektachem dry-slide technology.
9. Define the term *analytical run,* and describe how it affects quality control procedures.

Definitions

Automation: The process in which a task is accomplished by an apparatus with few steps performed by the operator. A completely automated system requires no operator once it is begun. Most clinical chemistry laboratory instrumentation is partially automated (semiautomated).

Bar Coding: A system in which information is encoded in a series of lines or bars. The spacing and thickness of these lines are sensed by a reader system, and this information is then relayed to and interpreted by a computer.

Bidirectional Interface: The hardware and software that enable an instrument's microcomputer to communicate with a laboratory information system computer. Information is uploaded to the instrument and downloaded to the laboratory computer. Data are often sent by using a standard computer communications protocol such as RS232.

Carryover: A sampling problem in which a small amount of one sample contaminates a subsequent sample. This can occur if sample pipet washing is incomplete. It is also an unavoidable feature of many continuous flow analyzers.

Discrete Analysis: Analysis in which each test is compartmentalized and separated from preceding and subsequent tests.

Ion-Selective Electrode (ISE):   An electrode with a unique phase that allows it to respond selectively to the concentration of a single ion in the presence of others.

Random Access: The ability to utilize any given reagent and/or any given sample at any time in any desired order.

Sequential Analysis: Analysis in which multiple tests on a given clinical specimen are performed one after another.

Simultaneous Analysis: Analysis in which multiple tests on a given clinical specimen are performed concurrently.

Throughput: The maximum number of tests or specimens that can be analyzed in a given time (usually per hour).

Turnaroud Time: The time between the receipt of a specimen and the reporting of analytic test result on that specimen.

Unidirectional Interface: The hardware and software that enable an instrument to download data to a computer.

Introduction

In preceeding chapters many types of clinical chemistry analyses have been discussed: spectrophotometric, turbidometric, fluorometric, nephelometric, potentiometric, coulometric, voltammetric, and so on. In this chapter we discuss automated instrument systems that employ one or more of these techniques. The term *automation* has become overused and abused. Automation is simply the process in which more tasks are performed by the mechanical or electronic system and fewer tasks are performed by the operator. Automation may be as simple as combining two switches into one or as complex as a computerized, roboticized, fully functional space exploration probe.

Clinical chemistry automation began with continuous flow technology in the 1950s. Technicon (now Miles Inc., Diagnostics Div., Tarrytown, NY 10591) developed the AutoAnalyzer® and then the SMA® 6/60 and SMA® 12/60 analyzers. These devices replaced repetitive manual benchtop analyses with partially automated ones. They were fast, precise, and labor-saving. Continuous flow analyzers moved samples and reagents through plastic tubing. Samples were separated only by air bubbles and wash solution. Carryover was a problem, especially with enzyme assays, where, for example, a sample with 2000 IU/L of aspartate aminotransferase (AST) could be followed by one with only 10 IU/L. Automated discrete analyzers were developed in the 1960s. The first were single analyte (at a time) batch analyzers. Discrete analyzers with random access to specimens and to reagents followed. Advances in technology and increased testing demands in the clinical laboratories led to the development of highly sophisticated, multichannel, discrete analyzers. These allow a high throughput of specimens and analyze only those tests that are actually requested on each specimen (unlike continuous flow analyzers that perform their entire test repertoire

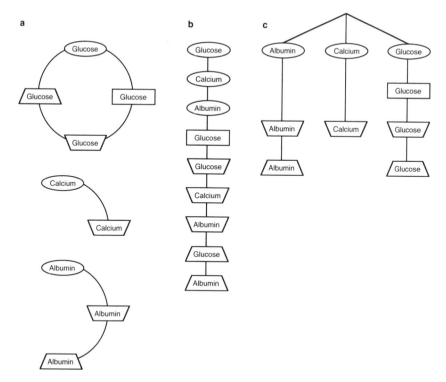

Figure 18-1. Automation schemes with three assays and four samples. (a) Batch analyses. (b) Sequential multianalyte analyses. (c) Simultaneous multianalyte analyses.

on every specimen). Today, the majority of clinical chemistry laboratory tests are performed on multichannel discrete analyzers.

We will first describe components common to all types of automated chemistry analyzers and then discuss three classes of automated instruments: discrete batch, discrete sequential multiple analyte, and discrete simultaneous multiple analyte analyzers. These types of analyzers are depicted in Figure 18-1.[1]

Principles and Components of Automation

There are many steps between specimen arrival at the bench and reporting of results. Any or all of these steps can be automated. The first component of automation in most systems is specimen sampling. Almost all modern clinical chemistry analyzers have automated samplers. Specimens are usually loaded onto carousels or racks. The instrument rotates the carousel or moves the racks to place each sample into the sampling position. Sampling probes aspirate specimen and deliver it to a reaction chamber. Some instruments have also automated sample identification with bar code readers. Bar code-labeled specimens are positively identified by the instrument.

This reduces laboratory errors due to inadvertent misplacement or misidentification of a specimen by the operator.

Reagent and diluent addition also are automated on most modern chemistry analyzers. Pumps or syringes commonly are used to add liquid reagents. Dry reagents come premeasured (see discussion of Ektachem and *aca*™ instruments).

Sample-diluent-reagent mixtures are placed into reaction vessel holders (if they are not already there). Reaction vessels automatically are moved into detection areas in most analyzers. Detector signals are processed and reported digitally or by computer. Modern analyzers contain microprocessors or complete microcomputers for signal processing, data analysis, and result reporting.

Discrete Batch Analyzers

Discrete batch analyzers perform only one type of assay at a time. Specimens requiring this analysis are processed in a group or batch. There are three common types of batch analyzers: centrifugal, immunoassay, and bichromatic analyzers. Bichromatic analyzers are no longer manufactured and will not be discussed in this chapter. Automated immunoassay systems are discussed in Chapter 19. In this chapter we discuss only centrifugal batch analyzers, using the MULTISTAT® III F/LS (Instrumentation Laboratory, Inc., Lexington, MA 02173) as an example.[2]

Centrifugal analyzers were developed in the late 1960s. They were popular throughout the 1970s and early 1980s but are less commonly used today. Few centrifugal analyzers are made today, having been displaced by more popular and versatile sequential random access or simultaneous multiple analyte instruments. However, Instrumentation Laboratory replaced the MULTISTAT® III with the random access IL Monarch®. It uses 24 cuvette wheels and functions as a multibatch analyzer. The IL Monarch® has an extensive test menu that includes electrolyte analyses by ion-selective electrodes (ISE).

PRINCIPLES AND COMPONENT PARTS OF CENTRIFUGAL ANALYZERS

Centrifugal analyzers employ a sample and reagent carousel or rotor. The rotor spins at various speeds to mix and move samples and reagents. In addition, the rotor is kept in a temperature-controlled environment. Finally, the rotor may also act as cuvettes that revolve past a fixed detection system.

Sampling System

The MULTISTAT® III F/LS uses a syringe to aspirate specimens through a sample probe. Each specimen is delivered to one of 20 sample wells on a disposable transparent plastic rotor. A separate probe/syringe system adds reagents to separate reagent wells on the rotor. Sample and reagent carryover are minimized by dipping the probes in a saline wash solution and repeatedly aspirating and expelling the saline. Sample volume can be as small as 1.25 μL. Maximum reagent volume is limited to 250 μL.

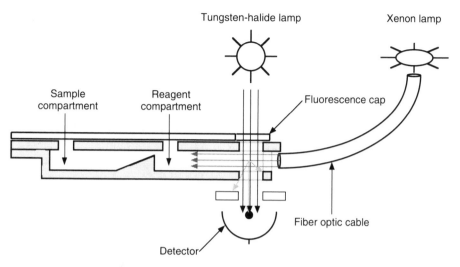

Figure 18-2. MULTISTAT® III disposable plastic rotor. The sample is initially separated from reagent by a ramp and mixes with reagent when centrifugal forces drives the fluid over the ramp into the reagent chamber. The reagent chamber functions as a cuvette. Light passes through it vertically for absorbance measurements. For fluorescent measurements a cap slides over the top absorbance window. Light from a xenon lamp is directed to the outer edge of the reagent chamber through a fiber optic cable (dark gray arrows). Fluorescence at 90° can reach the detector (light gray arrows).

Mixing and Incubation

The MULTISTAT® III F/LS rotor contains partially covered sample and reagent compartments separated by a barrier (Fig. 18-2).[2] These liquids are kept separated until all samples and reagents are dispensed and temperature equilibration is achieved. If a second reagent is required, it is added to the sample well. The rotor then is spun at moderate speed (4000 rpm). Centrifugal force drives the liquid in the sample wells into the adjacent reagent wells. Mixing occurs from turbulence when the rotor is suddenly stopped. After mixing, rotor speed is maintained at 1000 rpm. This keeps the reaction mixtures at the outer edges of the reagent wells, where detection occurs.

Detection

The MULTISTAT® III F/LS functions as a spectrophotometer or turbidimeter and as a fluorometer or nephelometer. The outer portions of the reagent wells function as cuvettes with 0.5-cm pathlengths (Fig. 18-2). In the spectrophotometric and turbidimetric modes, the tungsten-halide light source is located above the rotor. Light passes through each cuvette as it rotates past the detection area. A photodetector is located below the rotor. Transmittance is recorded for each cuvette by averaging the signals from at least 64 passes. The averaging corrects for variations in light intensity. At 60-millisecond intervals the light beam is directed to a reference detector, and a dark current (no light) measurement is made. This measurement corrects for photodetector noise.

In the fluorometric or nephelometric modes, a fiber optic cable directs light from a xenon lamp to the sides of the rotating cuvettes. Fluorescence or light scatter is measured 90° to the incident light.

Signal Processing and Reporting

Sophisticated electronics allows the MULTISTAT® III F/LS to correlate each detector measurement with the appropriate cuvette and to average signals from multiple passes of the rotor. Sophisticated data processing allows the MULTISTAT® III F/LS to perform linear and nonlinear curve fitting on multiple standards. The MULTISTAT® III F/LS supports equilibrium, endpoint, kinetic, EMIT, and fluorescence immunoassay analyses. In addition, the MULTISTAT® III F/LS is programmable by the operator. This allows customization of existing assays and in-house development of new assays.

Results can be printed or directed to a laboratory information system computer.

Discrete Sequential Multiple Analyte Analyzers

Discrete sequential multiple analyte analyzers are discrete because each specimen is totally separate from all other, sequential because tests are done one at a time, and multiple analyte because numerous tests can be performed on each sample (Fig. 18-1). Most analyzers of this type have some random-access capability: only desired tests are performed on each sample. A few have full random-access capability, allowing the operator to determine the order of testing (i.e., moving a stat test to the head of the line).

These analyzers are frequently more versatile than batch analyzers. Besides photometric assays they may also use ISEs. In this chapter we use four instruments as examples: DuPont *aca*™, Baxter Paramax®, Olympus DEMAND™, and Abbott Spectrum™.

PRINCIPLES AND COMPONENT PARTS OF SEQUENTIAL MULTIPLE ANALYTE ANALYZERS

Discrete sequential multiple analyte analyzers have the same types of components as batch analyzers. Samples are placed in carousels, racks, or trays. Individual, disposable cuvettes are common. These instruments may have more than one detection area. Signal processing and data analysis capabilities are generally greater than with batch analyzers. Some analyzers use bar coding to identify specimens; others require operator identification or downloading of a work list from a laboratory information system computer.

Sampling Systems and Specimen Identification

The DuPont *aca*™ (DuPont, Wilmington, DE 19880) is the least automated of the four analyzers considered in this section. Samples (serum, urine, cerebrospinal fluid, or other fluid) are manually placed into individual plastic sample wells (Fig. 18-3). The wells are covered with a pierceable plastic lid to minimize evaporation. A plastic

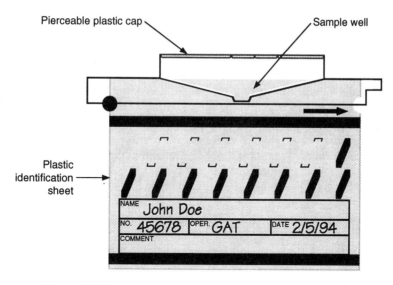

Figure 18-3. *aca*™ plastic tray and sample identification card.

card with specimen identification information (in pencil) is attached beneath the sample well. The sample well and card are slid onto a spring-driven loader. Bar-coded reagent packs for each analyte are placed behind each sample in any order. At the sampler, a needle probe pierces the sample well cover and aspirates specimen. The specimen and a diluent solution are injected into the plastic reagent packs through a plastic stopper. This is repeated for each reagent pack behind the specimen.

The Olympus DEMAND™ (Olympus Corp., Lake Success, NY 11042) and Baxter Paramax® (Baxter Healthcare Corp., Dade Div., Miami, FL 33152) use belts or chains to move samples. The Abbott Spectrum™ (Abbott Diagnostics, Abbott Park, IL 60064) uses specimen carousels. The Paramax® can sample directly from blood collection tubes. The DEMAND™ and Spectrum™ sample from disposable plastic cups. All these instruments use precision-bore syringes driven by stepping motors. Specimen identification on the DEMAND™ and Spectrum™ is by carousel or rack position. The operator can add test information by using a keyboard or touch-sensitive screen. The Paramax® uses bar code-labeled tubes for patient identification. The operator can interact with the system by using a light pen-sensitive monitor.

Reagent Addition, Mixing and Incubation, Detection
Dupont **aca**™ *V.*   After sample is added to the reagent pack, a chain moves it into a 37°C temperature-controlled air chamber. The sealed reagent compartments are broken and mixed with the specimen and diluent at one or both of two breaker-mixer stations. The liquid-filled plastic pack is molded into a cuvette, and spectro-photometric readings are taken at one or two wavelengths depending on the individual test. The first test result is available about 6 minutes after sampling, with an addi-

tional result every 37 seconds. Stat specimens can be manually introduced into the sampler at any time. The DuPont *aca*™ throughput is low—approximately 97 test results per hour. However, there are more than 50 different tests available for the DuPont *aca*™, many of which are unavailable on any other automated chemistry analyzer. The *aca*™ V can perform sodium and potassium analyses by ISEs.

Olympus Demand.   Reagents are stored in the analyzer console as a fivefold concentrate in a refrigerated compartment, allowing for reagent stability of 5 days. Concentrated reagents and serum are both diluted with four volumes of wash water when added to the reaction cuvette. All reagents are added at the beginning of the reaction. The disposable 1.0-cm pathlength plastic cuvettes, which also serve as reaction vessels, rotate on a cuvette wheel past 15 photometer stations. The cuvette wheel temperature is maintained at 37°C. All spectrophotometric measurements are made bichromatically. Three electrolytes are measured by ISEs if that option is added. The 72-position cuvette wheel advances one position every 9 seconds, and therefore requires almost 10 minutes for the first test result, followed by one result every 9 seconds.

***Abbott Spectrum*™.**   The reagent vessels are bar-coded for identification within the reagent carousel. Although reagents from manufacturers other than Abbott can be adapted to the Spectrum™, empty reagent containers must be purchased to have the proper bar-code. One of the unique features of this system is a linear photodiode array that, in conjunction with a holographic grating, can simultaneously monitor 16 different wavelengths. This feature, called polychromatic spectral mapping, allows the measurement of more than one analyte within a single reaction vessel. Another feature unique to the Spectrum™ is tandem access scheduling, in which the instrument's computer schedules the test sequence (based on the length of reaction for each assay) to yield the most rapid production of test results. With tandem access scheduling, the lag time for the first test result depends on the combination of tests that are requested. The Spectrum™ can also perform 20 different tests (23 tests with ISE) without changing reagents.

***American Dade Paramax*®.**   Reagents in the form of dry tablets are dispensed from a rotating reagent carousel. One tablet is dispensed into each reaction cuvette, diluent is added, and the reagent tablet is dissolved with the aid of an ultrasonic probe. Additional dispensers are provided so that user-determined liquid reagents may be used. Disposable cuvettes, which are also used as the reaction vessels, form a continuous belt and are incubated in a water bath set at either 30° or 37°C. The cuvettes advance one position every 5 seconds. The photometric unit uses fiber optic bundles connected to a single light source to transmit pulses of seven different wavelengths of light to eight separate photodetectors. One hundred absorbance readings are taken at each wavelength during the 5-second pause at the photodetector station. The readings are integrated and are used to produce bichromatic absorbance measurements as specified by the test parameters. The first result is available approximately 14 minutes after sampling, and with subsequent results every 5 seconds thereafter. The Paramax® can perform 32 different assays.

Data Analysis and Reporting

All the instruments described in this section are capable of bidirectional communication with a laboratory information system computer. They all can print or display results at the instrument. Data analyses and other tasks are performed by microprocessors or microcomputers. The Spectrum™ and Paramax® require more powerful processors because of the large numbers of tasks performed: specimen identification, tandem access scheduling or parallel processing, analyses of multiple readings at multiple wavelengths, signal integration and conversion to medically useful units, and bidirectional communications.

Discrete Simultaneous Multiple Analyte Analyzers

Discrete simultaneous multiple analyte analyzers are discrete because each specimen is totally separate from all others, simultaneous because many tests are done at the same time, and multiple analyte because numerous tests can be performed on each sample (Fig. 18-1). All the analyzers of this type have random-access capability: only ordered tests are performed on each sample. Most have full random-access capability, allowing the operator to determine the order of testing.

These analyzers generally have higher throughputs than sequential analyzers. In this chapter we use four instruments as examples: ASTRA™ (Beckman Inst., Brea, CA 92621), Parallel® (American Monitor, no longer in business), Hitachi 717 (Boehringer Mannheim Diagnostics, Indianapolis, IN 46250), and Ektachem (Eastman Kodak Co., Rochester, NY 14650). They were selected because of their uniqueness or acceptance in the clinical laboratory. Because the instruments are quite dissimilar, they will be discussed separately.

PRINCIPLES AND COMPONENT PARTS OF SIMULTANEOUS MULTIPLE ANALYTE ANALYZERS

Discrete simultaneous multiple analyte analyzers have the same type of components as the analyzers we described. Samples are placed in carousels, racks, or trays. Individual, disposable cuvettes or reaction chambers are common. These instruments have multiple detection areas that employ photometry, enzyme kinetic assays, and electrochemical assays such as ISEs. Signal processing and data analysis capabilities are high. Most analyzers of this type can use bar coding to identify specimens.

Beckman ASTRA™

The Beckman ASTRA™ (Automated Stat/Routine Analyzer) was introduced in the late 1970s. It originally came in two models. The ASTRA™ 4 is a benchtop model capable of containing four chemistry modules, and the ASTRA™ 8 can contain up to eight modules. The more recently introduced ASTRA™ IDEAL System links two ASTRA™ 8 instruments with a data-management system.

The ASTRA™ has four main functional areas: (1) a sampling area with specimen carousel; (2) the chemistry modules; (3) a microprocessor; and (4) a program keyboard interface.

Sampling System.   A 40-position carousel accepts various sizes of plastic sample cups. The carousel is controlled by the operator or by the computer. A plastic tray hood is provided to lessen specimen evaporation. Sampling is through dual stainless steel probes on a belt drive. Positive-displacement pumps driven by stepping motors are used to aspirate sample (Fig. 18-4a). The probes dip twice into each specimen cup while the sample pumps are drawing up sample. This creates two air slugs in each probe separated by about 9 μL of sample (Fig. 18-4b). The first sample slug clears any remaining wash solution from the probe and eliminates any bubbles. It is not used for testing. After the second air slug, a specimen for analysis is drawn into the probes. During sampling, a low-voltage ac signal is passed between the two sample probes. If this signal is interrupted during aspiration of the sample, the instrument will abort the assays on that sample and alert the operator.

After sampling, the probes are dipped into a wash cup to remove sample liquid clinging to the outside. The probes then separate, swing out over the reaction cups of the chemistry modules, and descend into the reaction cups where the appropriate

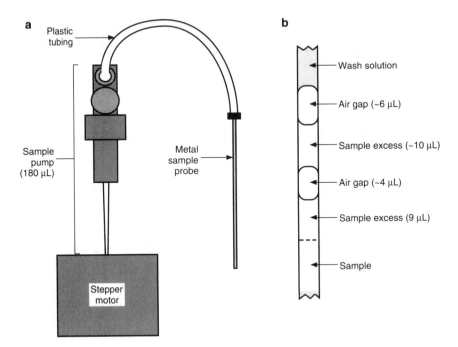

Figure 18-4.   ASTRA™ sampling system. (a) Pump and sample probe. (b) Enlargement of sample probe showing use of wash solution, air, and excess sample to clean inside of probe and minimize carryover.

amount of specimen is injected. If a particular analysis has not been ordered on a specimen, no sample is injected. The probes move to the next set of reaction modules and the process is repeated. After the final injection of sample, the sample transport mechanism returns the probes to the wash cup where wash solution is aspirated through the probes.

Chemistry Modules. Each self-contained module contains the pumps necessary for delivering reagents to the reaction cup as well as the electrochemical or colorimetric analysis system for each test (Fig. 18-5). Modules can be removed quickly and repaired or replaced to resolve a problem. Modules can also be removed to provide better access for maintenance. Reagents are mounted on a shelf and are not refrigerated. More than 24 analytes are available. Several of these analyses can be performed on urine; glucose, chloride, and protein can also be performed on cerebral spinal fluid.

Sodium and potassium are measured simultaneously in a single module with two ISEs. Fifty microliters of specimen are injected into the reaction cup that contains 1.3 mL of high-ionic-strength buffer. The large dilution minimizes protein interferences. The high ionic strength of the buffer ensures that the activity contribution of ions other than sodium or potassium is nearly constant from sample to sample.

The other modules of the ASTRA™ 4 (glucose, CO_2, and chloride) use electrochemical techniques. Glucose uses an oxygen electrode to measure oxygen consumed when glucose reacts with glucose oxidase. An electrode is also used to measure CO_2. Chloride is measured by the classic silver electrode amperometric titration method.

Creatinine is determined colorimetrically using an alkaline picrate methodology. Light from a tungsten lamp is directed through the reaction mixture, and the transmitted light is detected by a photodiode fitted with a 520-nm narrow bandpass filter. The ASTRA™ measures the rate of product formation at 25.6 s after sample injection (instead of waiting for the endpoint). This time was chosen to eliminate interferences from most other molecules that react with alkaline picrate.

Two modules are designed for enzyme assays. Each module can measure three enymes—two at 340 nm (aspartate aminotransferase [AST], alanine aminotransferase [ALT], lactate dehydrogenase [LD], or creatine kinase [CK]), and one measured at 405 nm (g-glutamyltransferase [GGT] or alkaline phosphatase [AP]). Temperatures of 30 and 37°C are available. Each module holds a carousel with 15 cuvettes. Reagents are dispensed into the cuvettes by syringes. One to three injections of each patient sample can be made per module. Thorough mixing occurs when a high-speed rotating rod dips into each cuvette after specimen injection. A sample blank is read shortly after injection. Ten absorbance measurements are taken in 30 seconds on each cuvette. A regression line is calculated on these points, and the slope of the line is used to calculate enzyme activity. Substrate depletion is monitored, and a system called Over-Range Detection and Correction (ORDAC) automatically resamples a reduced amount of specimen. After an initial delay of 2.5 minutes, the enzyme modules can generate six enzyme results per patient every 80 seconds.

Microprocessors. The microprocessor runs the operating system for the ASTRA™. The basic system consists of two 5¼ inch floppy disk drives and the Disk

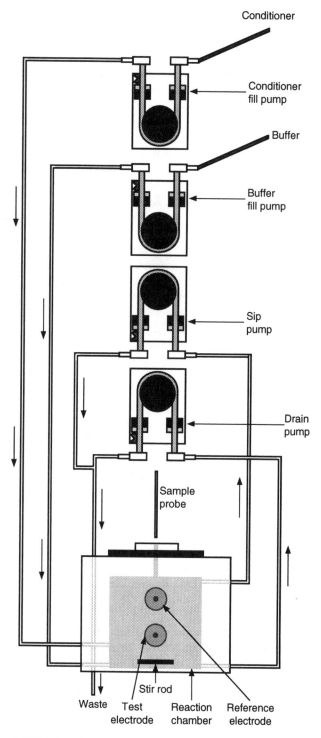

Figure 18-5. ASTRA™ module consisting of four peristaltic pumps and a reaction chamber.

338

Operating System (DOS). The more extensive Disk operating Reporting System (DoRS) has two additional disk drives and an off-line printer. DoRS is especially useful for laboratories that do not have a laboratory information systems computer. The basic operating system is loaded from two floppy disks. The operating system contains programs that control the carousel and sample probes; perform instrument setup, calibration, and diagnostics; process data from the analytical modules; and report results. The operating system can also report anion gap, blood urea nitrogen (BUN):creatinine ratio, and other user-requested calculations. The microprocessor sends calibration data to a thermal printer. Results can be printed or transmitted to a laboratory information system computer.

Keyboard Interface. The operator interacts with the instrument through a system program keyboard and video display screen. The keyboard contains three functional areas: system command selections, measurement channel selections, and numerical data entry selections. The system command keys control major system tasks such as calibration, prime reagents, and stop. The measurement channel selection keys allow the operator to select the analytes to be measured on a particular specimen. The numerical data entry keys are used to enter patient identification numbers or specimen location parameters such as carousel number and cup number.

Maintenance and Quality Assurance of the ASTRA™. A start-up procedure is performed daily. This includes adjusting the heights of the pick-up probes, checking reagent levels, inspecting tubing for leaks, priming the modules, checking the waste container, and cleaning the chloride module electrode, anode, reaction cup, stirrer, drain line, and outlet. Weekly maintenance includes cleaning tray and hood and inspecting inline filters for the sample pump and the Na/K and CO_2 modules. Every two weeks the sample pick-up probes, wash cup, lines, and stirrer must be cleaned. Monthly maintenance includes cleaning Na/K and CO_2 modules, replacing inline filters, and recharging the glucose electrode.

Quality assurance is based on periodic calibration and assaying controls. The ASTRA™ should be calibrated at least once each day of use. Controls should be run after calibration. The interval between recalibration and control runs on a given day should be determined by each laboratory. We recommend recalibration every 8 hours for instruments used throughout the day.

Summary of the ASTRA™. The Beckman ASTRA™ is a discrete random-access analyzer that is capable of performing a wide range of analyses. Its several sizes and configurations make it usable in both large and small laboratories, and its modular construction aids in maintenance and repair. Beckman has developed the Synchron CX™ line of instruments (CX3, CX4, CX5, and CX7) based on ASTRA™ technology and other technology. This line of instruments offers higher throughput, primary tube sampling, bar code sample identification, random sample access, bidirectional interface, bichromatic spectrophotometric assays to minimize interferences, and a greatly expanded test menu.

American Monitor Parallel®

The American Monitor Parallel® can process 240 samples with up to 7200 test results per hour, one of the highest throughputs available. This very large system (288 square feet of floor space and nearly 5000 pounds of shipping weight) obviously is not meant for small laboratories.

The analyzer consists of two main units: electronic and chemistry. The instrument also has three terminals, a high-speed printer, an optical card reader, an optional bar code–reader wand, and an air compressor. The chemistry unit contains the serum sampler mechanism, reagent storage and dispensing mechanism, reaction vessels, spectrophotometers, and a flame photometer. The electronic unit consists of two cabinets, one of which contains a DEC (Digital Equipment Corporation) PDP 11/23 processor and two 10 megabyte DEC hard disk drives. The other cabinet contains a Computer Automation minicomputer that controls the chemistry analyzer with instructions from the DEC computer.

The American Monitor Parallel® processes up to 30 test channels simultaneously. The key to understanding the chemistry unit is the 15-second cycle of the analyzer. During this 15-second cycle, numerous functions are occurring simultaneously in different areas of the instrument: (1) aliquots from up to 30 specimens are introduced into a set of reaction vials; (2) reagents are dispensed into reaction vials that received specimens in the previous cycle; (3) mixing occurs in reaction vials that received reagents in the previous cycle; (4) incubation of reaction vials that were mixed lasts for one or more 15-second cycles; (5) reaction mixtures are aspirated into spectrophotometer flow cells for absorbance determinations; and (6) reaction vials whose contents have been aspirated are washed three times with deionized water and evacuated during a series of cycles before reuse. Based on the 15-second cycle, the instrument is capable of processing 240 samples per hour for a theoretical test rate of 7200/hr if 30 tests per specimen are ordered. True throughput depends on the mean number of tests per specimen.

Chemistry Unit. Blood collection tubes or specimen cups with serum or plasma are loaded onto a continuous loop of 150 carriers. Specimens can be identified by bar code with encoded patient demographic and test selection information or by carrier position determined from a downloaded sample list from a laboratory computer. Alternatively, specimens may be scheduled via one of the terminals. Bar-coded samples can be loaded in any position.

Specimen aliquots are transferred to the reaction vials by way of a sample bar that contains 30 sample probes (Fig. 18-6). The sample bar moves out and over the sample transport chain, and the sample bar with probes is lowered into one to 30 sample tubes or cups, depending on chain position. Sample probes are connected to precision micro-syringes that are filled with deionized water down through the sample probe. During specimen transfer, the syringes aspirate a specific amount of sample that has been preset for that particular chemistry. The sample bar then moves over the reaction vials and dispenses the sample aliquot and a deionized water flush that washes out the probe. If one of the analytes is not ordered on a particular specimen, deionized water alone is dispensed to prevent air from being transferred to the spectrophotometer flow cells. The sample probes are then washed in a deionized water reservoir. These steps are all completed in one 15-second cycle. Specimen volume range is 1.0 to 100 μL and may be set by the operator.

The Parallel® has two sets of 34 bars (rows) of 30 reusable 2.0-mL-capacity

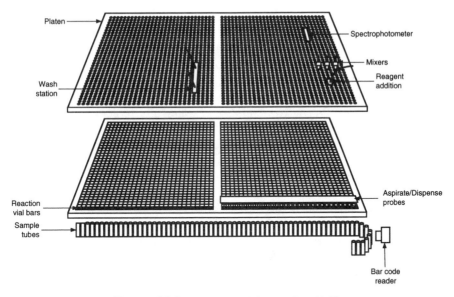

Figure 18-6. American Monitor Parallel®.

reaction vials (2040 total) in a 37°C bath (Fig. 18-6). During each 15-second cycle, a reaction vial bar with freshly washed and dried vials moves from the left set of bars to the first row of the right set of bars, adjacent to the sample rack. The reaction vial bar that had been filled with specimen in the previous cycle moves back one row in the right set of reaction vials. Reaction vials in the last row in the right set move to the back row of the left set, and then that bar moves forward one position. Because one reaction vial bar moves into position every 15 seconds, it takes 16 minutes for each bar to complete the counterclockwise rotation.

Mounted above the reaction vial bars is a fiberglass platen with circular holes over each reaction vial position (Fig. 18-6). The platen contains reagent dispensing lines, mixers, spectrophotometers, flame photometer, and tubes for aspirating and washing reagent vials. During each 15-second cycle, the platen is raised and lowered above the reaction vials. Depending on where a vial is in the cycle, it can be stirred, mixed, incubated, read for absorbance, or aspirated and washed.

Reagent dispensation is controlled by varying the time solenoid valves are held open while under constant pressure. Reagent volumes can vary from 50 to 1300 μL with a precision of ±0.2%. Reagent volumes are controlled by the computer and can be modified by the operator. One to six reagents can be dispensed into each vial. Reagents are stored in a cabinet at ambient temperature and or in a refrigerated cabinet.

Mixing is accomplished by motor-driven mixer blades. Each channel can have one to three mixers. The duration of mixing in each 15-second cycle is controlled by the computer.

Reaction mixtures are transferred to spectrophotometer flow cells after incubation by means of an air pressure-driven test transfer assembly. The spectrophotometers are mounted on the platens at appropriate positions depending on the incubation times needed for each analyte. Each spectrophotometer unit serves two channels and contains two 1.0-cm quartz flow-through cuvettes that hold 0.076 mL. A tungsten-halogen lamp serves as a light source for each spectrophotometer unit. Monochromatic light is achieved with narrow-bandpass (2.0-nm) interference filters. Lenses and a beam splitter focus transmitted light onto a test or a reference silicon photodetector. A feedback circuit from the reference detector adjusts the lamp power (Fig. 18-7). The spectrophotometers are linear from 0 to 2.0 absorbance units at 340 nm. The flow cell contents are aspirated to waste when the next reaction vial is aspirated. One of the 30 channels is for a sample blank. The absorbances of diluted samples are measured at 500, 546, and 650 nm. Corrections for icterus, hemolysis, and turbidity are applied to each assay.

The flame photometer simultaneously measures sodium and potassium from a single channel. Lithium is used for an internal reference. Two sets of lenses and a beam splitter direct the emitted light to the three photodetectors.

Electronic Unit and Minicomputer.   Almost every aspect of instrument operation is under some form of computer control or interaction. This is accomplished by a number of utility programs through which the operator can interact with the computer. These utilities control options such as result verification and data acceptance, specimen scheduling, quality control and standardization data review, printout format selection, and profile definition.

The Parallel® comes equipped with a bidirectional direct interface (RS232C) for communicating with a laboratory computer. An optional buffered interface is also available. Information concerning patient demographics and test ordering can be downloaded from the laboratory computer to the resident DEC computer in the

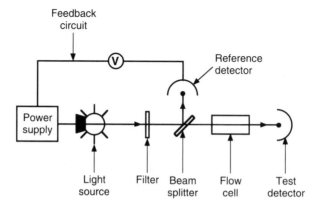

Figure 18-7.   American Monitor Parallel® spectrophotometer with lamp-power feedback circuit from reference detector.

Parallel®. Data transmission from the Parallel® to the laboratory computer usually consists of collated patient results.

The minicomputer also controls the Reflex Reschedule Delta Detection (R^2D^2) system. The R^2D^2 system consists of a panel of light-emitting diodes (LEDs) and switches mounted on the front of the instrument and a small printer. Software for the system resides in the DEC computer. The R^2D^2 panel has three sets of LEDs. The first displays the status of every chemistry channel and warns the operator that a particular channel may need attention. The second set of LEDs displays the status of individual samples. For instance, if a particular sample has a result that exceeds the linear dynamic range, this is indicated by a red LED on the panel. The operator may then request that the Parallel® dilute and reanalyze the specimen. The dilution ratio is calculated by the R^2D^2 software—the operator merely places the sample in an empty position and signals the instrument by pressing an LED. The instrument reads the bar code and automatically repeats the analysis on the diluted sample and calculates the value. The dilution factors for each test are determined in advance by the operator and are entered into the computer. Other combinations of LEDs alert the operator to other sample problems and allow the operator to interact with the samples before verifying and transmitting results. The third set of LEDs composes the stat pad. This combination of LEDs and switches allows the operator to schedule tests without interacting with a terminal. The printer is used to print an audit trail of the samples.

Maintenance and Quality Assurance of the Parallel®.   A start-up procedure is performed once a day and takes 30 to 40 minutes. This includes powering up the computer and verifying spectrophotometer function and water regulation. Standardization, also performed once every 24 hours, takes an additional 20 minutes. After these procedures, the instrument may be left in a standby status while not running samples. Shutdown is performed once per day as part of maintenance and takes about 25 minutes. Controls are run at least once per day.

Summary of the Parallel®.   The American Monitor Parallel® is a computerized, high-throughput instrument that is capable of performing multiple tests on a sample in a discrete test-selective manner. It is the best example of an automated chemistry analyzer using parallel processing. Its high throughput, small sample volume requirements, and minimal labor inputs make it a cost-effective instrument for high-volume laboratories.

Hitachi 747

The Boehringer Mannheim Diagnostics/Hitachi systems are discrete, random-access, multichannel chemistry analyzers. The members of the series include the 705, 704, 717, 736, 747-100, and 747-200. The Hitachi 747-100, which we will describe, has a large test menu that includes typical serum chemistry tests as well as therapeutic drugs, drugs of abuse in urine, and thyroid tests. Thirty-five different tests can be performed simultaneously. All tests except sodium, potassium, and chloride use liquid reagents in spectrophotometric assays. Ion-selective electrodes are used to measure these three electrolytes.

The Hitachi 747-100 can process up to 150 samples per hour and has a maximum test throughput of 3300 tests per hour. The 747-200 model uses two 747-100 analyzer units and can therefore process up to 300 samples and 6600 tests per hour. Hitachi 747 features include primary tube sampling, bar-code specimen identification, bidirectional communication with laboratory information system computers, and testing of serum, plasma, urine, cerebrospinal fluid, and other body fluids.

The Hitachi 747 consists of an analyzer unit, a control unit and printer, and a vacuum pump unit.[3] The analyzer unit includes the sampling system, reagent dispensing system with refrigerated storage area, incubator bath, reaction cells, photometric and electrometric detectors, and a wash station. The control unit consists of a Hewlett Packard Vectra QS/16S microcomputer, monitor, keyboard, and printer. The vacuum pump unit is connected to the rear of the analyzer unit. It removes waste fluid and rinse water from reaction cells.

Instrument Operation. Sample tubes or cups are placed in racks that hold up to five specimens. Up to 30 racks can be loaded into the supply area. A robotic arm moves the racks to a rack carrier, which moves the racks to a rack identification reader and then a bar code reader. The rack advances to a photometric test sampling area and then an ISE test sampling area. The photometric sampling area has four pipetters with liquid-level sensing probes. Piston-driven fluid-filled syringes control sample aspiration into the probes. An air slug separates water in the sample lines from aspirated sample fluid. After sample aspiration, the sampling arm moves over four reaction cells and dispenses sample. If more than four tests are ordered, the sampling arm returns to the specimen tube and aspirates more fluid (without an initial air slug). The ISE test sampler uses a single probe to aspirate sample fluid. Liquid-level sensing prevents excessive sample contamination of the outsides of the probes. Carryover is avoided by internal and external probe washes.

The core of the analyzer unit is the reaction area. A circular reaction disk holds 480 reaction cells (two rings of 240 cells) for photometric assays. There are two reagent-dispensing arms with 32 nozzles each. (Two refrigerated reagent solutions are available for each photometric test.) The arms are positioned over the reaction disk and move inward and outward to position different pairs of nozzles over four reaction cells (Fig. 18-8). The reaction disk rotates counterclockwise through 183° of arc at each 6-second half cycle, bringing two pairs of cuvettes into position each time. Stirring mechanism arms are adjacent to the reagent-dispensing arms. Each stirring mechanism has four paddles, one for each cuvette beneath arm.

Temperature in the reaction cells in maintained at 25, 30, or 37°C by a circular, water-filled incubation bath beneath the reaction disk. Incubation occurs from the time sample is dispensed. The incubation period between addition of the first reagent and the second reagent (if needed) is 72 seconds or 792 seconds (six cycles or 66 cycles). Total incubation time is variable, because photometric readings can be made every 12 seconds.

Reaction cells pass the photometric detection area once every 12 seconds. This enables kinetic determinations as well as measurements of water, sample, and reagent blanks. The Hitachi 747 has two photometers, one for each ring of cells on the reaction disk. The photometers use water-cooled tungsten halogen lamps. Dif-

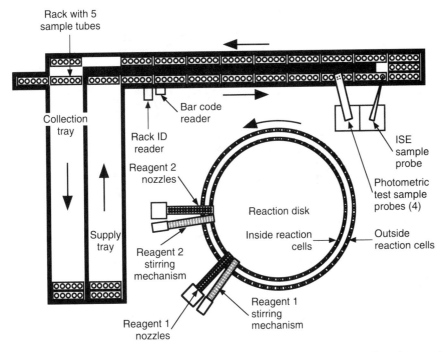

Figure 18-8.   Overhead schematic of Boehringer Mannheim/Hitachi 747 analyzer unit.

fraction grating monochrometers are used to select one of 12 available wavelengths between 340 and 800 nm. Transmitted light intensity is measured by photodiode arrays. Data are transmitted to the microcomputer for processing.

After all photometric measurements are completed, reaction cells move beneath the cell rinse mechanism. The first set of four dual probes aspirates the reaction mixtures and dispenses a cleaning solution. The second set of triple probes aspirates the cleaning solution, dispenses rinse water, and aspirates any water overflow. The third set of triple probes is identical to the second. The next set of four probes aspirates the rinse water and dries the reaction cells. Water is added for a water blank measurement by the fifth set of probes. A sixth set of probes removes the blank water and dries the reaction cells. The reaction cells are then ready for new samples.

Ion-selective electrode cartridges are used to measure sodium, potassium, and chloride. The ISE compartment is kept at $35°C$. Twenty microliters of sample fluid and $600\,\mu L$ of diluent are dispensed into a dilution vessel within the ISE compartment (Fig. 18-9). The ISE compartment contains five electrodes: Na^+, K^+, Cl^-, reference, and ground. A potassium chloride solution is used for the reference and ground electrodes. Diluted sample ($500\,\mu L$) is drawn past the three analyte electrodes. Analyte concentrations are related to the potential differences between the reference electrode and analyte electrodes. Calibration is maintained with an internal standard solution. After diluted sample is evacuated from the dilution vessel and electrode

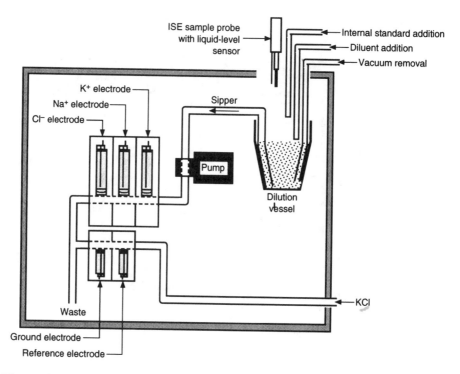

Figure 18-9.   Boehringer Mannheim/Hitachi 747 ion-selective electrode compartment.

flowpath, internal standard solution is used as a rinse solution. A second aliquot of internal standard is dispensed for calibration. This is removed just before the addition of the next sample.

Control Unit.   The control unit directs the analyzer unit and communicates with a laboratory computer and the printer. The operator interacts with the control unit through keyboard inputs. A color monitor displays menus and information. Sample identification and test requests can be entered manually. A STAT key allows quick identification of specimens needing urgent processing. Other tasks controlled by the microcomputer include instrument maintenance, test calibrations, quality control displays and evaluations, adjustment of assay parameters, and result verifications. The monitor can display patient and control data, absorbance versus time for selected reactions, and calibration curves.

The bidirectional interface allows uploading of patient information from and downloading of test results to a laboratory information system computer. Patient, control, and calibration results can also be directed to the printer.

Maintenance and Quality Assurance of the Hitachi 747.   The control unit handles daily routine maintenance functions. Reagent and sample degassers, water bath detergent, and sample probe cleaning solution minimize the maintenance needs for fluid-handling components of the analyzer. Quality control is necessary once each day or run. Ion-selective electrode tests need to be calibrated daily. Photometric test calibration intervals vary by assay.

Summary of the Hitachi 747. The Hitachi 747 is a versatile, moderately high-throughput analyzer suitable for medium- or high-volume laboratories. It has a broad test menu and can handle plasma, urine, and other body fluids. Startup and operation are simplified by a sophisticated computer control unit, primary tube sampling, and bar code specimen identification.

Kodak Ektachem

The Ektachem 700 is a discrete chemistry analyzer capable of simultaneous performance of a wide variety of analyses. The Ektachem 700 uses slides comprised of multiple layers of dry film (except for sodium, potassium, CO_2, and chloride) to perform clinical chemistry tests. The construction of the slides is an extension of technology developed in the photographic industry. The multiple-layered slide technology offers significant advantages in both sensitivity and selectivity over other commonly used chemistry analyzers.

The Ektachem 700 needs infrequent calibration and minimal maintenance. Quality controls are usually assayed only once per day. Maximum sample throughput is 300 per hour (with only one test per sample). Maximum test throughput is 540 per hour (750 per hour with the optional High-Volume Profiling Accessory C).

The Ektachem 700 consists of a main unit, a control unit, and a printer.[4] The main unit consists of a sampling area, two slide dispensing stations, three incubators, two reflectance spectrophotometers (reflectometers), a potentiometer (electrometer), and slide disposal containers (Fig. 18-10). The control unit consists of a keyboard, a monitor, a hard disk drive, and a floppy disk drive. Bidirectional communication between the control unit and a laboratory information system allows rapid transfer of patient and sample information.

Slide Technology. Most tests on the Ektachem are based on reflectance spectroscopy of colorimetric slides. Colorimetric slides are comprised of multiple layers above a transparent plastic backing: a spreading layer, one or more intermediate layers, and an indicator layer. The slides are designed to measure analytes accurately and to minimize interferences.[5,6] Some colorimetric reactions are similar to those used in wet chemistry analyzers; others are unique to the Ektachem. Interfering substances are handled in numerous ways: exclusion by a semipermeable membrane, immobilization in an upper layer with the analyte passing through to lower layers, or chemical alteration. Reflectance is achieved by incorporating a white, reflective chemical into the spreading layer or an intermediate layer.

The spreading layer is a highly porous polymer designed to permit rapid, uniform sample spreading horizontally from the point of application. This is essential for good analytical precision. The rate of horizontal spreading must be greater than the rate of vertical penetration to lower layers. Otherwise, there will be a concentration gradient from the center of application to the periphery of the spot. Rapid horizontal spreading occurs because of capillary action. Vertical penetration is delayed by an underlying gelatin layer—the gelatin must become hydrated by moisture from the sample before analytes can pass through.

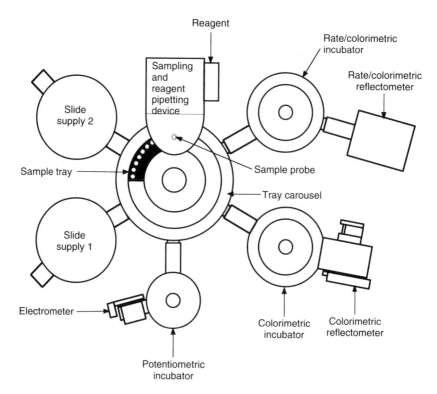

Figure 18-10.   Overhead schematic of Kodak Ektachem main unit.

The spreading layer may be made of cellulose acetate, microcrystalline cellulose, or plastic beads. Both the pore size and the thickness of the layer vary depending on the application. The spreading layer traps cells and cellular debris, crystals and other particulate matter, and (often) large protein molecules. The bottom of the spreading layer can be made reflective by the addition of TiO_2 or $BaSO_4$. This can mask colored constituents within the sample (e.g., erythrocytes) that are trapped by the spreading layer. In some applications, additional chemical and physical reactions take place in the spreading layer.

Beneath the spreading layer are intermediate layers designed to exclude or alter interfering materials and, if necessary, to convert the analyte into a product that will react stoichiometrically with the indicator. A wide variety of processes and reactions are used in the construction of the intermediate layers. Semipermeable membranes and gel permeation are used to exclude large molecules. Interferents can be trapped by ion-exchange resins or immunochemical reagents. Analytes are converted to reactive products (when necessary) by chemical reactions and enzymes. Reaction rates are increased by moving the slide to a 37°C incubator 12 seconds after application of the sample.

Chemicals in the indicator (dye) layer react with the analyte or the product

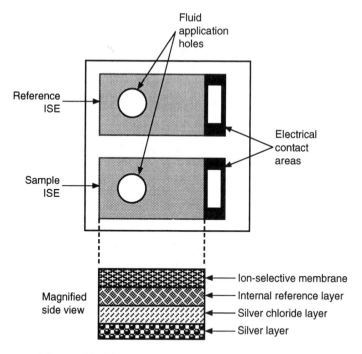

Figure 18-11. Kodak Ektachem potentiometric slide.

derived from the analyte and form a final colored product. The indicator layer also incorporates a mordant (a substance that combines with the dye and the substance to be dyed [the inert chemicals in the layer], thereby increasing dye binding).

The Ektachem 700 also performs kinetic (rate) analyses with enzymes as analyte or reagent. The slide is placed on a rotating disk in the 37°C rate incubator. A reflectometer is incorporated into the rate incubator. As the incubator disk rotates, a reading is taken of each slide as it passes over the read station.

Potentiometric slides used in the Ektachem contain two identical ISE half-cells (Fig. 18-11). The electrodes consist of four layers.[7] The top layer is an ion-selective membrane containing an ionophore. An internal reference layer, a silver chloride layer, and a silver layer lie below the ion-selective membrane. The two ISEs are connected by a paper bridge that forms a liquid junction. Undiluted sample fluid and reference fluid are simultaneously pipetted on separate halves of the slide. The slide is moved into a 25°C incubator for 3 minutes of equilibration. The slide then is moved into an electrometer that measures the potential difference between the two ISEs. Because the analyte concentration of the reference fluid is known, the analyte concentration in the sample can be calculated by using the Nernst equation.

Instrument Operation.[4]   One to 10 samples are loaded on curved trays. Four trays can be loaded at one time. Instruments with the Primary Container Sampling II option can sample from unstoppered tubes (special pierceable caps are available to prevent evaporation). Otherwise, sampling is from disposable plastic cups. Specimen identification is automatic if the Positive Sample Identification (bar code reader) option is in use. Otherwise, the operator uses the control unit to identify the sample by its tray number and tray position. Test selection is automatic if the orders were downloaded through the bidirectional interface. The operator can order tests manually by using the touch-screen monitor. After specimen loading, identification, and test ordering, the sample tray rack rotates clockwise. A sample probe picks up a disposable plastic tip and moves to the specimen. After insertion into the sample, the probe aspirates 30 or 40 μL of sample plus 10 μL for each colorimetric or potentiometric test or 11 μL for each rate/colorimetric test. A pressure transducer in the probe detects plugging, bubbles, or insufficient sample. The probe rotates to the dispensing area and dispenses sample to each slide. An optical wetness detector directs a light beam to the bottom of colorimetric slides. A change in reflectance indicates that fluid has wetted the slide. After all sample dispensing is completed, the probe moves to a tip-disposal area. The plastic tips are ejected into a disposal box.

The control unit coordinates slide dispensing. When multiple tests are ordered on a sample, slides are presented in a preprogrammed (operator-determined) order. This allows prioritization of tests when sample volume is inadequate for all tests ordered. Test slides are inserted into a slide block at the dispensing station. The slide supply stations are kept below 24°C. Relative humidity is kept between 25 and 45% with salt pads in station 1 and below 20% with desiccant packs in station 2.

After sample fluid is applied to a slide, it moves to one of three stations: a colorimetric incubator, a potentiometric incubator, or a rate/colorimetric incubator. Each incubator has a precondition station that quickly brings slide temperatures close to that of the incubator. Slides remain in the precondition stations for only 12 seconds (one instrument cycle). The colorimetric incubator is maintained at 37°C ±1°C by means of resistance heaters above and below the incubator disk. The potentiometric incubator is maintained at 25°C ±0.1°C by means of a thermoelectric heat pump that provides both heating and cooling. The rate/colorimetric incubator is maintained at 37°C ±0.1°C by means of a heater and a thermoelectric cooler located below the incubator disk.

For colorimetric assays, the slide is moved to a read station after incubation. Light from a tungsten-halogen lamp passes through one of seven narrow-band filters. The resultant monochromatic light is directed to the bottom of the slide at a 45° angle. The light passes through the clear plastic support and then the indicator layer. A photodetector positioned at a 90° angle from the slide measures the intensity of light reflected from an intermediate layer or the spreading layer. The reflection intensity correlates with analyte concentration in a nonlinear fashion. The observed signal undergoes linear data transformation, and analyte concentration is calculated and reported.

For rate/colorimetric assays, reflectance measurements are made every 6 seconds during the 5.5-minute incubation period. Calculation of enzyme activity requires a number of steps. First, the reflectance intensity of each reading is transformed to color density. Next, this piece of data is systematically manipulated to provide optimum results. This includes eliminating noise spikes, discarding early readings before steady-state conditions, and discarding late readings with decreasing slope due to substrate depletion. A linear "inside-out" regression method, which limits slope determinations to a central linear region, is applied to the remaining data points. Analyte concentration is calculated from the slope of the regression line or by using a third-order polynomial to calculate maximum rate. The analyzer can detect problems such as substrate depletion, too few data points in the linear region, multiple linear regions, and low signal-to-noise ratio.

After slides are read, they are ejected into one of three disposal boxes. These must be emptied by the operator.

Computer System.   The entire operation of the Ektachem analyzer is controlled by a complex computer system. The Ektachem 700 is driven by two microcomputers that communicate via a high-speed data bus. The Ektachem computer system supports bidirectional communications with a laboratory information system computer.

The master computer handles the operation of the analyzer as well as the data processing. The operator interacts with this unit through a keyboard and touch-sensitive monitor. Communications to printers, modems, or laboratory computers are also controlled by this unit. Sample identification and test selection, assay calibration, data manipulation and result calculation, error detection, test reporting, and data transfer to the internal hard disk or to floppy disks are all functions of this computer.

The mechanism computer coordinates and directs the mechanical and thermal components of the analyzer. Slide selection and ordering, mechanical operation synchronization, temperature maintenance, and transfer of reflectometer and electrometer readings to the master computer are controlled by 12 software modules in the mechanism computer.

Maintenance and Quality Assurance of the Ektachem.   The Ektachem needs little maintenance beyond emptying tip- and slide-disposal boxes and cleaning parts exposed to biological fluids. The disposable tip on the reference fluid pipette must be changed every 8 hours. The tip retainer, sleeve, and reference fluid reservoir must be cleaned daily.[8] Internal parts such as the sample probe, slide dispensers, precondition stations, and potentiometric read station need weekly cleaning.

Calibration is necessary with each new lot of slides. Calibration is stable for months. Two or more liquid calibrators are used for each assay. Calibrator values and algorithms are supplied by Kodak on floppy disks.[9] The master computer performs the calibrations using the supplied data.

Because the Ektachem is a random-access instrument, a run is usually defined as a time interval such as 8 or 24 hours. Quality control samples are assayed at least once per user-defined run. Control samples should also be analyzed after calibration, after detector or lamp service, or when ambient temperature has changed by 5°C or more. Quality control sample parameters can be entered into the master computer. The computer can display individual control results and standard deviation indices as well as control mean, standard deviation, and coefficient of variation over a specified time.

Summary of the Ektachem.   Dry-film slide technology makes the Ektachem a unique analyzer. Its sophisticated computers and touch-sensitive monitor simplify operation. Assay stability allows long runs and infrequent calibrations. These features and a moderately high throughput are the reasons why Ektachem analyzers are found in many clinical laboratories in North America.

Summary

Automated chemistry analyzers have greatly increased laboratory productivity since the 1950s. The degree of automation has increased steadily, making the analyzers faster, easier, and safer to operate. In this chapter we described discrete batch, discrete sequential multichannel, and discrete simultaneous multichannel chemistry analyzers. These three classes comprise the vast majority of analyzers in use today.

Although modern automated chemistry analyzers are extremely complex, they can be understood by looking at each major step or process: sampling and sample identification, combining sample and reagents, incubating mixtures, detecting analyte or its product, converting detector response data to concentration, and reporting results. Automation has affected all these processes. Future advances in chemistry analyzer automation will probably include widespread ability to sample from stoppered tubes, further decreases in sample volume requirements, and further reductions in analyzers' sizes.

References

1. Tanaka WK, Witte DL. Discrete chemistry analyzers, part I. In: Hicks MR, Haven MC, Schenken JR, McWhorter CA, eds. Laboratory instrumentation, 3rd ed. Philadelphia: JB Lippincott, 1987:280.
2. Pesce MA. Evaluation of the Multistat III fluorescence/light scatter centrifugal analyzer. J Clin Lab Autom 1983, 3:327-39.
3. Boerhinger Mannheim/Hitachi 747-100 Analyzer Operator's Manual. Indianapolis: Boehringer Mannheim Corporation, 1992:1-1 to 1-48.
4. Kodak Ektachem 700 Analyzer C Series. Rochester, NY: Kodak Clinical Products, 1993:1-1 to 1-14, 2-1 to 2-17.
5. Curme HG, Columbus RL, Dappen GM, Eder TW, Fellows WD, Figueras J, et al. Multilayer film elements for clinical analysis: General concepts. Clin Chem 1978, 24:1335-42.
6. Spayd RW, Bruschi B, Burdick BA, Dappen GM, Eikenberry JM, Esders TW, et al. Multilayer film elements for clinical analysis: Applications to representative chemical determinations. Clin Chem 1978, 24:1343-50.
7. Shirey TL. Development of a layered-coating technology for clinical chemistry. Clin Biochem 1983, 16:147-55.
8. Kodak Ektachem 700 Analyzer C Series. Rochester, NY: Kodak Clinical Products, 1993:16-1 to 16-41.
9. Ibid., 3-1 to 3-9.

Suggested Readings

Bradley CA. Centrifugal analysis in the clinical laboratory. In: Stefanini M, Gorstein F, Fink L, eds. Progress in clinical pathology, vol. IX. New York: Grune & Stratton, 1984:225-46.

19

AUTOMATED IMMUNOASSAY SYSTEMS

Lora L. Arnold
Maximillian D. Fiore

Objectives

After completing this chapter, the reader will be able to:

1. Define and discuss homogeneous and heterogeneous immunoassays.
2. Define and discuss competitive and immunometric immunoassays.
3. Describe common labels and reactions used in automated immunoassays.
4. Describe various separation techniques used in automated immunoassays.
5. Discuss the different ways current automated immunoassay instruments process samples.
6. List and discuss the component parts common to automated immunoassay instruments.
7. Formulate a quality assurance and maintenance program for automated immunoassay systems.

Definitions

Biotin: Water-soluble vitamin of the B-complex that binds to avidin and streptavidin.[1]
Biotinylated Antibody: An antibody coupled to biotin.
Conjugated: Chemically attached.
EMIT: Enzyme Multiplied Immunoassay Technique, a homogeneous enzyme immunoassay for small-molecular-weight proteins. Binding of the enzyme labeled antigen to the antibody affects the action of the enzyme on the substrate, either making the enzyme unavailable for reaction or enhancing the reaction.
Immunoassay: Any assay where an antibody binds an antigen and a second labeled antibody or antigen is used to detect the reaction.
Ligand: A molecule that binds to another molecule.

Paramagnetic Particles: Particles attracted by a magnet to a position parallel to the magnetic field.

Peltier Unit: A unit that can give off or absorb heat at the point where two dissimilar metals are joined and subject to an electrical current.

Radioimmunoassay (RIA):   Immunoassay in which the label is radioactive.

Stepper Motor: A precision motion control device that provides a precise rotational movement in response to a step command. The command consists of four simultaneous digital signals in a specific sequence. Stepper motor torque decreases as stepping rate increases. These motors are widely used when precise control of motions is required in relatively low-speed, low-torque applications. They are usually controlled by microprocessors.

Streptavidin: Tetrameric protein produced by *Streptomyces avidinii* with a high binding affinity for biotin.

Thermistor: A device constructed of solid semiconductor material, whose electrical resistance decreases with an increase in temperature.

Introduction

Radioimmunoassay (RIA) techniques have been used for more than 30 years to measure amounts of hormones and tumor markers, monitor therapeutic drug use, and detect infectious diseases. Growing concerns about the use of radioactivity and increasing regulations concerning its disposal led to the development of nonisotopic labels such as enzymes, fluorescent substances, and substances capable of chemiluminescence. These new immunoassay techniques were still manual and labor-intensive. During the 1980s the shortage of medical technologists made it necessary for laboratories to consolidate workstations. At the same time there was an increasing demand for the immunoassay laboratory to decrease turnaround time so that hospital stays could be shortened and outpatient results reported in a more timely manner. The automation of immunoassay techniques meets both of these needs, but immunoassay techniques have proved difficult to automate. Over the past 5 to 7 years manufacturers have made significant progress in this area resulting in a variety of automated immunoassay instruments in a wide range of formats.[1-4]

Principles

ASSAY DESIGN

Immunoassays are either homogeneous or heterogeneous. *Homogeneous assays* do not require separation of the bound and unbound antigen because the unbound antigen can be distinguished from the bound antigen. Homogeneous techniques are easier to automate and are compatible with many current chemistry analyzers, but have disadvantages. These assays are limited to small-molecular-weight analytes because the differentiation between free and bound is usually based on the small "free" antigen giving off a different signal from the larger antigen-antibody complex. These assays are also subject to interference from endogenous substances in the patient specimen because the bound portion is not separated from the sample before measurement. Homogeneous assays are also less sensitive than heterogeneous assays.

Homogeneous assay methodology has made possible the automation of small-molecular-weight analytes such as therapeutic drugs, thyroid markers, and drugs of abuse. Fluorescence polarization (FPIA) and Syva Company's (Palo Alto, CA 94303) enzyme multiplied immunoassay technique (EMIT) are the most widely used homogeneous immunoassays. The former is used by Abbott Laboratories (Abbott Park, IL 60064) on the TDx®, ADx®, and some IMx® assays; EMIT assays have been adapted to various centrifugal and random-access chemistry analyzers.

Heterogeneous assays do require separation of the bound from the free, and this is usually accomplished by complexing the bound portion to a solid phase in some manner and washing away the unbound portion. The need for separation makes a heterogeneous assay more difficult to automate, but a wide range of analytes, both large- and small-molecular-weight, can be measured with excellent sensitivity. Most automated immunoassay instruments use heterogeneous assays and have addressed the problem of separating bound from unbound in a variety of ways.

Immunoassays are further characterized as competitive or immunometric assays, also referred to as *sandwich assays*. In a *competitive binding assay* the amount of antibody available for binding is limited. The unlabeled antigen, present in the patient's serum, and a known amount of labeled antigen "compete" for binding sites on the limited antibody. The amount of analyte present in the sample is indirectly proportional to the signal generated by the bound labeled antigen. In an *immunometric assay* two antibodies are used, one of which is labeled. The labeled antibody is in excess. The analyte is bound at different sites by both antibodies, so it is "sandwiched" between the two antibodies. In this design the relationship between analyte concentration and signal generated is direct. Sandwich assays can measure minute amounts of large molecules, such as thyroid stimulating hormone, with excellent sensitivity.[1-3]

TYPE OF LABEL

The most common labels used in the automated instruments available today are enzymes and chemiluminescent labels. *Enzyme immunoassays (EIA)* have traditionally been done manually by using a technique called *enzyme-linked immunosorbent assay (ELISA)* where one of the reaction components is adsorbed to a solid phase, usually a $\frac{1}{4}''$ polystyrene bead or a microtiter plate well.

Figure 19-1 shows an example of a typical sandwich EIA reaction sequence. In step 1, the first reagent consists of an antibody that has been adsorbed on to a solid phase. The sample containing the analyte is incubated for a given time, at a precisely controlled temperature, with the antibody-coated solid phase. The analyte (antigen in this example) binds with the antibody on the solid phase in proportion to the concentration of the analyte in the sample. In step 2, the unbound analyte is washed away, leaving the antibody-analyte complex attached to the solid phase. A second reagent is incubated with the antibody-analyte complex on the bead in step 3. The second reagent typically consists of another antibody that is conjugated to an enzyme. During the incubation with the antibody-analyte complex on the solid phase, the conjugated antibody attaches to another antigenic site on the analyte. In

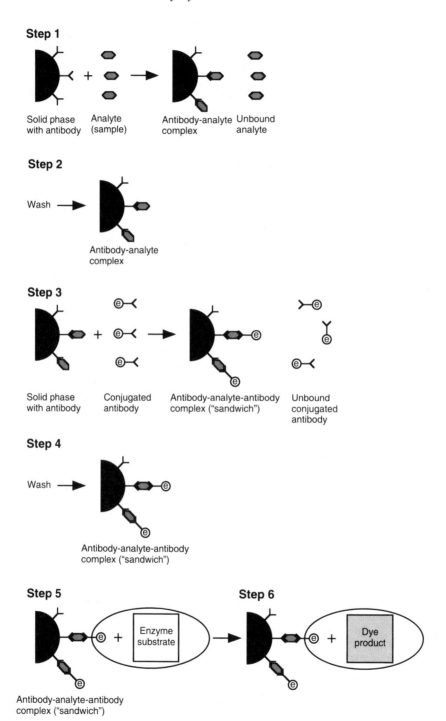

Figure 19-1. Manual enzyme immunoassay reaction sequence.

step 4 the new antibody-analyte-antibody/conjugate complex is washed, and the unbound antibody/conjugate is removed. Finally, an enzyme substrate is added as the third reagent. This substrate is incubated with the sandwich complex (step 5). The enzyme catalyzes a chemical reaction that oxidizes the substrate to form a colored dye product (step 6). The intensity of the colored product is then measured in a spectrophotometer and is proportional to the number of sandwich complexes attached to the solid phase.

The common enzymes used to label antibody or antigen for manual EIAs, horseradish peroxidase and alkaline phosphatase, are also used in the automated EIAs. Horseradish peroxidase is the enzyme label used by Boehringer Mannheim Diagnostics' (Indianapolis, IN 46250-0100) ES 300. The horseradish peroxidase acts on a patented substrate, ABTS, to produce a color reaction.[5] Many automated EIAs use substrates that produce a fluorescent product, not a colored product. The change to fluorescence has increased the dynamic range of the assays and improved their sensitivity. Abbott Diagnostics' IMx® and Tosoh Medics, Inc.'s (San Francisco, CA 94080-7021) AIA-1200™ and AIA-600™ use alkaline phosphatase as the conjugate, and the substrate is 4-methyumbelliferyl phosphate (4-MUP). Alkaline phosphatase catalyzes the reaction to remove a phosphate group and a fluorescent product, 4-methyumbelliferone, is formed and measured (Fig. 19-2).[6-8]

Chemiluminescent immunoassays were developed in the late 1970s. They showed excellent sensitivity with a wide range of analytes, and the reaction time was short. For a more detailed discussion of chemiluminescence, see Chapter 10.

Ciba Corning Diagnostics Corp.'s (East Walpole, MA 02032-1516) ACS:180™ and Diagnostic Products Corp.'s (Los Angeles, CA 90045-5597) Immulite® use chemiluminescence but in different ways. The label, conjugated to the antigen (competitive) or antibody (sandwich), used on the ACS:180™ is dimethyl acridinium ester. After the binding portion of the reaction has taken place, hydrogen peroxide (H_2O_2) in acidic solution is added. The sample is moved in front of the luminometer where sodium hydroxide is added. An oxidation reaction is produced by the alkaline H_2O_2, and an intermediate compound is formed that decomposes to the chemiluminescent compound, n-methyl acridone (Fig. 19-3).[9-11] The Immulite® uses an EIA with alkaline phosphatase as the label for antigen or antibody. The substrate is adamantyl dioxetane phosphate. The alkaline phosphatase hydrolyzes the phosphate group on adamentyl dioxetane, producing adamantyl dioxetane, the chemiluminescent molecule (Fig. 19-4).[12,13]

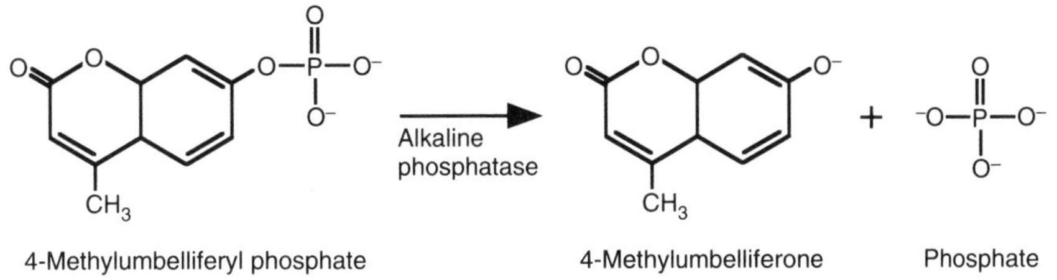

4-Methylumbelliferyl phosphate   →   Alkaline phosphatase   →   4-Methylumbelliferone   +   Phosphate

Figure 19-2. Reaction of 4-methylumbelliferyl phosphate and alkaline phosphatase.

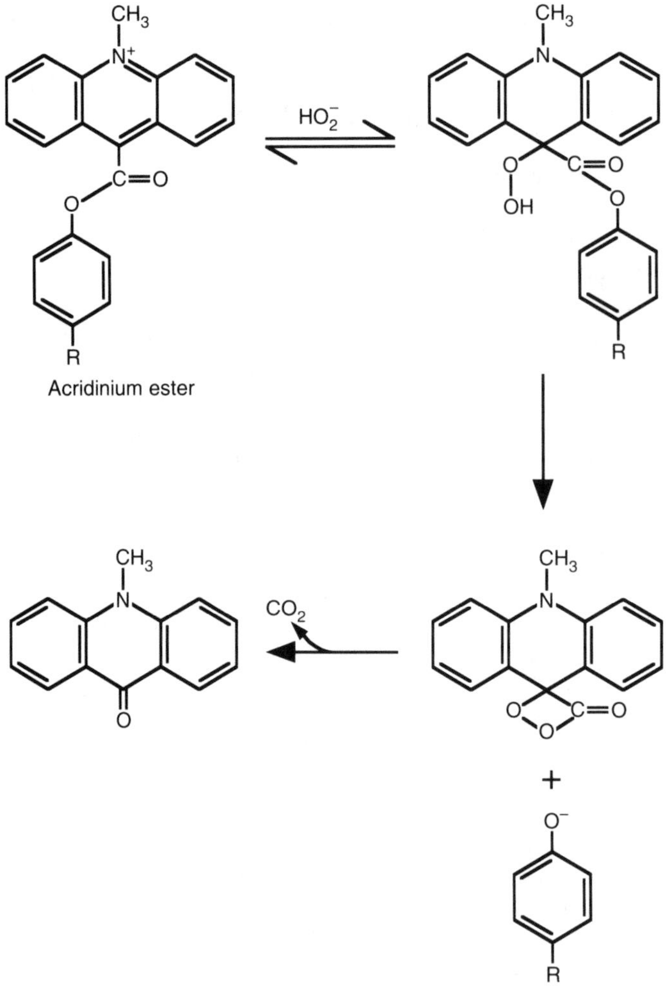

Figure 19-3.   Acridinium ester chemiluminescent reaction.

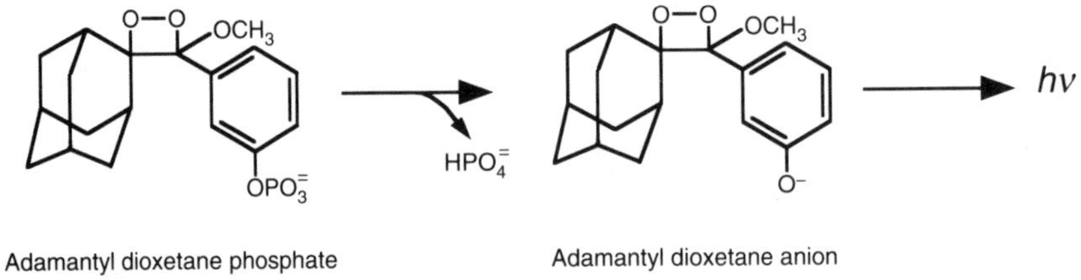

Figure 19-4.   Action of alkaline phosphatase on adamantyl dioxetane phosphate.

SEPARATION METHODS

The solid phases used in separating bound from unbound in the automated heterogeneous assays are quite varied and include antibody-coated tubes and beads, magnetic particles and beads, and other unique methods. In these assays the solid phase is coated with an antibody or some other molecule that in some way binds the analyte being measured. The instrument must then separate the liquid phase, containing unbound components, from the solid phase, containing the bound components. In manual immunoassays, centrifugation and decanting of the liquid phase or aspiration of the liquid phase are the most common methods of separating bound from unbound. Aspiration has proven to be the most adaptable to automation.

Tubes, coated on the inside with antibody, have been used as the solid phase in manual RIAs and EIAs for many years. The ES 300 uses antibody-coated tubes and aspiration of the liquid phase for most of the assays performed on the instrument. Boehringer Mannheim has added a modification of this methodology for three of the analytes on the ES 300, TSH, estradiol, and progesterone. The tubes for these assays are coated with streptavidin, which has a high binding affinity for biotin. Biotinylated antibodies and patient sample are added to the tube. The analyte binds to the biotinylated antibody, which binds to the streptavidin on the wall of the tube. The rest of the reaction proceeds as in any EIA (Fig. 19-5). Using streptavidin instead of antibody to coat the tubes provides an excess of binding sites, because streptavidin can bind four molecules of biotin.[5] An excess of binding sites negates any effects that imperfections in the wall of the tube might have on assay precision. This technique also improves the sensitivity of a coated-tube assay, making it possible to measure very small amounts of hormones.[5,14,15]

The IMx® uses antibody-coated latex microparticles as the solid phase. The microparticles increase the surface area used for binding, which increases the kinetics of the reaction and decreases the reaction time. A glass-fiber matrix, contained in the reaction cell, adsorbs the microparticles (Fig. 19-6). The affinity of the glass fibers for the latex particles is not well understood but appears to be irreversible. With the microparticles held fast to the fibers, unbound species are easily rinsed into an underlying blotter layer by pipetting wash solution onto the matrix.[7,8]

A special patented tube design (Fig. 19-7) allows for quick and efficient separation in the Immulite®. The solid phase is an antibody-coated, ¼″ polystyrene bead contained in the bottom of the special tube. The design of the tube and its small mass allow it to be rapidly spun, forcing transfer of the liquid phase and repeated washings into a sump chamber around the top of the tube.[12]

Antibody-coated paramagnetic particles are the solid phase in Ciba Corning's ACS:180™, and antibody-coated magnetized beads are used in Tosoh's AIA-1200™ and AIA-600™, but the magnetic characteristic of the particles and of the beads is used in a different manner in the two manufacturers' instrument designs. The paramagnetic particles of the ACS:180™ system are micron sized, which increases kinetics and decreases incubation time due to the increase in binding surface. After the binding reaction, the reaction tube is passed through a magnetic field and the particles are pulled to the back wall of the tube. The liquid phase, containing free

First antibody reaction

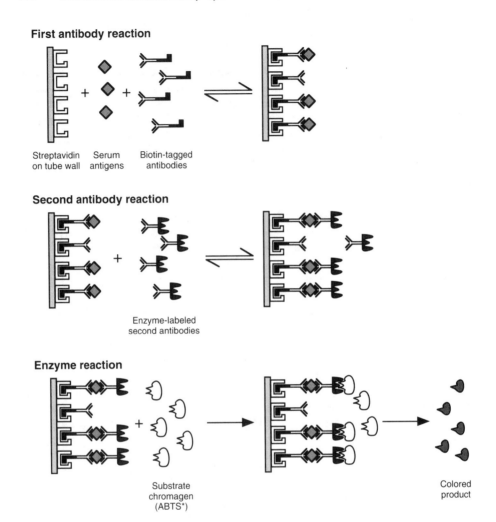

Second antibody reaction

Enzyme reaction

Figure 19-5. Reaction in a streptavidin-coated tube.

components, is aspirated and the paramagnetic particles are thoroughly washed and aspirated again before the chemiluminescent reaction is initiated.[10,11] In the AIA-1200™ and AIA-600™ the antibody-coated beads are subjected to a magnetic field during incubation. This causes constant mixing of the beads in the incubation mixture that helps to speed the reaction. At the end of the incubation time the test cup is moved out of the magnetic field and the liquid phase is aspirated by a probe programmed to remain above the level of the magnetic beads.[6]

Radial partition immunoassay, used on the Stratus II® from Baxter Diagnostics Inc. (Miami, FL 33152-0672), employs a separation technique based on chromatographic principles (described in Chapter 13). The solid phase is a glass-fiber filter

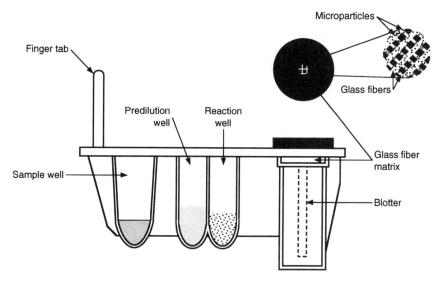

Figure 19-6. IMx® reaction cell.

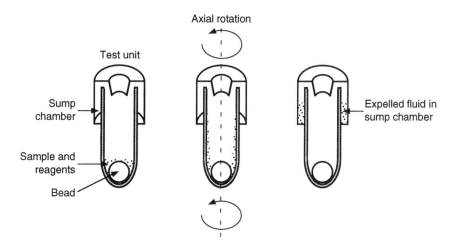

Figure 19-7. Immulite® test unit.

paper coated with immobilized antibody. After the antigen-antibody reaction on the filter paper, the "mobile phase" (a substrate wash solution) is added. The solution radially elutes or partitions the unbound enzyme-labeled antigen (competitive assays) or enzyme-labeled antibody (sandwich assays) away from the bound complexes (Fig. 19-8).[16,17]

The OPUS® immunoassay analyzer, manufactured by PB Diagnostics (Westwood,

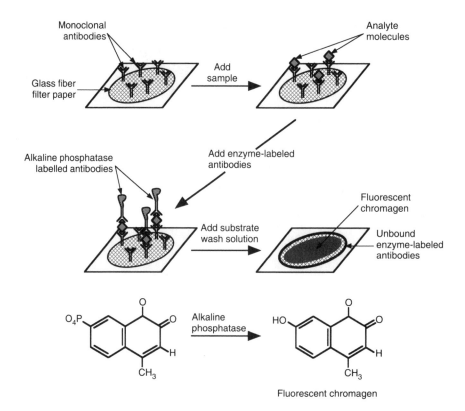

Figure 19-8. Radial partition immunoassay.

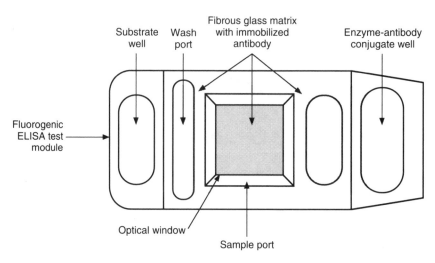

Figure 19-9. Opus® EIA test module.

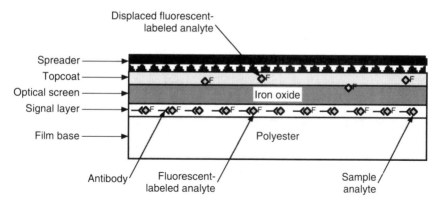

Spreader
Topcoat
Optical screen
Signal layer
Film base

Displaced fluorescent-labeled analyte

Iron oxide

Polyester

Antibody
Fluorescent-labeled analyte
Sample analyte

Figure 19-10. Opus® multilayer film test module.

MA 02090-2306), uses plastic, ready-to-use modules with two different separation techniques. The modules contain all reagents necessary for the immunoassay. The module type used primarily for assaying large molecules has a glass-fiber matrix for a solid phase. Unbound enzyme conjugate is washed away by substrate as it moves through the glass-fiber matrix by capillary action. The unbound conjugate is absorbed into a medium positioned away from the solid phase (Fig. 19-9).[18,19]

The second module, used for small-molecular-weight analytes and some thyroid assays, uses a methodology called *multilayer film assay.* The solid phase is a film chip coated with antibody bound to a fluorescent antigen in the bottom layer of the module. An iron oxide layer is above this and then a layer of dry reagents necessary for the immunoassay. The sample is added to the top of the module. Large molecules are prevented from diffusing down by the reagent layer. Smaller molecules move downward to the solid phase, and a competitive reaction occurs. Displaced fluorescent antigen diffuses upward, and the iron oxide layer blocks it from the fluorescent reading (Fig. 19-10).[18,19]

Instrumentation

INSTRUMENT TYPE

Manual immunoassays are expensive and time-consuming, so they are usually not done more than once a day, and certain assays may be performed only once a week or less. This allows for a batch of specimens to be assayed by using a single standard curve, which optimizes the standard-to-sample ratio. Cutoff times must be established and specimens drawn before the cutoff times are run. Specimens drawn after the cutoff are stored until the next scheduled run. Stat testing or setting up extra runs at a clinician's request are expensive and impractical. Many automated instruments have been designed around this batch concept, but others are more characteristic of the automated chemistry analyzers. Today's automated immunoassay instruments can be divided into three categories based on the way they process samples: batch, batch random access, and continuous random access.

Batch processing is the easiest to automate; consequently, the first automated immunoassay instruments developed were *batch analyzers*. The IMx® and Stratus® II are among the earliest and most popular batch analyzers. These instruments can assay for one analyte at a time on a limited number of samples. Once a run is started the instrument must assay all samples in the run or abort all samples before starting a different assay. Batch immunoassay analyzers, for the most part, have shorter incubation times compared to manual immunoassays, but it is still more economical to run assays on a batch of specimens because quality control and in some cases one or more calibrators should be assayed with each batch. Cutoff times and scheduling of tests on different days are still necessary because the instrument can only perform so many runs a day because of the incubation time of each run. Analytes, such as CK-MB or β-hCG, can be performed on a stat basis on these instruments, but in most cases results will be considerably delayed if the instrument is already processing a batch when the stat request is received. One exception to this is the Stratus® II that, when assaying the analyte requested stat, can be paused, the stat sample added, and the run restarted.

Random-access batch instrumentation is designed to run different assays at the same time on one sample or a group of samples. The samples are still batched, and once the instrument is started the run must go to completion. The ES 300 and Abbott Diagnostics' TDxFLx® and IMx® Select are examples of this type of instrument. The capability to perform random-access processing does decrease the technologist's time because specimens are only loaded onto the instrument once and several different assays incubate at the same time, but the turnaround time for stat testing is not improved.

Continuous random-access immunoassay instruments have been the most difficult to develop. These instruments not only assay more than one analyte at a time but also allow specimens to be added while the instrument is processing other specimens. With this design immunoassay tests can be performed as they are requested (whether they are stat or not) instead of being batched and performed on certain days. The management of multiple samples, multiple assays, and pauses to add on new samples requires sophisticated software and hardware, which has slowed their development. The Immulite®, ACS:180™, and the AIA-1200™ and AIA-600™ are continuous random-access immunoassay instruments.

COMPONENT PARTS

Although there is great variety among the automated immunoassay instruments, the basic functions that must be automated on an analyzer are the same, and the instruments share some common parts. These functions are control of instrument functions; data input; pipetting sample, reagents, and wash; transport of the reaction vessel; temperature control; signal detection; and data processing.

Control of Instrument Functions

The *control of instrument functions* is handled by microprocessors which form the central control entity in all of the instruments. The microprocessor system has the capability to generate commands. The instruction processing system of the chip operates in a sequential fashion that is precisely timed based on the vibrations of a quartz crystal. It is this intrinsic accuracy of timing that gives the microprocessor its capability to control processes in a very precise and repeatable fashion. The microprocessor(s) sends commands to input–output boards that contain small, specialized microprocessors that decode the commands into the basic sequential commands that are sent to the various parts of the instruments. Information from internal monitors and from the detection system is sent back to the microprocessor for evaluation of instrument performance and data reduction.

Data Entry

Data entry into the instruments can occur in several different ways. Several instruments have either a touch screen or computer keyboard to input patient identification and assay to be performed. Most instruments also have bidirectional interface capabilities so information can be downloaded and results uploaded from a mainframe computer.

Internal bar-code readers are used to provide various types of information in most of the instruments. On the ACS:180™ bar-coded samples can be loaded in any order, and a bar code reader informs the instrument of the sample location. Bar-code readers are also used to scan for assay identification and reagent lot number, which are coded on the pack or test unit. Bar-code wands are used on some instruments to input this information.

Pipetting

For *pipetting,* several instruments, such as the IMx® and Immulite®, use one probe for sample, reagent, and wash pipetting. Other instruments, such as the ACS:180™ and Stratus® II, use a dedicated probe for sample pipetting and multiple probes for reagent pipetting and wash. The probes are mounted in one of two ways: on a robotic arm or a stationary bar. The movement of the robotic arm or of the probe across the base is controlled by stepper motors. The amount of liquid aspirated and dispensed is controlled by various arrangements of syringes or valves that provide precise pipetting of samples and reagents. The probes are equipped with liquid level sensors that alert the operator to low sample or reagent volume. Capacitance liquid level sensing is the most common, but the AIA-1200™ uses an optical sensor to verify the presence of sufficient sample, and the AIA-600™ uses radio frequency.

Carryover between samples is a major problem for many analytes, such as tumor markers and β-hCG, measured by immunoassay instruments. An abnormal sample may have an analyte concentration 100,000 times greater than a normal sample. Instruments using one probe to pipet all samples must have a system of probe washing between each sample to ensure minimal sample carryover. The probes are washed inside and out, using either instrument-specific buffers or deionized water. The interior of the probe is cleansed by rapidly dispensing wash solution through it at a specially designed wash station (unique for each instrument). The exterior is cleaned as wash solution is forced across the outside of the probe by the geometry of the wash station. Capacitance liquid level sensing helps to limit the exterior area of the probe contaminated with specimen. The AIA-1200™ and the OPUS® solved the problem of carryover by using individual sample tips for each specimen.

Transport

The reaction vessels must be *transported* to positions where sample and reagent can be added, to an incubation area, to a signal detection area, and finally to a biohazardous waste reservoir. The timing of the movements must be precise, and stepper motors are again used. The reagent tabs in the Stratus® II and the reaction cells in the IMx® are arranged in a circular fashion on a carousel that rotates the tabs or cells to the various positions. In the ACS:180™, the AIA-600™, and the Immulite® the reaction tube is placed by the operator of the instrument, on a conveyor belt, that then moves the tube to the various positions within the instrument. Unique to the AIA-1200™, a robotic arm with a vacuum mechanism picks up the test cups and places them on a transport block. The transport block then moves through the instrument in an assembly line fashion.[6]

Temperature Control

Temperature control is critical for accurate and precise immunoassays. The analyte-antibody reaction and the enzyme reaction in an EIA are very temperature sensitive. The most common reaction temperature used by the automated instruments is 37°C, and reagents are usually preheated to this temperature before addition to the reaction vessel. The instruments use a variety of heating techniques. The IMx® uses three different heating systems. Reagents are placed in a heating block that preheats them to a set temperature, buffers are heated when they pass through a flow-through heater block, and the reaction cells are warmed and maintained at the correct temperature by a forced air heating system.[7,8] The ES 300 uses Peltier units, located under an incubation carousel, to heat or cool the temperature during reaction. The AIA-1200™ uses electric heating pads to warm the transport blocks holding the reaction cups. One or more thermistors are used to monitor the internal temperature.

Signal Detection

The method of *signal detection* is, of course, dependent on the label used. Instruments using fluorometric EIA have internal fluorometers. The Immulite® and ACS:180™, with chemiluminescent reactions, house luminometers. The ES 300 has a photometer to read the intensity of the color developed. More detailed descriptions of fluorometers, luminometers, and photometers can be found in Chapters 9, 10, and 6, respectively.

Data Processing

Data processing is programmed into each instrument. Various methods for data reduction are used by the automated immunoassay instruments to calculate a standard curve. Some instruments use more than one method depending on assay type, and others use a single method for all assays. The methods used include least-square linear reduction, cubic spline, and, most frequently, a four-parameter logistic method.

All the instruments also include some quality control functions, and some even have a limited capacity for archiving patient data.

REAGENT CONFIGURATION

Reagents for the automated immunoassay instruments are packaged in two different formats. Instruments such as the OPUS®, Immulite®, and AIA-1200™ and AIA-600™ have individual reagent packs used for one test only, although the OPUS® test module is the only one containing all reagents necessary for assaying the sample. With this arrangement the operator must load the patient sample and a test cup or module for every assay being performed. The ACS:180™, Stratus® II, IMx®, and ES 300 supply their reagents in bulk packs that can be used for a number of tests. Reagent loading is simplified with this arrangement, but the disadvantages are a shortened outdate after opening, and either the instrument or the operator must maintain an inventory of how much reagent is left.

CALIBRATION

One of the major advantages of automated immunoassays is long-term storage of a *calibration curve*. A significant cost of manual immunoassay is setting up a calibration curve with each batch of samples, whether the batch is one specimen or 100. Precise pipetting, temperature control, and control of incubation time on automated instrumentation allows a calibration curve to be stored and used to assay specimens on several runs. For most instruments, calibrators (usually six or seven levels) from the manufacturer are assayed, and the curve is calculated and stored. Some batch instruments require one or more of the calibrators to be assayed with each run of samples, so minor adjustments can be made to the curve. The IMx® uses this technique with some assays. One calibrator, specified by the manufacturer, is run with each batch of specimens. The software automatically adjusts the curve based on the reading of this calibrator, and sample values are calculated from this adjusted curve. The Immulite® and ACS:180™ use a master curve supplied by the manufacturer. The manufacturer runs several calibrator curves with each new lot of reagents and determines the "best fit" curve. The parameters of this curve are entered into the instrument by the operator. Subsequent calibrations are done by running two calibrators to adjust the master curve.[10-12]

Maintenance and Quality Assurance

The maintenance for the various instruments is a combination of system performance checks and housekeeping and the time needed varies from a few minutes to 2 hours. The ES 300 has no specified daily and weekly maintenance because the instrument primes cleaning solution and rinses with distilled water at the beginning and end of each run. The OPUS® is one of the most maintenance-free instruments with a monthly detector lamp check, monthly and weekly cleaning of various parts of the instrument, and daily restocking of supplies and emptying of used pipet and module waste. In contrast, the AIA-1200™ requires 2 hours for recommended monthly maintenance that includes monthly standardization of the five fluorescent detectors and recalibration of the assays.[6] Several instruments have internal start-up checks to determine if the performance of the detector and instrument temperature are within specified range, but some, like the IMx®, also require scheduled operator checks using calibrated thermometers and optical standards. Maintenance tasks performed on many of the instruments include daily priming for instruments with tubing, restocking universal reagents, such as wash buffers or substrate, and emptying liquid waste reservoirs.

Quality control for batch instrumentation is the same as for manual immunoassays. Bilevel or trilevel controls, with ranges in different parts of the calibration curve, should be run with each batch of specimens. The decision of how often quality control samples should be run on continuous random-access instruments is somewhat more difficult because there are no discrete runs. Most manufacturers recommend running quality control for all assays daily, but many operators run controls more often, at least once per shift.

Summary

The majority of automated immunoassay instruments available today use heterogeneous competitive and immunometric immunoassay techniques. Heterogeneous immunoassays can measure a wider range of analytes than homogeneous assays and offer better sensitivity. Chemiluminescent and enzyme immunoassays are the most popular methods used in these instruments. The type of solid phase varies but includes coated tubes, beads, and magnetic particles.

Automating manual immunoassays on batch and random-access batch instrumentation improves turnaround time and decreases the technologist's time, but specimens must still be run in a group. During batch processing, the instrument is unavailable for other testing. Continuous random-access instruments can assay routine and stat specimens as they are received in the laboratory.

The immunoassay instruments have common functions that manufacturers have automated in various ways. The common functions are data input, pipetting, transporting the reaction vessel, temperature control, signal detection, and data processing. These functions are controlled by one or more microprocessors.

One of the expenses associated with manual immunoassays is the necessity to run a standard curve each time the assay is set up. The precision of the automated immunoassay instruments makes it possible to use a stored standard curve.

Significant progress has been made in automating immunoassays. More and more tests are being automated on existing analyzers, and new instruments are in development. The future will probably see an increase in the number of instruments using chemiluminescent assays and more emphasis on continuous random-access capability.

References

1. Butler JE, ed. Immunochemistry of solid-phase immunoassay. Boca Raton, FL: CRC Press, 1991:300.
2. Chan DW. Automation of immunoassay. In: Chan DW, ed. Immunoassay automation: A practical guide. San Diego, CA: Harcourt Brace Jovanovich, 1992:9-21.
3. Gosling JP. A decade of development in immunoassay methodology. Clin Chem 1990, 36:1408-27.
4. Ng RH. Immunoassay automation. J Clin Immunoassay 1991, 14:59.
5. Sagona MA, Collinsworth WE, Gadsden RH. ES-300 immunoassay system. In: Chan DW, ed. Immunoassay automation: A practical guide. San Diego, CA: Harcourt Brace Jovanovich, 1992:191-202.
6. Anderson FP. A hospital laboratory's experience with the TOSOH AIA-1200. J Clin Immunoassay 1992, 15:222-28.
7. Keller CH, Fitzgerald KL, Barnes A. The Abbott IMx® and IMx Select™ systems. J Clin Immunoassay 1991, 14:115-19.
8. Sasse EA. The Abbott IMx and IMx SELECT: A user's perspective. J Clin Immunoassay 1992, 15:229-34.
9. Dudley RF. Chemiluminescence immunoassay: An alternative to RIA. Laboratory Medicine 1990, 21:216-22.
10. Dudley RF. The Ciba Corning ACS:180™ automated immunoassay system. J Clin Immunoassay 1991, 14:77-82.
11. Smart JB. The CIBA Corning ACS:180-a user's perspective. J Clin Immunoassay 1992, 15:246-51.
12. Babson AL. The Cirrus IMMULITE™ automated immunoassay system. J Clin Immunoassay 1991, 14:83-88.
13. Schaap AP, Akhavan H, Romano LJ. Chemiluminescent substrates for alkaline phosphatase: Application to ultrasensitive enzyme-linked immunoassays and DNA probes. Clin Chem 1989, 35:1863-64.
14. Duncan T, Engelberth L, LaBrash B. The Boehringer Mannheim ES 300 immunoassay system. J Clin Immunoassay 1991, 14:105-10.
15. Sheehan M. The Boehringer Mannheim ES 300 immunoassay system: A user's perspective. J Clin Immunoassay 1992, 15:205-12.
16. Austin L, Johnson C. Clinical experiences with the Baxter Stratus II. J Clin Immunoassay 1992, 15:218-21.
17. Plaut DS, McLellan WN. The Baxter Diagnostics Inc., Dade Stratus® II automated fluorometric immunoassay system. J Clin Immunoassay 1991, 14:120-25.
18. Olive C. PB Diagnostics' OPUS® immunoassay system. J Clin Immunoassay 1991, 14:126-32.
19. Velazquez FR. The P.B. Diagnostics' OPUS immunoassay systems. J Clin Immunoassay 1992, 15:235-41.

Suggested Readings

Chan DW, ed. Immunoassay automation: A practical guide. San Diego: Academic Press, 1992.

Product Comparison System. Enzyme immunoassay analyzers; fluorescence immunoassay analyzers; chemiluminescence immunoassay analyzers. International Laboratory Equipment Encyclopedia and Purchasing Guide. Plymouth Meeting, PA; ECRI, 1993.

20

AUTOMATED HEMATOLOGY SYSTEMS

Linda L. Fell

Objectives

After completing this chapter, the reader will be able to:

1. Describe the principle of the electrical impedance method of counting and describing blood cells.
2. Describe the principle of high-frequency radio waves in counting and describing cells.
3. Describe the principle of optical scattering of light by cells illuminated by a laser.
4. Describe the principle of peroxidase staining of leukocytes.
5. Describe the applications of the listed principles in hematology instrumentation.
6. Discuss histogram and scattergram generation and the role of computer analysis in hematology instrumentation.
7. Describe the principles and applications used in the Coulter® STKS, the Sysmex NE-8000, the Abbott Cell-Dyn®, and the Technicon H•2™.
8. Describe the technology used in the dedicated reticulocyte counter, the Sysmex R-3000.
9. Discuss quality control applications in hematology instrumentation.

Definitions

Aperture: An orifice through which cells pass to be counted.
CBC: Complete blood count.
Coincidence Counts: Cells that pass through the aperture together but are counted as one cell.
Femtoliter (fl): A unit of volume equal to one-quadrillionth of a liter (10^{-15}). It is the

recommended unit for expressing mean cell volume (MCV) and is equal to the formerly used measure, the cubic micron.

Hct: Hematocrit.

Hgb: Hemoglobin.

Histogram: A bar chart with equal width to each bar, often depicting the number of cells in a particular size range.

Hydrodynamic Focusing: Centering something (cells) with the use of sheath fluids around the sample.

Impedance: Opposition to flow of electrical current, fluid, or sound waves.

Laser: The acronym for light amplification by stimulated emission of radiation.

MCH: Mean cell hemoglobin.

MCHC: Mean cell hemoglobin concentration.

MCV: Mean cell volume.

Mean: Arithmetic average.

MN: Mononuclear cell.

MPV: Mean platelet volume.

Noise: Any unwanted disturbance or spurious signal within an electronic component. Noise is an unintended addition to the needed signal independent of the signal's presence.

PDW: Platelet distribution width. It indicates size variation.

Photodiode: A detector that converts photon energy to electrical energy (emf).

Plt: Platelet.

PMN: Polymorphonuclear leukocyte.

RBC: Red blood cell, or erythrocyte.

RDW: Red cell distribution width.

Scattergram (scatterplot): A graph plotting different measurements that represent cells. Often, a scattergram is three-dimensional and plots two histograms.

Software: The programs or instructions that cause data to be processed in a computer, and their associated documentation.

Threshold: An electronically set size limit above which the pulse is analyzed and below which it is ignored.

WBC: White blood cell, or leukocyte.

Introduction

Instrumentation in hematology has advanced from simple automated cell counters to complex automated cell counters with five-part differentials in a remarkably short time. Today, virtually all hospital laboratories and large clinics have multiparameter instruments that measure, derive, and/or calculate at least 20 complete blood count (CBC) parameters. In addition to white blood cells (WBCs), red blood cells (RBCs), and platelets measured in the past, instruments now provide information on anisocytosis (red cell distribution width—RDW), hemoglobin, mean platelet volume (MPV), and relative and absolute values for the five types of leukocytes normally seen in peripheral blood. Alert messages are generated when the presence of abnormal cells is suspected. Histograms and scatterplots are also standard features.

Manual differential analysis of the leukocytes is a time-consuming procedure in hematology. The differential includes not only the identification and structure of the leukocytes, but also a description of the erythrocytes and an estimation of the platelet count. For a differential instrument to be of value in the laboratory, these three components must be included. An automated differential must also be able to identify specimens with abnormal WBCs, RBCs, and platelets.

The new multiparameter instruments are autodiluting (the operator does not have to make dilutions before entering the specimen into the system). All can sample blood from stoppered tubes, thereby decreasing the operator's risk of infection. All the instruments discussed in this chapter also include a bar-coding feature that minimizes error in handling large numbers of samples.

Principles

Cell detection in hematology instrumentation is based on three principles: increased electrical impedance, deflection of radio waves, and optical scattering of a laser beam. Peroxidase staining is also used in differentiation of WBCs.

ELECTRICAL IMPEDANCE

Electrical impedance detection was first introduced by Wallace Coulter in 1956.[1] This method is based on the electrical conductivity (see Chapter 11) difference between a cell and its diluent. Cells act as insulators, whereas the diluent acts as a conductor. Cells suspended in an electrolyte solution pass through a small aperture (Fig. 20-1). A constant-strength direct current passes through the aperture between two electrodes, one inside and one outside. The passage of a cell through the aperture increases the resistance of the electrical path between the two electrodes. A higher voltage is needed to maintain constant current in the face of increased electrical resistance. An electrical pulse proportional to the voltage increase is generated by the instrument. The number of pulses yields the particle count. The amplitude of each electrical pulse correlates with cell size. Different cell types can be distinguished by sorting the pulses.

Thresholds or discriminators, preset in earlier cell counters, are now floating or automatic in many instruments. In instruments with automatic discriminators, a circuit is incorporated that disregards all signals below a threshold level. A computer then automatically adjusts the threshold position to the optimum levels for each sample. Discriminators float between ranges that exclude electrical noise, erythrocyte fragments, microcytic erythrocytes, or clumped platelets.

A histogram, a bar chart with equal width to each bar, is often used to depict the number of cells in a particular size range (Fig. 20-2). A typical histogram plots cell size versus number of pulses. By applying thresholds based on size, cells can be differentiated as leukocytes, erythrocytes, or platelets (Fig. 20-3).

A potential problem with impedance counters is two or more cells passing through an aperture at the same time (coincidence). This coincidence is statistically predictable, however, and instrument computers can correct for it when reporting cell counts.

An added feature in some instruments using direct current is the adaptation of

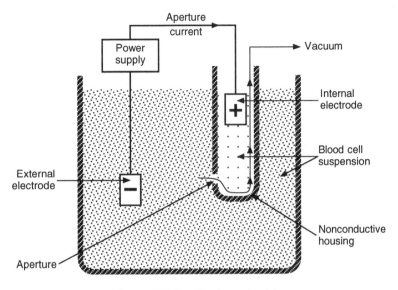

Figure 20-1.   Coulter principle.

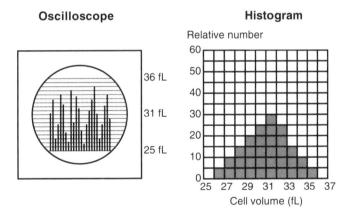

Figure 20-2.   Histogram—a distributional plot of cell size.

hydrodynamic focusing (see Chapter 17). Hydrodynamic focusing reduces coincidence (cell volume error due to two cells being measured at the same time), pulse variations due to different paths taken through the aperture, and recirculation of cells as they are carried away from the aperture into the waste flow.[2] A sample stream is injected into the center of a sheath stream and enters a flow cell. The pressurized sheath fluid focuses the sample stream. The high-speed flow of the sample keeps cells in single file.

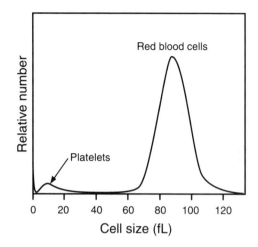

Figure 20-3.   Normal platelet and RBC distribution.

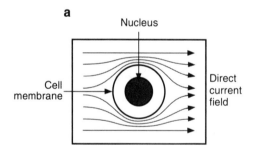

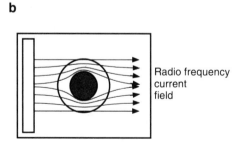

Figure 20-4.   (a) Leukocyte in a direct current field. Cell membrane resists flow of current. Voltage must increase to maintain constant current flow. (b) Leukocyte in a radio frequency field. Dense nucleus impedes radio waves. Again, voltage must increase to maintain constant current flow.

Deflection of Radio Waves

The current impedance method has been adapted to use another kind of current: high-frequency, or radio waves. In this technology, high-frequency, alternating current sine waves generated by a crystal oscillator are superimposed on the direct current. Cells increase the impedance of the system in proportion to their average density. The cell membrane and cytoplasm usually contribute little to impedance. Nuclear size, nuclear density, and cytoplasmic granularity are the biggest contributors to cell density and, therefore, *radio wave impedance.*[3] In this system, the alternating current is held constant. Increased impedance therefore needs a higher voltage to maintain the same alternating current flow (Voltage = Current times Impedance). The strength of the voltage pulse generated when the cell passes through the current is related to nuclear characteristics and cytoplasmic granularity (Fig. 20-4).

LIGHT SCATTER

The second basic principle is that of *light scattering* by a particle as it moves through a laser beam[4] (see Chapters 17 and 8 for discussions of flow cytometry and light scatter, respectively). Cells in a flow cytometer pass through the beam of a helium-neon laser. The laser beam is tightly focused on the sample stream. As a cell passes through the beam, light is scattered in all directions. In the original technology, only the presence of cells was detected. Modern instruments take advantage of the fact that the intensity of forward angle light scatter is proportional to cell size. The scattered light intensity is measured by a photodetector that generates a voltage pulse for each cell. Each pulse is compared to threshold requirements, and the cell is classified by size.

Orthogonal (90°) light scatter provides information about cytoplasmic granularity and nuclear characteristics such as density and shape. It is also known that some cells cause polarized light scattered at 90° to depolarize. The ability to depolarize light scattered orthogonally is related to the type of granules in a leukocyte: eosinophils strongly depolarize light, whereas neutrophils do not.

Orthogonal light scatter intensity is measured with a photomultiplier tube. Lymphocytes, monocytes, and granulocytes can be differentiated by combining measurements of forward, polarized orthogonal, and nonpolarized orthogonal light scatter intensities. Refinements of this technology are now used to differentiate WBCs and to generate scattergrams (see Computer Analysis section).

PEROXIDASE STAINING

The Technicon (Miles Diagnostic Division, Miles, Inc., Tarrytown, NY 10591) instruments use enzyme activity to differentiate WBCs. This will be discussed in the section on the Technicon H·2™.

HEMOGLOBIN DETERMINATION

Cell counter systems also measure hemoglobin concentrations. All instruments use a modification of the cyanmethemoglobin method, in which a blood sample is diluted with potassium ferricyanide to form methemoglobin and then cyanmethemo-globin.[5] Cyanmethemoglobin is measured photometrically at its peak absorbance of 540 nm.

COMPUTER ANALYSIS

Sophisticated computer analysis converts the detector data from all the particles in a sample into usable information. The computer software instantly classifies cells based on their light scattering properties. This information is collected for the entire sample. The computer then reports cell counts and cell indices and prepares histograms and scattergrams (see later in the chapter). The reports and graphs enable the operator to interpret the data and provide clinically relevant information to physicians and other health care workers.

A *histogram* is a bar chart of frequency distribution. Each bar is of uniform width and represents a range of data or a classification. The height of a bar represents the number of items with that classification. In automated hematology systems, histograms are usually of cell size ranges. This type of histogram is useful for showing the size distributions of erythrocytes, leukocytes, and platelets. A two-dimensional *scattergram* (scatterplot) plots two different measurements on many items. Blood cell scattergrams of forward and orthogonal light scatter aid in the interpretation of hematological data. A scattergram of this type is also known as a *cytogram*. Three-dimensional scattergrams can add a third measured parameter such as nonpolarized orthogonal light scatter. Histograms and scattergrams aid in the detection and enumeration of abnormal cells. Many types of abnormal cells can be identified visually from the graphs.

Histograms of cell size, based on information gathered from either electrical impedance or measurement of light scatter by a laser, yield partial (two or three part) WBC differentials. Populations of lymphocytes, monocytes, and granulocytes can be differentiated. Eosinophils and basophils are included in the granulocyte area of this histogram. Newer systems measure more parameters and provide better WBC differentials.

DERIVED PARAMETERS

Some instruments report cell counts that are derived from a histogram by selecting some of the bars and applying algorithms to "smooth" the curve. The Coulter® STKS, for example, derives the platelet count from the cell volume histogram. The count is obtained by smoothing histogram values with cell volumes between 2 and 20 fL. This provides a more accurate count of low-volume platelets. The MCV is derived from the RBC histogram in some instruments. The MPV, platelet distribution width (PDW), and RDW are also derived from histograms.

CALCULATED PARAMETERS

The mean cell hemoglobin (MCH) and MCH concentration (MCHC) are calculated in all instruments. Other parameters, such as hematocrit and absolute numbers of WBCs, are calculated by some automated hematology systems.

Automated Systems

COULTER® STKS

The Coulter® STKS is the latest hematology instrument by Coulter Diagnostics (Coulter Corp., Miami, FL 33196), the developer of the electrical impedance method of counting cells. In the STKS, RBCs and WBCs are enumerated directly by using this electrical impedance principle. Hemoglobin is measured photometrically at 525 nm using an incandescent lamp.

Other CBC parameters (mean cell volume [MCV], RDW, platelet [Plt], and MPV) are derived from histograms that are in turn developed from data using the Coulter principle. The MCV and RDW are derived from the RBC histogram. The RBCs are counted and categorized by size based on the strength of the voltage pulse generated by each cell. A pulse-height analyzer (described in Chapter 10) sorts the pulses into volume categories (channels) and generates a histogram. A moving average method is used to "smooth" the data on the histogram. The MCV is the average size of all the cells in the histogram above 36 fL. The RDW is the coefficient of variation of erythrocyte size on the histogram. The platelet count and MPV are derived from the cell size histogram by looking at volumes between 2 and 20 fL. This allows the instrument to report an accurate platelet count in the presence of microcytic erythrocytes. The MPV is also derived from the platelet size histogram. The hematocrit, MCH, and MCHC are calculated from measured parameters.

Leukocytes are also detected and counted by electrical impedance. The WBC differential is assessed by the *VCS system,* which combines measurements of Volume, Conductivity, and Light Scatter. A three-dimensional plot of the measurements differentiates neutrophils, lymphocytes, monocytes, eosinophils, and basophils.[6] Cells are analyzed in their native state (without stains or dyes).

Volume, conductivity, and light scatter are measured simultaneously at the flow cell in the triple transducer. Cell volume is calculated from the increased resistance to low-frequency direct current (Coulter principle). Conductivity to direct current radio frequency waves varies with nuclear size, nuclear density, and the presence of cytoplasmic granules. Small lymphocytes with large nuclear:cytoplasmic (N:C) ratios and basophils with numerous large cytoplasmic granules exhibit large differences in radio wave conductivities. Low- and high-angle light scatter of monochromic light from a helium-neon laser are also measured. The scattered light intensities provide information on cell structure, shape, and reflectivity. For example, low-angle light scatter is greater in eosinophils than in neutrophils because of the large eosinophilic granules just beneath the cell membrane.

The data analyzer generates a three-dimensional plot of light scatter (*x* axis), conductivity (*y* axis), and volume (*z* axis) (Fig. 20-5). If only volume and light scatter are plotted, four cell populations can still be distinguished: neutrophils, lymphocytes, monocytes, and eosinophils (Fig. 20-6). The addition of radio wave deflection (conductivity) allows identification of basophils. Abnormal cell populations are readily detected from the scattergrams. "Suspect" flags are automatically generated for immature granulocytes, variant lymphocytes or blasts, and nucleated RBCs. A "Review WBC" alert is sent whenever leukocyte distribution is abnormal.

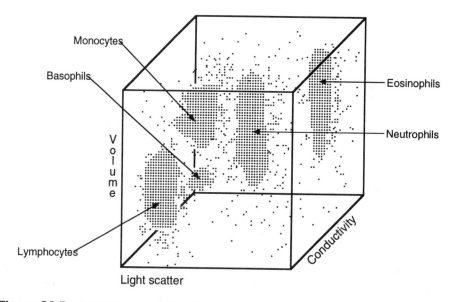

Figure 20-5. VCS Technology, Coulter® STKS—a three-dimensional measurement; light scatter on the x axis, volume of the y axis, and conductivity plotted on the z axis.

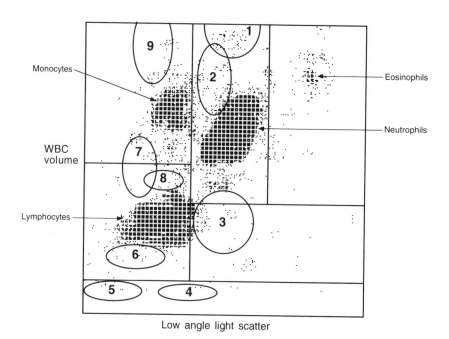

Figure 20-6. Coulter® STKS plot of cell volume versus low-angle light scatter for WBCs. Normal lymphocytes, monocytes, neutrophils, and eosinophils are labeled. The numbered regions correspond to abnormal cell populations: (1) blasts, (2) immature granulocytes, (3) aged or damaged neutrophils, (4) giant platelets, (5) nucleated RBCs, (6) atypical lymphocytes, (7) blasts, (8) atypical lymphocytes, and (9) blasts.

378

Coulter Diagnostics has nine other models of automated hematology analyzers available. They all use one or more of the methods we described for counting, sizing, and classifying blood cells.

SYSMEX NE-8000

The Sysmex NE-8000 is a multichannel hematology analyzer that reports 23 parameters and generates five histograms and one scattergram. The system uses five separate detectors, four that measure direct current or alternating radio frequency electrical impedance, and one that measures light transmittance. One impedance detector enumerates erythrocytes and platelets. Its results are used to calculate MCV, RDW, MPV, and PDW. A second impedance detector counts total leukocytes and differentiates lymphocytes, monocytes, and granulocytes. The other two impedance detectors are for eosinophils and basophils. Hemoglobin is measured photometrically at 540 nm.

There are two basic technologies used by the NE-8000. The primary method uses direct current electrical impedance. Platelets and RBCs are counted and sized by this method. Their enumeration includes use of *hydrodynamic focusing* to improve accuracy and precision of counts. The NE-8000 uses automatic discriminators to separate RBCs from platelets.

Differential and WBC technologies in the NE-8000 are based on two principles: direct current impedance, and the use of high-frequency alternating current. The use of a radio frequency to assess nuclear characteristics was patented by TOA Medical Electronics in 1968. In the WBC (lymphocytes, monocytes, granulocytes) detection system, a gentle lysing agent is added that increases WBC membrane permeability without destroying the cell membrane. The lysing agent releases some of the cytoplasm and causes some shrinking of the nucleus.

Each altered cell passes through an aperture to the detector block where it is counted (by resistance to direct current). Cell volume is calculated from the amplitude of the direct current voltage pulse. The computer analyzes these pulses and sorts them into size categories.

The second technology uses high-frequency alternating current (radio frequency [RF] waves) generated by a crystal oscillator. The high-frequency ac signal is overlaid on a dc signal. Impedance to radio waves depends mostly on nuclear size, nuclear density, and number of large cytoplasmic granules. The ac voltage pulse resulting from the impedance is proportional to the size and density of the nucleus and the granularity of the cell.

After each cell has been detected and characterized by both methods, a scattergram of dc pulse amplitude versus rf pulse amplitude is plotted. Lymphocytes, monocytes, and granulocytes are identifiable (Fig. 20-7). Abnormal cells (nucleated red blood cells [NRBC], atypical lymphocytes, blasts, immature granulocytes) can also be identified from their location on the scattergram.

Eosinophils and basophils are included in the granulocyte cluster and must be further differentiated. The NE-8000 treats whole blood with two special lysing agents, each at a *p*H that causes all cells except eosinophils or basophils to lyse or shrink. The

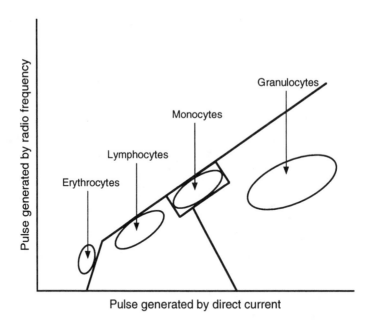

Pulse generated by radio frequency

Granulocytes

Monocytes

Lymphocytes

Erythrocytes

Pulse generated by direct current

Figure 20-7.   WBC scattergram, Sysmex NE-8000.

blood dilutions are sent to separate detectors that use direct current electrical impedance. The intact, unshrunken eosinophils or basophils produce larger voltage pulses than other granulocytes. Histograms for each cell type are generated. Neutrophils are then calculated by subtracting eosinophils and basophils from the total granulocyte count.

A recently introduced module for the NE-8000 is a slide maker with user-defined parameters for automated generation of a wedge smear. The slide is labeled with a bar code.

CELL-DYN® 3000

The Abbott Cell-Dyn® 3000 is a 22-parameter hematology analyzer. The Cell-Dyn® 3000 counts RBCs and platelets by using direct current electrical impedance. One channel is dedicated to these two parameters. A second channel measures hemoglobin, and a third channel counts and differentiates WBCs.

The WBC and differential channel uses the MAPSS (Multi-Angle Polarized Scatter Separation) system (Fig. 20-8). A vertically polarized, helium-neon laser beam passes through the flow cell. Hydrodynamic focusing allows only single cells to enter the flow cell. Forward (0°) light scatter and low angle (10°) light scatter are detected by separate silicon photodiodes. Polarized and nonpolarized orthogonal light scattering are detected by two different photomultiplier tubes.

The computer analyzes these four measurements of light scatter. Forward light scatter is used to count cells, and its intensity is used to estimate the *size*. Low-angle

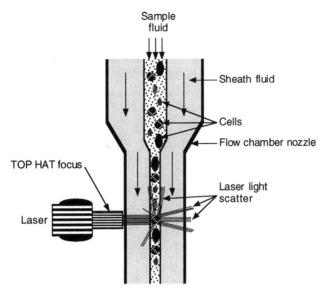

Figure 20-8. Multiangle polarized scatter separation (MAPSS) technology, Abbot Cell-Dyn®.

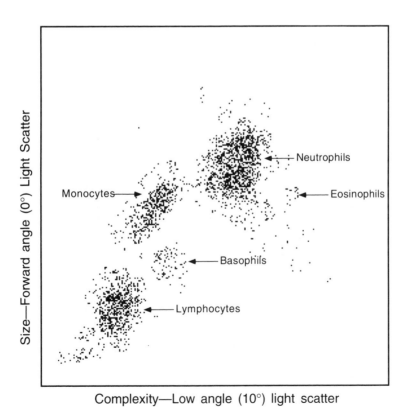

Figure 20-9. WBC scattergram, Abbott Cell-Dyn®.

light scatter intensity predicts cellular *complexity* (internal structure). Polarized orthogonal light scatter intensity correlates with cellular *lobularity.* Depolarized orthogonal light scatter intensity correlates with cellular *granularity.*

Different WBC clusters or populations can be visualized and enumerated from scattergrams. Plots of 0° light scatter intensity (size) versus 10° light scatter intensity (complexity) allow identification of lymphocytes, monocytes, neutrophils, and basophils (Fig. 20-9). Plots of 90° polarized light scatter (lobularity) versus 10° light scatter (complexity) allow better separations of granulocytes and mononuclear cells. Plots of 90° polarized light scatter (lobularity) versus 90° depolarized light scatter allow identification of eosinophils that can then be subtracted from the polymorphonuclear (PMN) population.

These scatterplots will also detect the presence of abnormal cells such as immature granulocytes, large lymphocytes, and blasts. Alert flags are generated to trigger manual review of stained smears.

Smaller 16-parameter (Cell-Dyn® 1600cs) and 8-parameter (Cell-Dyn® 1400) hematology instruments are also available. They use the same principles as the Cell-Dyn® 3000 for the parameters measured in each system.

TECHNICON H·2™

The Technicon H·2™ hematology analyzer (Miles Diagnostic Division, Miles Inc., Tarrytown, NY 10591) uses peroxidase activity to differentiate WBCs. It also uses laser technology to count and size RBCs and platelets and to distinguish basophils and lobularity of cells. The H·2™ system is the larger of two systems manufactured by Miles Diagnostics. Both systems use the same principles and reagents.

The instrument has four channels: hemoglobin, RBC/plt, peroxidase, and basophil/lobularity. Hemoglobin is converted to cyanmethemoglobin and measured photometrically at 546 nm.

Flow cytometry and laser light scatter are used to count and differentiate cells. Light scatter measurements are evaluated by computer algorithms to provide the reported parameters.

The peroxidase channel is unique to Technicon instrumentation. The WBCs are fixed and then are stained for peroxidase activity by the addition of a chromogen and hydrogen peroxide solution. Peroxidase in the cells reacts with the solution and forms a dark precipitate that stains the cells. Staining intensity is proportional to peroxidase activity. Eosinophils have strong peroxidase activity; neutrophils have moderate activity; and monocytes have weak activity. Peroxidase is not present in lymphocytes. The stained cells are directed into a flow chamber illuminated by a tungsten lamp. Two detectors are used. One measures low-angle light scatter to count cells and estimate their volumes (Fig. 20-10). The other detector measures absorbance by the stain. The scattergram of absorbance versus light scatter allows identification and enumeration of neutrophils, monocytes, lymphocytes, and eosinophils (Fig. 20-11).

Basophils are not distinguished from lymphocytes in the scheme we described; therefore, another detector system enumerates basophils and provides information

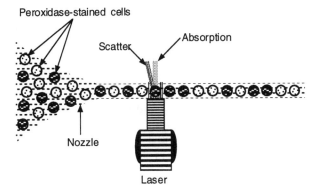

Figure 20-10.   Peroxidase Technology, Technicon H·2™.

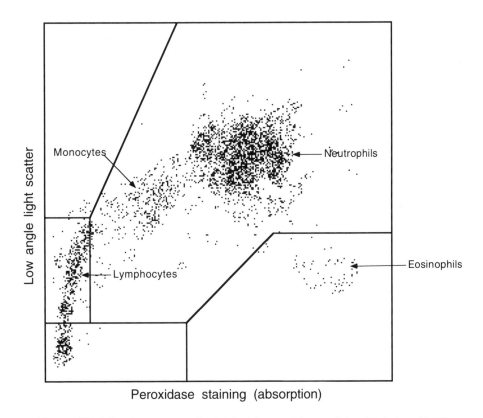

Figure 20-11.   Scattergram obtained with peroxidase staining, Technicon H·2™.

on the lobularity of WBCs. The WBCs are exposed to a surfactant at low pH that strips the cytoplasm from all cells except basophils. This channel uses a helium-neon red laser. Low-angle (0-5°) and high-angle (5-15°) light scatter intensities are measured (Fig. 20-12). Low-angle light scatter measures WBC size, so that intact basophils can be distinguished from the smaller cytoplasm-stripped WBCs. High-angle light scatter intensity increases with increasing nuclear lobularity. A plot of low-angle versus high-angle light scatter separates mononuclear cells from PMNs (Fig. 20-13).

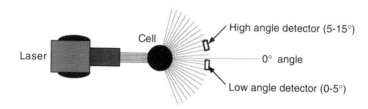

Figure 20-12.   Basophil/lobularity channel, Technicon H·2™.

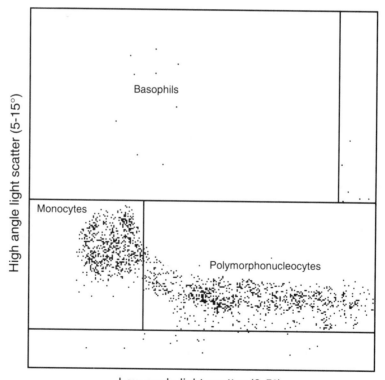

Figure 20-13.   Detection of basophils on Technicon H·2™.

The ratio of PMNs to mononuclear cells (MN), or lobularity index (LI), correlates with the degree of PMN segmentation. Therefore, a "left shift" (the presence of neutrophilic bands) can be detected. Other abnormal cells can be estimated by the location of clusters on the cytogram.

The RBC/plt channel also uses the helium-neon laser system. In the Technicon methodology, RBCs and platelets are made spherical without changing their volumes and then are passed through the laser. Two angles of light scatter (low [2° to 3° of arc] and high [5° to 15° of arc]) are measured simultaneously.[7] This combination measures cell size (volume) and optical density (that correlates to hemoglobin concentration within each RBC). The cellular hemoglobin concentration mean (CHCM) is assessed by the refractive index application of the Mie theory of light scatter. (The Mie theory states that for every pair of low-angle and high-angle scatter signals by a RBC, only one volume and one hemoglobin correspond.)[7] These signals have been mapped, and values are compared to the standard. Computer analysis generates a cytogram with hemoglobin concentration versus volume. MCV, RDW, and CHCM values are derived from these histograms. Hematocrit (hct), MCH, MCHC values are calculated from the measured hemoglobin (hgb), RBC, and MCV values.

Platelets are detected using only the measurements of high-angle light scatter. The MPV is derived from the measured platelet volume.

RETICULOCYTE COUNTING

A dedicated reticulocyte counter has been introduced by TOA Medical Electronics, Inc. (Los Alamitos, CA 90720). The Sysmex R-3000 is a benchtop flow cytometer that measures RBC count, relative reticulocyte value, and absolute reticulocyte count. Reticulocytes, unlike mature erythrocytes, still have ribonucleic acid (RNA) in their cytoplasm. Increased numbers of reticulocytes are seen in conditions associated with increased RBC production. Decreased numbers of reticulocytes are seen in aplastic conditions and nutritional deficiencies.

The R-3000 has automated specimen aspiration and dilution. The RBCs are stained with a fluorescent dye, Auramine O, that binds to nucleic acids. The stained cells pass through a flow cell and are illuminated with an argon laser (Fig. 20-14). Two measurements are taken simultaneously: forward angle scatter and fluorescence detected at 90°. The scattered light is proportional to cell size. The fluorescence intensity is proportional to cellular RNA content. More than 30,000 cells are analyzed per specimen.

A scattergram displays the 90° fluorescence intensity versus forward angle light scatter intensity. Each cell is plotted as a single dot on the scattergram. The scattergram depicts mature RBCs, reticulocytes, and platelets. Discriminator lines separate these cell populations. The reticulocyte area of the scattergram is subdivided into low-, middle-, and high-fluorescence intensity regions. Only the total reticulocyte values are reported in the United States at this time (Fig. 20-15).

The RBC count and relative reticulocytes (percentage) are measured directly; the absolute reticulocyte count is calculated.

Quality control material is available from Sysmex. The instrument's quality

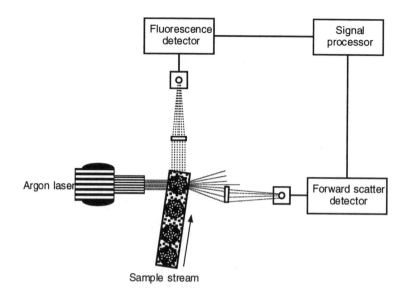

Figure 20-14. Flow cytometer, Sysmex R-3000.

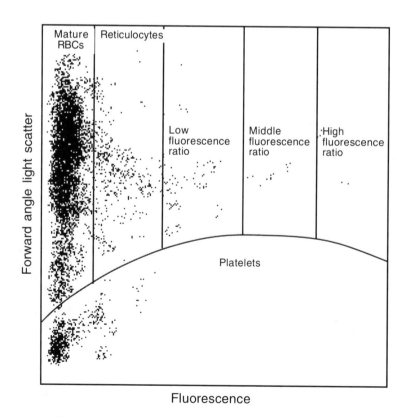

Figure 20-15. Reticulocyte Scattergram, Sysmex R-3000.

control system includes the mean and standard deviation with Levey-Jennings charts, as well as weighted moving averages.

Maintenance and Quality Assurance

QUALITY CONTROL

Automated hematology instruments offer sophisticated databases for quality control. Computer data storage for patient samples and quality control results is standard. Most hematology analyzers use three control liquids (low, normal, and high) that include a 5-part differential.[8] Control liquids are purchased from instrument manufacturers or from other companies. Most whole-blood controls have shelf lives of 30 to 60 days. They must be warmed and mixed carefully to achieve reproducible results.

Many laboratories also use a patient's blood sample as a 1-day control. The sample is reassayed numerous times in a 24-hour period. This control verifies stable instrument functioning.

Multiparameter instruments have computer data libraries for storing control results. Control parameters can be displayed on Levey-Jennings charts and assessed for accuracy and precision. The operator can set control means and ranges. Control results are "flagged" when they fall outside the range. Standard deviation and coefficient of variation are computed for each parameter.

All the instruments also monitor the moving averages of patient samples. Brian Bull first proposed the use of moving averages to assess accuracy of blood counts and measurements.[9] The moving average method compares a smoothed, weighted average from a group of 20 samples to the average of the patient population. The most recent results are weighted more heavily than earlier results. The moving average formula also gives less weight to outliers and smoothes the average by incorporating information from the previous batch of 20 patient samples. This improves early detection of systematic errors. When the smoothed average exceeds set limits, an error message is generated. This is done most often for the RBC indices: MCV, MCH, and MCHC.

For example, the MCV of the hospital's patient population is established. This mean is the target value. Then, as each sample is processed, its red cell indices are subtracted from the corresponding means of the previous set of samples. The square roots of the differences between these means are stored. After 20 patient samples have been processed, the sums of these square roots are divided by 20. These values are squared to obtain the average (mean) deviation. The deviations carry a positive or negative sign, so they can be added to or subtracted from the corresponding previous means. The resulting new means are then used for the next batch of 20 samples. This produces smoothed means. The smoothed means are compared to the predetermined population means. A change in the moving average of a parameter reflects either a change in the patient population or a systematic error. The weighted moving average is referred to as $\overline{X}_b$ (read X bar B) analysis.

A 3% limit of acceptability is often used with Bull's moving average method. After a mean for the patient population has been established, the smoothed average should be within 3% of that mean. The computer analysis program can also alert the operator when other limits of acceptability are exceeded by using the moving average method. For example, if a 3% acceptability standard is used for the moving average, an alert message can be generated when the last three moving averages exceed 2% limits.

As stated, the moving average method is useful in early detection of trends. This method works well for high-volume hematology instruments. In situations where only a few samples are analyzed, the moving averages are calculated too infrequently to detect a problem promptly.

MANUAL REVIEW

Automated differential instruments evaluate thousands of cells from each sample and have better precision than traditional 100-cell manual differentials. Each laboratory must establish criteria for review of automated results based on the patient population. The instruments have preset alert messages for the presence of cells that fall outside prescribed areas on a histogram or scattergram. The operator can also define the limits of tolerance for many parameters. Manual screening of a Wright-stained smear is indicated whenever "alert" messages are generated for suspected abnormal WBCs, platelet clumping, or size and distribution abnormalities of RBCs, WBCs, and platelets. The technologist must be able to understand and interpret alert messages, so that the CBC with differential is reported correctly.

CALIBRATION

Calibration of the multiparameter instruments is done first at the factory and again at installation. Calibration must be verified every 6 months or at intervals recommended by the manufacturer. Calibration materials must be appropriate for the methodology and should be traceable to a reference method or reference material.

MAINTENANCE

Automated hematology analyzers have preprogrammed system checks that are activated daily. The automatic checks include a cleaning cycle, background counts, hemoglobin blank readings, temperature and pressure monitoring, and determination of reagent and waste volumes. Special cleaning procedures of apertures and tubing are done less frequently. The manufacturers' specified routine maintenance schedules should be followed. Laser light sources should *always* be handled by a trained factory service engineer.

Summary

Current hematology analyzers use variations of four technologies in counting and differentiating blood cells (Table 20-1). Electrical impedance can be used to count and size WBCs, RBCs, and platelets. When used in conjunction with radio

Table 20-1
Principles of Automated Hematology Analyzers

	Electrical Impedance	Radiowaves	Light Scatter	Peroxidase/ Absorbance
Coulter STKS®	X	X	X	
Sysmex NE-8000	X	X		
Abbott Cell-Dyn®	X		X	
Technicon H·2™			X	X

wave deflection or optical scattering, blood cells can be differentiated according to cellular characteristics. Optical scatter can also be used to count and size cells. Peroxidase staining of WBCs is also used to differentiate WBCs.

Computer-generated histograms and scattergrams improve the understanding and interpretation of the measurements derived through these technologies.

Computer storage and sophisticated analyses of quality control data including Levey-Jennings plots and Bull's moving averages are also standard.

Future automated hematology instruments may incorporate flow cytometric reticulocyte counters similar to the Sysmex R-3000's. New technologies and new combinations of existing technologies will allow accurate identification and quantitation of abnormal cell populations.

References

1. Coulter WH. High speed automatic blood cell counter and cell size analyzer. Proc Natl Electronic Conf 1956, 12:1034-40.
2. Jones AR. Counting and sizing of blood cells using aperture-impedance systems. In: van Assendelft OW, England JM, eds. Advances in hematological methods: The blood count. Boca Raton, FL: CRC Press, 1982:50-72.
3. Leif RC, Schwartz S. Rodiguez CM, Pell-Fernandez L, Groves M, Leif SB, et al. Two-dimensional impedance studies of BSA buoyant density separated human erythrocytes. Cytometry 1985, 6:13-21.
4. Salzman GC, Crowell JM, Martin JC, Trujillo TT, Romero A, Mullaney PR, LaBaume PM. Cell classification by laser light scattering: Identification and separation of unstained leukocytes. Acta Cytol 1975, 19:374-77.
5. van Kampen EJ, Zijlstra WG. Standardization of hemoglobinometry. II. The hemoglobincyanide method. Clin Chim Acta 1961, 6:538-44.
6. Hall R, Malia RG. Automated blood-cell analysis in medical laboratory haematology, 2nd ed. Oxford: Butterworth Heinemann, 1991:193-218.
7. Mohandas N, Kim YR, Tycko DH, Orlik J, Wyatt J, Groner W. Accurate and independent measurement of volume and hemoglobin concentration of individual red cells by laser light scattering. Blood 1986; 68(2):506-13.
8. National Committee for Clinical Laboratory Standards (NCCLS) Pub. No. H26-P. Performance goals for the internal quality control of multichannel hematology analyzers; Proposed standard. Villanova, PA 1989.
9. Bull BS, Elashoff RM, Heilbron DC, Couperus J. A study of various estimators for the derivation of quality control procedures from patient erythrocyte indices. Am J Clin Pathol 1974, 61:473-81.

Suggested Readings

Harmening DM. Clinical hematology and fundamentals of hemostasis, 2nd ed. Philadelphia: FA Davis, 1992.

Koepke JA, ed. Practical laboratory hematology. New York: Churchill Livingstone, 1991.

Lotspeich-Steininger CA, Stiene-Martin EA, Koepke JA. Clinical hematology principles, procedures, correlations. Philadelphia: JB Lippincott, 1992.

Mares JF. Automated Hematology Systems. In: Hicks MR, Haven MC, Schenken JR, McWhorter CA, eds. Laboratory instrumentation, 3rd ed. Philadelphia: JB Lippincott, 1987.

21

AUTOMATED COAGULATION SYSTEMS

John D. Olson
Beverly J. Pennell

Objectives

After completing this chapter, the reader will be able to:

1. Discuss the basic concepts of coagulation testing.
2. Understand plasma coagulation detection methods.
3. Compare whole-blood coagulation detection methods with plasma coagulation detection methods.
4. Discuss fibrinolytic/anticoagulant assay methods.
5. Outline platelet function analysis.

Definitions

Conductivity: The ability of a substance to conduct an electric current.

Elasticity: The property that enables a substance to change its shape in response to a force and then to recover its original shape when the force is removed.

Impedance: The ratio of the force on a system undergoing harmonic motion to the velocity of the fluid in the system.

Monomer: A simple unpolymerized form of a compound.

Polymerization: The combination of similar modules to form a more complex, higher-molecular-weight product.

Synthetic Substrate: A compound made in a laboratory that can act as a substrate for one or more enzymes. As used in this chapter, the synthetic substrate contains a chromogenic or fluorogenic component that is released by enzymatic cleavage.

Tensile Strength: The greatest longitudinal stress a substance can bear without tearing apart.

Viscosity: The property of a fluid that resist the forces tending to cause it to flow.

Introduction

Hemostasis is the mechanism by which we protect ourselves from exsanguination following an injury. The mechanism involves the complex interaction of the blood vessel, the blood platelet, and plasma coagulation factors. The formation of a clot after blood is placed in a container and the time for hemostasis to occur when the skin is lacerated are observations that have been made by clinicians for more than a century. Instrumentation began facilitating this laboratory practice in the 1940s and 1950s and has been increasing in sophistication continually.

Some knowledge of platelet function and the coagulation mechanism is needed to understand the operation of the instruments to be described. The simplest definition of blood coagulation is the solidification of blood by converting the soluble molecule fibrinogen to its insoluble polymer, fibrin. The formation of the polymer is a two-step reaction. First, fibrinopeptides are cleaved from the fibrinogen molecule by the enzyme thrombin to form fibrin monomer. The second step is the polymerization of fibrin monomer into a highly organized, structured fiber. This polymer of fibrin monomers (clot) is strong enough to withstand low levels of mechanical stress, thus allowing its formation to be measured mechanically. Formation of the stable, covalently linked fibrin clot depends on a second enzymatic reaction catalyzed by a plasma transaminase, Factor XIII (fibrin stabilizing factor). Once Factor XIII has carried out its function, cross-linking the fibrin molecule, the fibrin clot has very high tensile strength and is resistant to high mechanical stress.

Instruments that measure the coagulation mechanism depend in general on the formation of the enzyme thrombin, and subsequently measure the polymerization of the endogenous fibrin monomer (i.e., the fibrin monomer derived from fibrinogen in the patient's plasma). The formation of cross-linked fibrin (which depends on the activated form of Factor XIII) is usually not measured well by these instruments.

Platelet functions can be described briefly as follows: (1) adhesion—the ability of activated platelets to stick to a foreign surface; (2) aggregation—the ability of activated platelets to stick to each other; (3) the release of granular contents—the secretion of proteins and other compounds stored in platelet granules; (4) clot retraction—the contractibility of activated platelets that cause the shrinkage of the fibrin clot; (5) support of plasma coagulation—the role the platelet plays in the generation of thrombin, providing the surface on which this activation occurs; and (6) endothelial cell support—the "rescue" of the damaged endothelial cell by platelet fusion with the endothelial cell membrane. Most of these platelet functions are best assayed in the laboratory by manual techniques. There are, however, some instruments that are involved in the measurement of the platelet aggregation and the release reaction.

The mechanisms for the measurement of coagulation and platelet functions can be categorized as follows: (1) conductivity; (2) elastic modulus or mechanical resistance; (3) turbidity; (4) absorbance spectroscopy; and (5) fluorescence spectroscopy. We address the role of each of these methodologies in coagulation and platelet function testing.

Plasma Coagulation

Specimen collection technique is critical for the accurate evaluation of plasma coagulation. The venipuncture should be made with as little trauma as possible, and the first 2 ml of blood should be discarded. Platelet-poor plasma (as clear as it can be prepared) is critical for these measurements.

The challenge is to design instruments which can detect the generation of the enzyme thrombin. In most cases, as fibrin monomer polymerizes, the increasing optical density of the specimen, its increasing viscosity, or the formation of the fiber have been exploited. In addition, substrates that, when activated by thrombin or other coagulent enzymes, generate a color, have been used.

END-POINT MEASUREMENT

Mechanical endpoints detect the fiber formation by monitoring a physical change in the signal being generated. One of these devices uses electrical conductivity between the ends of two probes submerged in the reaction cup. At approximately 0.5-second intervals one of the probes is mechanically lifted above the surface of the plasma, interrupting the current. This action continues until the tensile strength of the fibrin clot is sufficient to maintain the conductivity. This stops the timer, thus recording the seconds required for the reaction to occur. The electrodes are easily accessible to allow for effective cleaning. Figure 21-1 shows the components of such an instrument, which includes: (1) a stationary electrode; (2) an electrode with a cycling up and down motion; (3) a motor for cycling the mobile electrode; (4) a switching device; (5) a timer; (6) a temperature control block for the specimen container; and (7) the specimen. Reaction in this instrument is started by simultaneously activating the start switch and adding the activation material to the specimen. During the reaction, the motor cycles the mobile electrode in and out of the specimen, continually breaking the current between electrodes 1 and 2 at about 0.5-second intervals. When fibrin monomer polymerization occurs, the fibrin polymer attaches to the mobile electrode and maintains the electrical conductivity between electrodes 1 and 2 throughout the entire cycle of the mobile electrode; this action activates the switch that shuts off the motor and stops the timer.

The interruption of a magnetic field by fibrin monomer polymerization is another mechanical end-point detection method. Iron spheres in the reaction vessel or microscopic iron particles embedded in solid phase reagents are put into motion by an oscillating magnetic field. When motion is restricted by fibrin formation, the timer stops. An example of electromagnetic measurement of the coagulation endpoint[1] is found in Figure 21-2. A metal shot is placed into the plasma specimen in the cuvette. The shot is put in motion by the isolation of electromagnets on either side of the specimen. The shot moves back and forth in the specimen until its motion is resisted by increased viscosity of fibrin monomer polymerization. The resistance to the motion of shot is detected and timer stopped.

Many laboratory instruments use photo-optical detection methods to determine clot formation. These instruments detect the increase in optical density (decrease in

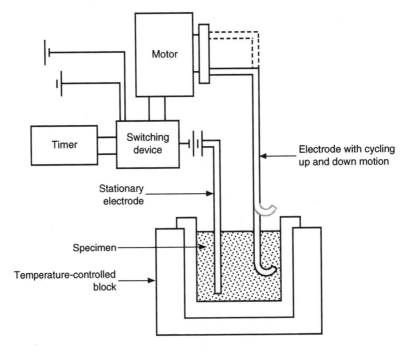

Figure 21-1. Mechanical coagulation end-point measurement using conductivity.

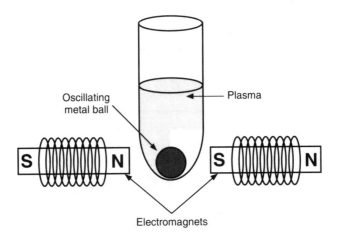

Figure 21-2. Electromagnetic measurement of the coagulation endpoint.

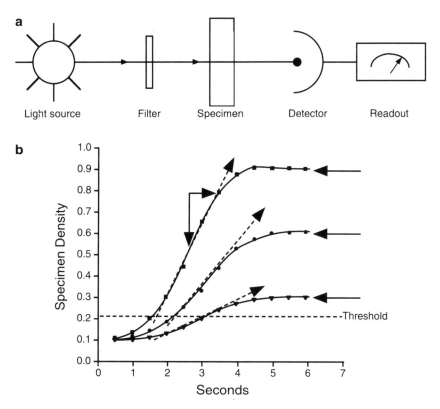

Figure 21-3. (a) Spectrophotometric measurement. (b) Specimen density as a function of time.

light transmitted) or light scatter produced as the fibrin monomer polymerizes to form the clot. Most instruments determine the time required to reach a threshold change from a baseline measurement of the patient specimen. The maximum light scatter of the patient's specimen can be compared to appropriate standards to determine the concentration of fibrinogen. In the instrument diagrammed in Figure 21-3, filtered light shines continuously through the cuvette containing the plasma specimen. The timer is started at the addition of the coagulation activator. Light is detected by a photocell and recorded continuously on a chart recorder or in a computer. A predetermined threshold for the coagulation endpoint is determined, and when the absorbed (or scattered) light reaches that threshold, the timer stops. The plot of specimen density as a function of time depicts alternate methods for quantifying functional fibrinogen. The rate of fibrin monomer polymerization reflected by the rate of change in specimen density or the total extent of density when the specimen reaches equilibrium can be quantified.

Synthetic substrates can also be used to measure plasma coagulation. With these methods the enzyme in the coagulation process (i.e., thrombin, Factor Xa, plasmin, and others) reacts with a specific chromogenic substrate producing color at a rate proportional to the amount of enzyme generated. In contrast to the other devices discussed, which monitor fibrin monomer polymerization, these instruments can specifically measure the generation of thrombin. These methods have been adapted to a variety of automated spectrophotometric instruments.

HIGH-VOLUME TESTING

Most high-volume instruments use the change in optical characteristics to detect the endpoint. These instruments also incorporate specimen identification methods, sample and reagent handling systems, and a variety of methods to handle and process data. Keyboard entry of patient identifiers, bar-code reading from the specimen collection tube, and downloading of this information from the host computer are available.

Most high-volume devices now offer both sample and reagent pipetting mechanisms. Positive displacement syringes or peristaltic pumps are used to deliver reagents to the reaction vessel. Specimen handling is usually with positive displacement; however, some high-volume instruments still require the operator to manually pipette the specimen into the reaction vessel. The increased precision of the automated fluid-handling methods has greatly increased the precision of the pipetting steps and allowed many laboratories to perform single rather than duplicate analysis. This saves both reagent cost and technologist time.

Temperature control is achieved by a platen or chamber heated to 37°C. Most of these instruments also are capable of maintaining the reagent reservoirs at 4°C, providing increased reagent stability. Reagents are warmed in-line immediately prior to pipetting.

To calculate the endpoint for routine coagulation testing, most instruments use the time required to achieve a preset change in optical density. A reading is taken immediately after the activating reagent is added and the optical density monitored until the threshold is met. Some instruments are also capable of continuously monitoring the change in optical density, calculating the first and second derivative of the resulting curve.

The overall change in the optical density in the prothrombin time (PT) reaction can be correlated to the fibrinogen concentration by extrapolation from a stored standard curve. Instruments that measure the optical density of the clot can exploit this piece of data to measure the fibrinogen concentration in each PT determination (Fig. 21-3). These instruments have throughput of approximately 100 specimens/hour when both a PT and an activated partial thromboplastin time (aPTT) have been requested.

LOW-VOLUME TESTING

Low-volume instruments require more operator time and attention. They usually require manual pipetting of sample and reagents, and often manual timing of incubation steps. The throughput is much lower, and more reagent is required because of larger volumes and duplicate testing.

These instruments have a variety of detection methods. Most of the mechanical end-point devices[2] fit into this category, however, optical methods similar to the higher volume instruments are used. Devices using conductivity and magnetic endpoints are commonly used.

These instruments are flexible, economical, and easy to operate. New models, with software that stores standard curves and conversion factors, automatically report results in a variety of formats (i.e., PT ratio, International Normalized Ratio, seconds).

Whole-Blood Coagulation and Fibrinolysis

In general, two types of instruments use whole-blood specimens. One is designed to determine PT and aPTT plasma equivalent results from whole blood in a clinic or bedside environment. The other type[3] has been adapted to critical care areas such as intensive care units or surgery suites where the analysis is done either to monitor the dose of heparin being used or to evaluate the more global view of coagulation and fibrinolysis.

These devices are designed to be used with fingerstick specimens or may require the phlebotomist to place the blood in specific reagent tubes unique to the testing device.

The detection methods used by these instruments are varied and innovative, as described. In general, the clotting times of whole blood are slightly longer than those of plasma.

LASER OPTICS

Laser optics instruments[4] are used in the Biotrack® Coagulation Monitor (Biotrack, Inc., Medfield, MA 02052) which has dry reagent in a disposable cartridge that is placed into the instrument and equilibrated to 37°C. This device (Fig. 21-4), devel-

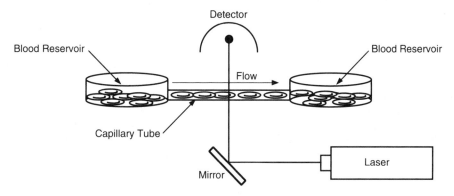

Figure 21-4. Whole-blood coagulation measured by laser optics.

oped for bedside testing, uses a cartridge that accepts a drop of blood into a blood reservoir. The blood will flow by capillary action through the tube into a receiving reservoir. Activating agents for the PT and aPTT are on the surface of the reservoir. The laser beam passes through the specimen in the capillary tube to a detector, detecting the motion of red blood cells. With fibrin monomer polymerization, the viscosity increases and the motion of the red blood cells slows and stops, stopping the timer.

MAGNETIC

The COAG-1™ (Cardiovascular Diagnostics, Inc., Research Triangle Park, NC 27709), uses instrument-specific cartridges with dry reagents in which paramagnetic iron oxide particles (PIOPs) are embedded.[5] When the blood specimen is placed into the sample well, it is drawn by capillary action into the reagent chamber, rehydrates the reagent, and frees the PIOPs. The PIOPs are then set in motion under the influence of an oscillating magnetic field produced in the instrument. The oscillation amplitude of the particles is monitored optically. The decay in the amplitude corresponds to the onset of fibrin monomer polymerization. This instrument also reports the results in calculated plasma PT and aPTT equivalent times.

Performance of the activated clotting time on whole blood with the Hemachron® (International Technidyne Corp., Edison, NJ 08820) requires a specific collection tube that contains reagent and a magnet. When this tube is placed into the instrument, the magnet is aligned with a magnetic detector. As the test proceeds, the tube rotates as the magnet remains aligned. As the clot forms, the magnet is forced out of alignment and can no longer be detected. The time from placement of the tube in the instrument to detection of the endpoint is then displayed.

MECHANICAL/OPTICAL

The optical system in the ACT (Automated Coagulation Timer) (Hemotec, Inc., Englewood, CO 80112) detects the mechanical impedance created by clot formation in the reaction vessel. The instrument-specific cartridge contains the reagent and a flag attached to a plunger device. As the analysis proceeds, the plunger is raised by a lift mechanism at a set time interval. The rate at which the plunger falls is reduced as clot formation occurs. This reduced rate is detected by the optical system of the instrument and the time displayed.

Another clever approach to measuring the fibrin endpoint, the Hepcon® HMS (Hemostasis Management System) (Hemotec, Inc., Englewood, CO 80112) uses air continuously bubbling through the specimen. The specimen is placed in a small cuvette with an air intake tube at the base (Fig. 21-5). Air pressure is applied, creating bubbles in the liquid specimen. As fibrin monomer polymerization occurs, the bubbles cannot pass through the specimen, and the air pressure forces the clot into the light beam stopping the timer. This whole-blood methodology uses no agonists. A detector continuously monitors a light beam located above the level of the specimen.

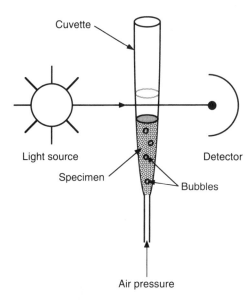

Light source

Detector

Specimen

Bubbles

Air pressure

Figure 21-5.   Whole-blood coagulation measured by a mechanical optical method.

This instrument is used mainly in the operating room to monitor heparin therapy during cardiopulmonary bypass.

CHANGE IN SPECIMEN VISCOSITY

The detection principle in another group of instruments is based on changes in the viscosity of blood as the clotting/lysing process proceeds. Viscosity changes are detected by electromagnetic resistance, mechanical impedance, and pressure changes.

Mechanical impedance caused by the increasing viscosity can be measured with a piston-cylinder viscometer. In the Elvi Bioclot 816 Thromboelastrograph (Logos Scientific, Henderson, NV 89015) (Fig. 21-6), the whole-blood sample is placed in a metal cup. A sensing piston connected to a magnet is then lowered into the specimen. The cup alternately rotates clockwise and counterclockwise about 5 degrees. The piston initially doesn't rotate because of low viscosity of the unclotted blood and the attraction of an electromagnetic field around the piston's magnet. As the clot forms, the increased fluid viscosity produces increased drag on the piston. Eventually, viscosity and drag increase enough to turn the piston. The movement of the piston's magnet within the electromagnetic field alters the current and produces an electrical signal. This whole process generates a graphic output of the coagulation and fibrinolytic process.

The increasing resistance to sound transmission is also used to measure the change in viscosity as fibrin monomer polymerizes in the Sonoclot® (Siencor®, Inc.,

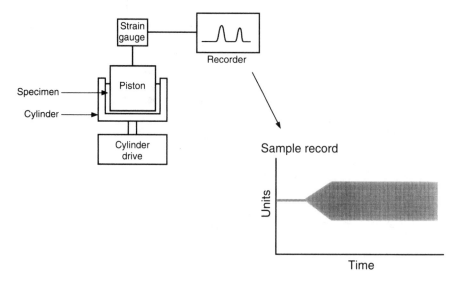

Figure 21-6.   Piston and cylinder viscometer.

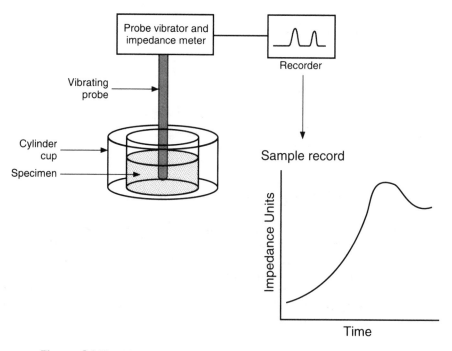

Figure 21-7.   Viscosity measurement by mechanical impedance (sonar).

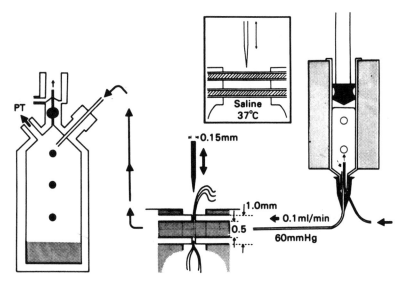

Figure 21-8. Principal parts of the hemostatometer. *Right.* Syringe with the blood sample, inserted into a heated black. *Arrows* show the infusion of paraffin oil into the blood and the displacement of the latter through the polyethylene tubing threaded through the punching device. *Center.* Mechanical punching device with the needle and the punched polyethylene tubing, from which the blood flows into saline. *Inset.* Arrangement with the two-channel apparatus. *Left.* Reservoir to collect the blood and to measure the pressure by a transducer (PT). *(Reprinted with permission. Kovacs IB, Hutton RA, Kernoff PB. Hemostatic evaluation in bleeding disorders from native blood. Am J Clin Pathol 1989, 91:271-79.)*

Morrison, CO 80465).[6] A plastic probe is placed in the specimen and vibrated at a frequency of approximately 200 Hz. As coagulation occurs, the viscosity and elasticity of the specimen increase, providing increasing resistance to the vibration of the probe. This increasing resistance is detected, and the energy to the vibrator is increased to maintain a constant vibration. The increasing energy input required is sent to a recorder and plotted (Fig. 21-7).

The change in viscosity can also be reflected by the pressure changes in an enclosed flowing system—the CSA® (Clot Signature Analyzer) (Xylum Corp., Scarsdale, NY 10583). Nonanticoagulated blood is pumped through polyethylene tubing at a constant rate and pressure. A piercing needle makes a standardized hole in the tube, resulting in a pressure drop. The pressure is restored because of hemostatic plug formation. The pressure change is graphed, generating a "clot signature" (Fig. 21-8). This methodology is somewhat unique in its reflection of platelet plug as well as fibrin formation and appears to be sensitive to platelet function disorders.[7]

These instruments produce a graphic representation of the entire process. The many clotting components functioning in concert make interpretation by trained personnel a necessity.

Plasma Procoagulant/Fibrinolytic/ Anticoagulant Assays

In the preceding section we reviewed the instrumentation used in the evaluation of plasma coagulation. Many assays required for hemostatic evaluation are low-volume, labor-intensive procedures that use many of the types of instruments described ments described here and elsewhere in this book. We now summarize briefly the application of these previously described instruments to the more sophisticated assays of hemostasis. Because we focus on instrumentation we will group the assay descriptions by the instruments that can be used.

FIBRIN ENDPOINT

Most of the instruments that perform both low- and high-volume tests of coagulation depend on fibrin monomer polymerization for the measurement of the endpoint. They are designed primarily for the performance of the PT and aPTT. The same instruments can measure levels of specific coagulation factors, using the same methodologies.

Measurement of fibrinogen is most frequently performed by examining the rate at which clot formation occurs or the total density of the fibrin clot formed (Fig. 21-3). The amount of fibrinogen can be quantified accurately by determining the rate of clot formation in the presence of a constant amount of thrombin (the method of Clauss[8]). This has become the standard method in most coagulation laboratories. The endpoints in these measurements can be determined by any of the instruments we described, but it is generally most successfully performed with instruments using a mechanical endpoint. More recently, the instruments that measure fibrin formation by specimen density or light scatter endpoints have been able to quantify fibrinogen at the same time the PT is performed. By continuing the measurement of the density of clot formation after the prothrombin time measurement until it is constant, the final density can then be compared to the density of standard of known fibrinogen concentration. This methodology provides an accurate and timesaving method for quantifying fibrinogen in most cases.

Assay of other coagulation factors is performed by mixing normal plasma with plasma known to be deficient in the factor to be assayed, followed by the performance of the aPTT or PT, depending on the factor to be analyzed. These endpoints are measured by using the various described instruments that detect the formation of the fibrin clot.

Some coagulation factor assays (prothrombin) and other coagulation tests are performed by using snake venoms. The venoms activate various proteins in the coagulation cascade, leading ultimately to the generation of the fibrin clot.

Although not frequently used in the clinical setting, assays for coagulation factor inhibitors (Protein C, Protein S, and Antithrombin III) depend on the rate of the fibrin clot formation. These natural anticoagulants are more frequently measured by alternative techniques described next.

SYNTHETIC SUBSTRATES

A variety of synthetic substrates have been developed for use in coagulation testing. Many of these substrates are nearly monospecific for an enzyme in the coagulation cascade. Most frequently used are substrates that reflect the activity of Factor Xa, thrombin, and plasmin. The cleavage of these substrates by their respective active enzymes are measured by the same spectrophotometric and fluorometric techniques described elsewhere in this book. With the growth in the prevalence of these assays and the varied number of synthetic substrates being developed, many of the major coagulation instrument manufacturers are developing instruments that will accommodate this technology. Even the measurement of aPTT and PT can now be made using synthetic substrates; however, the cost still makes routine use of these methodologies impractical.

IMMUNOLOGICAL METHODOLOGIES

In nearly all cases, the factors of interest in the coagulation and fibrinolytic mechanisms are proteins. Assays for these proteins have been developed by using the entire spectrum of immunological methods available, including enzyme-linked immunosorbent assay (ELISA), enzyme multiplied immunoassay technique (EMIT), immunoradiometric assay (IRMA), latex agglutination, and, as will be described, Laurell rocket immunoelectrophoresis. The instruments (nephelometer, microtiter plate reader, and others) used for measuring these immunological reactions are described elsewhere in this book. The methodologies are applied widely in the field of hemostasis. The comparison of the quantity of protein measured immunologically with the functional activity of the protein has led to the diagnosis of many syndromes of the production of abnormal coagulation, fibrinolytic, or inhibitory proteins.

ELECTROPHORETIC TECHNIQUES

The separation of proteins by electrophoretic methodologies is described in Chapter 12. The same methods have been exploited in the quantification of protein as originally described by Laurell.[9] The principle is one of electrophoresing the antigen (usually a protein in the plasma) into agarose, which contains a monospecific antibody to the antigen in question. As the antigen moves through the antibody-containing agarose, antigen-antibody complexes form. At the equivalence zone these complexes precipitate in a rocket formation that can be visualized after staining. The amount of antigen is quantified by measuring rocket heights and comparing them to a standard curve.

Another immunoelectrophoretic technique is crossed-immunoelectrophoresis. In this technique the specimen containing the antigen in question is first electrophoresed into plain agarose in one direction. The plate is then turned 90° and the specimen is electrophoresed into antibody-containing agarose in the second direction.

Plate A   **Plate B**

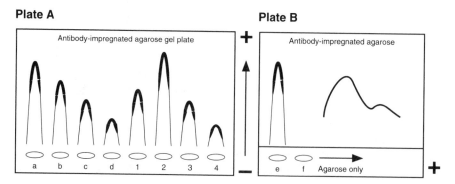

Figure 21-9. Electrophoretic immunoprecipitation to quantify antigen. Plate A. Specimens a, b, c, and d are control dilutions. Specimens 1, 2, 3, and 4 are examples of patient specimens. Plate B. Specimen f is first electrophoresized to the right without antibody, then antibody is added and the plate electrophoresized again. Specimen e is only added for the second electrophoresis.

With this methodology it is possible to determine different forms of the antigen based on the relative mobility and therefore molecular weight of the antigen in question. This technique is valuable to identify antigen bound to carrier protein (to identify free and bound Protein S) or to identify variable sizes of antigen (multimeric forms of von Willebrand antigen).

The method of Laurell, illustrated in Figure 21-9, is a single-dimensional electrophoresis of the specimen into thin layer of agarose containing monospecific antibody directed at the antigen in question. As electrophoresis proceeds, the concentration of antigen decreases until the ratio of antigen and antibody is appropriate for precipitation of antigen-antibody complexes in the rockets indicated. Specimens a, b, c, and d (Fig. 21-9, Plate A) are control dilutions of normal plasma from which a standard curve can be derived from the height of the rocket. Specimens 1, 2, 3, and 4 (Fig. 21-9, Plate A) are examples of patient specimens whose rocket heights are compared to the standard curve. A variation on this approach utilizes cross-immunoelectrophoresis in which the specimen is first electrophoresized to the right from well *f* (Fig. 21-9, Plate B) in agarose containing no antibody, distributing protein by size. Agarose containing antibody is then poured in the upper part of the plate, and the specimen is electrophoresed into the agarose-containing antibody. Well *e* (Fig. 21-9, Plate B) contains a sample that is added at the time of the second electrophoretic procedure. The resulting precipitin arc demonstrates the relative mobility of the specimen *e* at the left with a corresponding distribution of the molecular weight of the same molecule in the plasma when separated by its molecular size in the first dimension of electrophoresis. The example (Fig. 21-9, Plate B) shown indicates a significant portion of antigen at high molecular weight with moderate mobility to the right and a smaller proportion of lower-molecular-weight antigen with greater mobility. Crossed immuno-

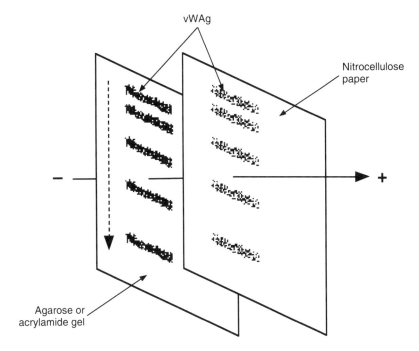

Figure 21-10.   Electrophoresis followed by blotting.

electrophoresis is used for determining varying sizes of the Willebrand factor molecule as well as generating semiquantitative information concerning bound and free molecules in the plasma.

The electrophoretic plates can be visualized by stains or by blotting techniques.[9] With blotting techniques the proteins electrophoresed into agarose can be transferred (also by electrophoresis) to nitrocellulose paper. The antigen on the surface of the nitrocellulose paper then reacts with a monospecific antibody that is radiolabeled or linked to an enzyme (peroxidase or alkaline phosphatase). A specific substrate for the enzyme can be used for subsequent color development and visualization of the protein. With radiolabeled identification, an autoradiogram can be developed. This methodology is useful for identifying and quantitating proteins (Fig. 21-10). Electrophoresis of antigen into slab agarose or acrylamide gel can separate varying antigens according to their size. A second electrophoretic procedure can then transfer these antigens to nitrocellulose paper. The presence of the antigen and its distribution in the nitrocellulose paper can then be detected by (1) incubation with radiolabeled antibody that recognizes the antigen followed by autoradiography; or (2) incubation with antibody linked to an enzyme (peroxidase or alkaline phosphatase) and the addition of substrate for the enzyme that will develop color at the site of the antibody.

These methodologies are used for determination of DNA (Southern blot), RNA (Northern blot), and protein (Western blot) in specimens.

Measurement of Platelet Function

Platelets often initiate hemostatic mechanisms. Most laboratory evaluations of platelet function are performed manually. The only two significant uses of instrumentation are the evaluation of platelet aggregation with the platelet release reaction and platelet support of plasma coagulation.

PLATELET AGGREGOMETRY

In general *platelet aggregation* is performed by using the platelet-rich plasma (PRP) isolated from a specimen of citrated whole blood. The Payton Aggregometer (Payton Scientific, Inc., Buffalo, NY 14202) is one of several instruments that uses a photodetector to measure light transmission through a cuvette containing PRP. The amount of light transmitted through the specimen is recorded as a function of time as illustrated in Figure 21-11. The PRP specimen cuvette is incubated at 37°C and stirred at a constant rate. Agonist is added to the specimen, and the light transmitted is measured continuously. The detector signal is displayed on a chart recorder or computer. Platelets response to the agonist has two phases. The primary phase produces increased light transmittance. The release of active components from the platelet triggers the secondary phase of aggregation and greater light transmittance (a few aggregates block less light than many individual platelets).

An additional feature on both the Chronolog and Payton instruments measures the release of platelet granules. This is accomplished by incorporating a fluorometer into the instrument.[10] Firefly luciferin and luciferase are added to the cuvette prior to platelet activation. As activation occurs, ADP is released from the platelet granules into the supernatant. The ADP allows the catalysis of luciferin by luciferase. Activated luciferin releases photons detected by the fluorometer. The instruments generate a plot of luminescence versus time. The same principles have been applied to quantify calcium mobilization within the platelets by using fluorescent compounds sensitive to free calcium.

Platelet aggregation is also successfully measured in whole blood by impedance of electrical current between two electrodes. With the whole blood Lumi-Aggregometer (Chronolog Corp., Havertown, PA 19083), whole blood is added to a cuvette containing positive and negative electrodes. A constant current is passed between the electrodes. The agonist is added, and as activation of the platelet occurs, platelets adhere to and aggregate on the surface of the cathode, impeding the flow of current between the two electrodes. This change in electrical current (the impedance of the current) is displayed on a chart recorder and reflects the aggregation of platelets in the whole-blood specimen (Fig. 21-12). The advantage of this methodology is the reduced time required for specimen preparation.

Most of the instrumentation in platelet aggregation provides data in the form of manually recorded charts. Technology is now moving into an era of reading analog

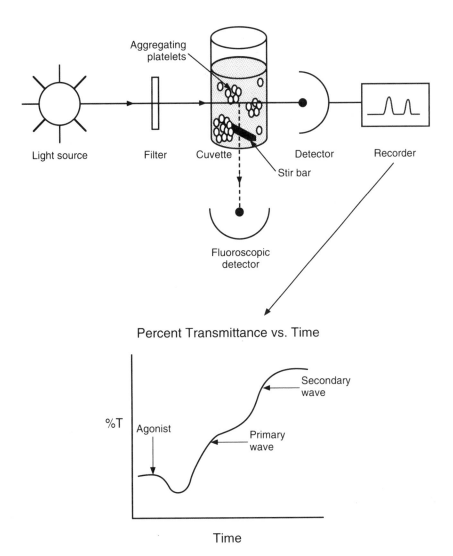

Figure 21-11. Platelet aggregometry by light transmittance and fluorescence.

data off to a computer, allowing for more sophisticated analyses of the aggregation curves.

PLATELET SUPPORT OF PLASMA COAGULATION

Two instruments described above, which measure the change of viscosity by impedance of sound (Sonoclot®) or elastic modulus (Thromboelastograph), display graphs of the entire process of fibrin clot formation. The rate and the nature of the

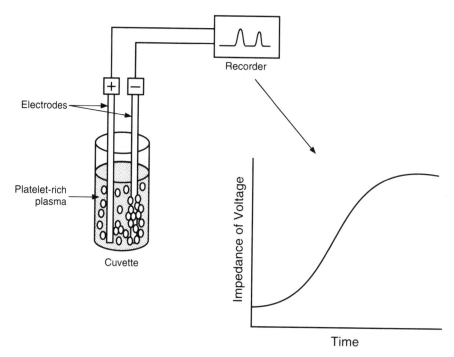

Figure 21-12.   Platelet aggregation by electrical impedance.

clot formed reflect the effect of platelet contribution to fibrin formation. Though not quantitative, these qualitative findings can be of value in determining the number and relative function of platelets at the bedside.

Maintenance and Quality Assurance

All instruments need to be maintained according to manufacturers' recommendations. Routine preventative maintenance procedures are necessary to ensure proper functioning. Due to the diversity of these instruments, the user needs to follow the specific manufacturers' instructions for each instrument. Quality control samples of the same specimen type (whole blood, plasma, etc.), in both the normal and abnormal ranges, should be analyzed with each run of patient specimens. Results should fall within predetermined ranges before patient results are accepted and reported.

Instruments that test unanticoagulated whole blood present a unique problem in both calibration and control. This is a problem that has not been adequately addressed in the literature. If many of these instruments (of the same model) are used in an institution, methods may be developed to compare the performance of each instrument against the group.

Summary

Since the 1970s there have been significant advances made in the instrumentation used in the evaluation of hemostasis. These instruments make possible the rapid and accurate determination of overall tests of coagulation such as the PT and aPTT. They can also measure specific factors of coagulation, fibrinolysis, anticoagulants, and platelet function. The sophistication of these devices makes possible detailed measurements of hemostasis in smaller laboratories and at the bedside. This creates new and interesting problems in satisfactory quality control of these devices.

References

1. Ledford MR, Kaczor DA. Evaluation of the ST4 clot detection instrument. Lab Med 1992, 23:172-75.
2. Reich DL, Zahl K, Perucho MH, Thys DM. An evaluation of two activated clotting time monitors during cardiac surgery. J Clin Monit 1992, 8:33-36.
3. Stead SW. Comparison of two methods for heparin monitoring: A semi-automated heparin monitoring device and activated clotting time during extracorporeal circulation. Int J Clin Monit Comput 1989, 6:247-54.
4. Lucas FV, Duncan A, Jay R, Coleman R, Craft P, Chan B, et al. A novel whole blood capillary technic for measuring the prothrombin time. Am J Clin Pathol 1987, 88:442-46.
5. Oberhardt BJ, Dermott SC, Taylor M, Alkadi ZY, Abruzzini AF, Gresalfi NJ. Dry reagent technology for rapid, convenient measurements of blood coagulation and fibrinolysis. Clin Chem 1991, 37:520-26.
6. Tuman KJ, Spiess BD, McCarthy RJ, Ivankovich AD. Comparison of viscoelastic measures of coagulation after cardiopulmonary bypass. Anestha analg 1989, 69:69-75.
7. Kovacs IB, Hutton RA, Kernoff PB. Hemostatic evaluation in bleeding disorders from native blood: Clinical experience with the hemostatometer. Am J Clin Pathol 1989, 91:271-79.
8. Clauss A. Gerinnungsphysiologische Schnellmethod zur Bestimmung des Fibrinogens. Acta Haematol 1957, 17:237-46.
9. Laurell CB. Quantitative estimation of proteins by electrophoresis in agarose gel containing antibodies. Anal Biochem 1966, 15:45-52.
10. Ingerman-Wojenski CM, Silver MF. A quick method for screening platelet dysfunctions using the whole blood lumi-aggregometer. Thromb Haemostas 1984, 51:154-56.

Suggested Readings

Colman RW, Hirsh J, Marder VJ, Salzman EW. Hemostasis and thrombosis: Basic principles and clinical practice, 2nd ed. Philadelphia: JB Lippincott, 1982.
Lotspeich-Steininger CA, Stiene-Martin EA, Koepke JA. Clinical hematology: Principles, procedures, correlations. Philadelphia: JB Lippincott, 1992.

22

AUTOMATED MICROBIOLOGY SYSTEMS

Dianne M. Kelly

Objectives

After completing this chapter, the reader will be able to:

1. List the types of automated microbiology systems available.
2. Describe the use of carbon dioxide quantitation to detect microorganism growth.
3. Describe the BACTEC and BacT/Alert systems for detecting microorganisms in blood or other body fluids.
4. Explain the basic principles of microorganism identification using biochemical reactions.
5. Explain the basic principles of antimicrobial sensitivity determinations.
6. Describe the Vitek® and MicroScan systems for identifying microorganisms and determining their antimicrobial susceptibilities.
7. Describe the VIDAS® system for detecting microorganism antigens and host antibodies in serum and other specimens.
8. List new technologies with the potential to provide rapid microorganism detection and identification.

Definitions

Abbott Cartridge: A plastic cuvette system with a linear arrangement of chambers, each containing a biochemical medium or an antibiotic for the performance of microbial identification or susceptibility testing.
ATCC: American Type Culture Collection.
Colorimetry: Detection of metabolic endpoints by means of color reactions.
DMS: Data Management System.
ELISA: Enzyme-Linked Immunosorbent Assay.

Fluorescence: Emission of light by a substance (or a microscopic preparation) shortly after excitation by radiant energy.

HEPA: High Efficiency Particulate Air filter. A filter used in biological safety cabinets to trap pathogenic organisms.

Kirby-Bauer Susceptibility Test: Test to determine antimicrobial susceptibility by addition of an antimicrobial-impregnated paper disk to a culture plate streaked with the microorganism of interest. Diffusion of the antimicrobial will prevent the growth of susceptible organisms around the disk.

McFarland Standard: A barium chloride turbidity solution used to standardize bacterial inocula.

MIC: Minimal Inhibitory Concentration. The lowest dilution of an antibiotic that inhibits visible bacterial growth.

Nephelometry: Determination of the degree of turbidity by measuring the amount of light scatter.

Nucleic Acid Probe: A piece of labeled single-stranded DNA used to detect complementary DNA in clinical material or culture. It specifically identifies the presence of an organism in these materials that is identical to that used to make the probe.

PCR: Polymerase Chain Reaction. A method for expanding small discrete sections of DNA by binding DNA primers to sections at the ends of the DNA to be expanded and using cycles of heat and cooling to create new sections of DNA between the primer ends.

UniScept® Strip: A disposable plastic carrier and strip of small cups containing biochemical and antimicrobial test materials.

Vitek® Test Card: A thin rectangular plastic card containing biochemical media or dilutions of antimicrobial agents in test wells for the performance of microbial identification and enumeration or for susceptibility testing.

Introduction

The microbiology section of the clinical laboratory is a more recent adopter of automation than either chemistry or hematology.[1] The two main tasks of clinical microbiology laboratories are to identify the causative agents of infection and to determine antibiotic susceptibilities. Traditionally, these have been accomplished with test-tube biochemical reactions and agar diffusion plates. In the 1960s and 1970s, microorganism identification kits became popular. The kits contain small cups of media and indicators that react with cultured organisms. Identifications are made manually by reading these biochemical tests. The success of these kits led to the development of fully automated systems that use similar techniques.

During the 1960s and 1970s, Kirby-Bauer antimicrobial susceptibility testing was done manually in most microbiology laboratories. In the 1980s and 1990s, automated susceptibility testing systems founded on the principles of nephelometry, spectrophotometry, fluorometry, and radiometry were introduced to microbiology laboratories. The advantages and disadvantages of rapid automated systems compared with traditional manual methods are summarized in Table 22-1.

It should be noted that microbiology automation is not just for large hospitals or reference laboratories. Microbiological procedures may take several days to complete and may therefore involve more than one worker for each sample. The workload can be reduced or evened out by using automated instruments. Automated

Table 22-1

Comparison of Automated Microbiology Systems with Manual Methods

Advantages	Disadvantages
Rapid results	High initial capital expenses
Labor efficiency	Possible mechanical failures
Objective endpoints (better control of human error)	Lack of flexibility in choice of antibiotic panels
Cost-savings when performing multiple test/organisms	Increased test cost if total volume is low
Reproducibility	
Interface with computer and/or LIS	

microbiology methods are usually easier to master than manual ones. This can be particularly important in smaller laboratories where workers cover more than one section of the laboratory and may not have time to develop the expertise needed for manual microbiology procedures.

In this chapter we describe two automated systems for detecting microorganisms in blood or other body fluids (Becton-Dickinson Microbiology Systems' BACTEC and Organon Teknika's BacT/Alert), four systems for identifying bacteria and their antibiotic susceptibilities (bioMerieux's Vitek®; MicroScan's TouchScan® and auto-Scan®; Abbott Diagnostics' MS-2, Quantum II, and Avantage; and Analytab Products' ALADIN), and one automated immunoassay system for identifying organisms' antigens and host antibodies (bioMerieux's VIDAS®).

BACTEC Systems for Detecting Microorganisms in Blood

The BACTEC series of automated instruments for the detection of microorganisms in blood has been dramatically improved and enhanced since the introduction of the BACTEC 460 in the early 1970s. Johnston Laboratories, early pioneers in the automation of blood culture systems, was acquired by the much larger Becton-Dickinson Microbiology Systems (Cockeysville, MD). Additional development and expansion of this unique system have rapidly taken place. A brief chronology follows, with pertinent information regarding each major component of BACTEC systems.

BACTEC 460

The BACTEC 460[2,3] is based on the automated measurement of carbon dioxide produced by growing microorganisms. The system uses four components: disposable culture vials inoculated with blood, the BACTEC instrument that continually tests vials to assess microbial growth, culture gas and adaptors to regulate gas flow, and a shaker to agitate the vials. The BACTEC 460 has a reading capacity of 60 vials. The culture medium in these vials contains carbon 14-labeled glucose and other substrates. Microorganisms break down the labeled chemicals and release ^{14}C-labeled carbon dioxide. Detection of radioactive carbon dioxide indicates growth of bacteria, mycobacteria, or fungi.

Aerobic and anaerobic culture bottles are incubated off-line in a standard microbiology incubator. The aerobic bottles are placed on the BACTEC shaker for the first 24 hours, which stimulates faster organism growth. The BACTEC systems use a wide variety of continually improved blood culture media. The familiar casein formulation is available in small and large vials. Fungal media with antibiotics, lytic media, and mycobacterial enrichment media are available for special needs.

Blood culture vials are placed on the BACTEC instrument in four-vial racks. The vials' tops are sterilized with alcohol. The instrument can automatically test up to 60 vials in one hour by aspirating the headspace gas above the culture medium. The radioactivity in the gas is quantitated, and a growth index (GI) number is computed and printed. If the radioactivity exceeds a preset growth threshold, a red indicator is illuminated on the front panel of the instrument. The numbered indicator light corresponds with the vial tested.

Testing of a vial begins with a pump producing a partial vacuum in the ion chamber (Fig. 22-1). Twin 18-gauge needles are heat-sterilized while the ion chamber is being evacuated. Next, the movable test head is lowered, which drives the needles through the rubber septum of the vial. The ion chamber outlet valve closes, its inlet

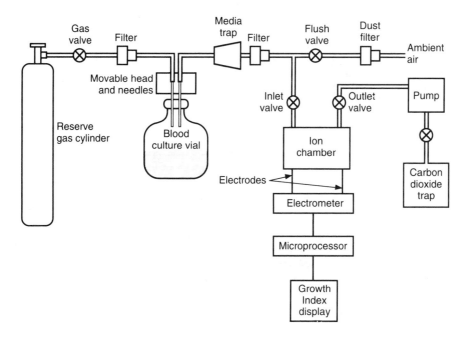

Figure 22-1.   BACTEC 460.

valve opens, and gas from a reserve cylinder passes through a filter and then through the culture vial. This flushes the gases above the culture broth into the ion chamber.

The ion chamber contains positive and negative poles from an electrometer. Radioactivity in the gas changes the impedance between the poles. The change in impedance is converted into a growth index (GI) number. The GI number is displayed on a front panel and printed on a paper tape. If the GI number exceeds the threshold value, a red light illuminates. This identifies the vial with growing organisms so that it may be removed for identification tests.

After the impedance change has been measured, the test head rises, and the needles leave the vial. The head, flush, and ion chamber outlet valves then are opened. Ambient air is pumped through the filter and then the ion chamber. The radioactive carbon dioxide is retained in the soda-lime trap. This prepares the ion chamber and electrometer for the next reading cycle.

The BACTEC 460 now is used almost exclusively in the mycobacteria section of the microbiology laboratory. A negative-pressure safety hood with ultraviolet light provides high-efficiency particulate air (HEPA) filtered to the instrument. Special media and the carbon dioxide replacement gas enhance growth of these fastidious organisms.

Quality Control and Maintenance of the BACTEC 460

A performance test is conducted daily to confirm proper instrument function. A ^{14}C-labeled carbonate solution is injected into a vial containing acid. Both solutions are provided by the manufacturer. The acidification of carbonate releases carbon dioxide. After the reaction is completed, the radioactivity is quantitated and converted to a GI number. Correct instrument operation is indicated by a GI number within a specified range.

Preventive maintenance is important to any automated microbiology system. Daily maintenance includes checking the display lights, examining the needles, and changing the tubing. Monthly, semiannual, and annual maintenance tasks include filter, needle, and needle heater replacements.

BACTEC NR 660

The four major improvements of the BACTEC NR 660[4] compared with the BACTEC 460 are (1) totally computerized data handling and retrieval system; (2) infrared CO_2 detection (NR indicates nonradiometric); (3) ability to process 600 blood culture vials (ten 60-vial trays); and (4) an internal incubator-shaker combination.

The basic operation of the 660 is similar to the 460: Microbial growth is detected by metabolism of substrates and subsequent release of carbon dioxide. Instead of an ion chamber and electrometer, carbon dioxide gas is quantitated by infrared spectroscopy. Absorbance of infrared light by carbon dioxide is measured by a photodiode detector. The computer then generates a Growth Value (GV) from each absorbance reading. A delta GV is also calculated from two consecutive readings. The data management system (DMS) compares GV and delta GV from each vial to defined threshold values. Results are displayed and printed.

The status of all the vials is printed after testing on a 60-vial tray is completed. The DMS stores all results and generates a summary report at midnight. Each patient's results can be viewed on the monitor. Complete histories of all pending and completed blood cultures can be displayed. The computer also prompts the operator to load new trays and displays the next available vial location and accession number. Mono- and bidirectional interfaces to laboratory information systems are available.

Aerobic vials are tested twice on days 1 and 2, and once a day thereafter. Anaerobic vials are tested once a day. Vials are incubated for 5 or 7 days, depending on the laboratory's protocol.

Quality control and maintenance procedures are similar to those for the 460. The biggest difference is that there is a spectrophotometer lamp to check and replace.

BACTEC NR 730

This instrument is smaller, less automated, and less expensive than the BACTEC NR 660. The 730 processes 30-vial trays in the same manner as the 660. However, the delta GVs are calculated manually, and the more limited DMS stores results only from the previously read tray.

BACTEC NR 860

The BACTEC NR 860 is a more automated blood culture system than the NR 660. The major advancement is a computer-controlled mechanism that transports the trays between the incubator storage drawers and the testing area. The robotic arms transport technology allows for continual unattended monitoring of the culture vials. The BACTEC 860 will automatically test vials and print a list of all positive samples for followup.

An additional feature is bar-code sample identification. A unique sequence number is assigned to each vial and is linked to patient identification information when the vial is accessioned.

The BACTEC NR 860 detects positive cultures more rapidly than the NR 660.

BACTEC 9240[5]

The BACTEC 9240[5] was introduced in 1992. The 9240 does not use infrared spectroscopy to detect carbon dioxide. Instead, at the bottom of each vial is a fluorometric carbon dioxide sensor. The incubator, shaker, and detection system are integrated. The BACTEC 9240 holds six 40-vial racks. A fluorometric detector is present at each vial position. The racks rock continuously at 60 cycles per minute.

The sensor bonded to the bottom of each vial is separated from the broth medium by a membrane permeable to carbon dioxide (Fig. 22-2). Carbon dioxide acidifies the sensor, which increases its fluorescence output. Fluorescence is triggered by filtered light from a light-emitting diode (LED). A second filter admits only the longer-wavelength fluorescent light to a photodiode detector.

Vials are tested every 10 minutes. All vials have bar-code labels for internal tracking and patient sample identification. Quality control checks are performed continually. Visual and audible alarms are triggered when a problem is detected.

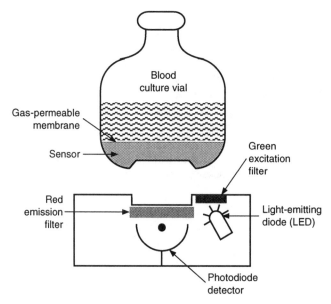

Figure 22-2.   BACTEC 9240 carbon dioxide detection system.

BacT/Alert System for Detecting Microorganisms in Blood

The BacT/Alert is an automated blood culture detection system.[6] It was introduced in the late 1980s by Organon Teknika (Durham, NC). The system is based on the colorimetric detection of carbon dioxide. The BacT/Alert is an integrated system composed of a detection unit, an incubator/shaker, a microcomputer, and unique blood culture bottles.

Each blood culture bottle has a carbon dioxide sensor bonded to its base. A gas-permeable membrane separates the sensor from the broth medium. The tryptic soy broth medium is supplemented with amino acids and carbohydrates. This mixture supports growth and high carbon dioxide production. The sensor consists of a pad impregnated with water that entered as a vapor when the bottle was autoclaved during manufacture. Carbon dioxide produced by growing organisms diffuses through the membrane and dissolves in the water. The CO_2 is converted to carbonic acid and lowers the pH of the sensor solution. Hydrogen ions turn the sensor's indicator from dark blue-green to lighter green and eventually to yellow. Reflectance photometry is used to quantitate CO_2 production. The reflection of red light increases as blue-green color decreases.

The instrument can hold 10 blocks with 24 wells each. The blocks are suspended at both ends and are continuously rocked (one cycle per second). The temperature within the module is held between 35 and 37°C. Each well contains a colorimetric

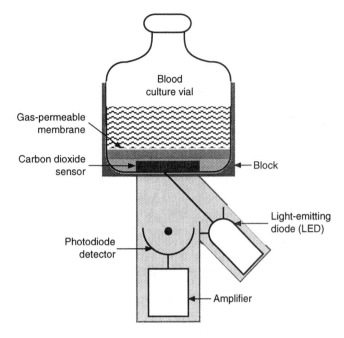

Figure 22-3. BacT/Alert carbon dioxide detection system.

detection system. The detection system consists of a red LED and a photodiode detector (Fig. 22-3). Light emitted from the diode enters the blood culture bottle. Some of the light is reflected from the sensor onto the photodiode, which produces a voltage signal proportional to the intensity of the reflected light. After amplification and filtering, voltage signals are digitized and transmitted to a microcomputer for analysis.

BacT/Alert tests for carbon dioxide production in each bottle 144 times per day. A growth curve results from the plot of reflectance units versus time. Growth detection is based on analysis of the rate of change of carbon dioxide concentration (not on absolute CO_2 concentration).

Blood culture bottles are logged into the system by entering the sample accession number and patient identification number into the computer or by using a wand to read specimen bar-coded labels. The DMS assigns each bottle a tray and well position. The loading position is also indicated by a small green light at the designated well. The light goes off after the bottle is placed in the well. The DMS records the time that each bottle is loaded. One BacT/Alert module has 240 wells. One to four modules can be linked electronically to one DMS.

When analysis reveals microorganism growth, the computer prints the following information: patient identification, sample accession number, well number, time growth was detected, and elapsed culture time. The corresponding bottle position is marked with a small light. After the bottle is removed for microorganism identification studies, the light goes off and the well is available for a new sample. Bottles may be returned to the instrument for further incubation and monitoring (if no microorganisms were seen after microscopic examination of a drop of stained broth).

The computer generates a list of bottles with no detectable growth after 5 or 7 days, depending on the laboratory's protocol.

BacT/Alert culture bottles can accommodate up to 10 mL of blood. Pedi-BacT bottles are suitable for smaller sample volumes ($\leq$4 mL). Bottles for blood from patients receiving antimicrobial drugs and bottles for processed specimens of suspected mycobacterial infections are being developed.

Minimal daily maintenance is needed. An internal quality control system provides immediate identification of all system problems. Instrument problems can be diagnosed by technical services at Organon Teknika through a modem link.

Vitek® Automicrobic System for Microorganism Identification and Susceptibility Testing

The Vitek® AMS automicrobic system is a true "space age" product.[7] It was developed in the late 1960s by McDonnell Douglas at the request of the National Aeronautics and Space Administration (NASA). The system was designed for use in gravity-free environments. In the late 1970s, McDonnell Douglas began selling the Vitek® to clinical microbiology laboratories. This was a difficult undertaking, given the company's inexperience in the laboratory market and most microbiologists' skepticism about the reliability of automated instruments. The venture was successful, and in 1988 McDonnell Douglas sold its Vitek® product rights to bioMerieux, which continues to modify and improve the Vitek® line.

The Vitek® AMS is designed to detect, enumerate, and identify microorganisms and establish their antibiotic susceptibilities. This highly automated system is available in several configurations. The most common one consists of a filler-sealer module, a reader-incubator, a computer control module, a data terminal, and a printer. Along with the modules, specially designed and manufactured test cards are an integral part of the system.

VITEK TEST CARDS

Test cards are clear plastic plates measuring 2.25 by 3.5 inches (Fig. 22-4). They consist of 16, 20, or 30 wells that contain small amounts of either conventional or novel dried test media. The cards are sealed with special tapes that control aeration of the underlying wells. Channels molded onto the card connect all the wells to the injection port. The test kit assembly (card, transfer tube, and sample) is placed into a chamber that is sealed and then evacuated. The test card wells are inoculated and hydrated in the filling module. This occurs by releasing the vacuum and aspirating diluted specimen through the injection port and channels. Each well has a trap to capture any air bubbles formed in the filling process. After inoculation, the card is

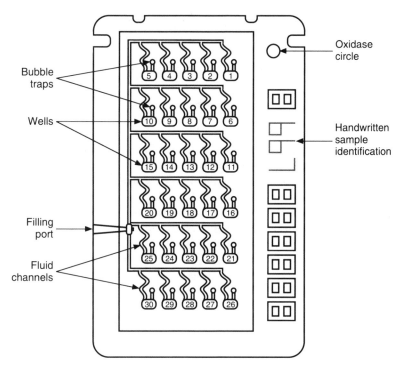

Figure 22-4.   Vitek® microorganism identification test card.

transferred from the filling module to the sealing apparatus. Here the plastic transfer tube is cut and sealed at the surface of the test card's injector port.

Each test card is coded to identify its type (identification or susceptibility). The operator must mark the card (with block-style numbers) to allow isolate identification when the card is being scanned by the reader head.

After coding, filling, and sealing, the test cards are transferred to the reader-incubator module. Reading is done continually until the system is shut down. Each microorganism isolate needs an identification card and a susceptibility card. If both cards are in the same tray, the Vitek® microcomputer will use the organism's growth response data in the evaluation of susceptibility.

READER-INCUBATOR MODULE

The reader-incubator module is a temperature-controlled chamber that contains electromechanical devices for processing the inoculated test cards. Test card trays are mounted on a carousel within the chamber. Each tray is processed by the AMS once each hour. Every 15 minutes, the carousel rotates 90° and aligns a different tray with the reader head. Vertical and horizontal drive mechanisms slide the tray into the processing position. Optical detectors ensure proper alignment of the reader head with the card. The reader head then extracts the card from the tray and sequentially reads each row of wells.

The processing of one tray (30 cards) takes 6 minutes. During tray processing, the system automatically closes the carousel access door to minimize stray light and to prevent aberrations of the reading process due to mechanical movement. Access for insertion or removal of cards is allowed at all other times.

The optical system consists of five LEDs and corresponding detectors. The LEDs emit red light (660 nm) that passes through the test card wells. Detector units measure transmitted light. Each detector unit is composed of four separate phototransistor detectors. This design allows the system to obtain a correct reading even if a small air bubble is trapped in the well. (The reading from the detector "seeing" the air bubble will be discarded.) The amount of light transmitted to the detector unit varies with the amount of bacterial growth (turbidity) or the color change in the well. Detector signals are processed and stored in the DMS.

The 30 wells in the identification test cards contain 29 biochemical broths and one growth control broth. The latter serves as a quality control check on the organism's viability. Most of the biochemical tests are conventional ones in which a substrate is converted to a colored product by a direct chemical reaction, a dye becomes colored due to a pH change, or bacterial growth (turbidity) is affected by inhibitors. Separate test card types are available for gram-negative and gram-positive organisms. This system can even detect fastidious organisms such as *Haemophilus influenzae.*

Susceptibility testing also begins with card inoculation and filling. Numerous panels are available for gram-negative and gram-positive organism susceptibilities to serum antibiotic levels and for gram-negative organism susceptibilities to urine antibiotic levels. Each laboratory must determine which panels are appropriate for its patient population. Each susceptibility card contains 29 wells with multiple dilutions of antibiotics and one well with growth control broth. After inoculation and placement in the reader-incubator, the cards are read hourly. When bacterial growth occurs at levels equal to or greater than a predetermined cutoff, regression analysis yields the minimum inhibitory concentration (MIC) value for each antimicrobial agent. If, during a 4- to 6-hour period, the organism in the growth control well reaches the threshold for an accurate sensitivity determination, the final report status is automatically printed. If the growth threshold in the control well is not reached in 10 hours, the final status is given as "insufficient growth in positive control well."

The inoculum for identification and susceptibility testing is prepared by placing isolated, morphologically identical colonies into 1.8 mL of 0.45% sterile saline. The suspension should have the same turbidity as a particular McFarland standard. The appropriate turbidity standard depends on the type of organism.

COMPUTER MODULE

The Vitek® AMS microcomputer uses a software program to control instrument functions and parameters. A 50-megabyte hard disk drive stores all the software and the test card data. Data storage for a particular test card begins after the first reading process. The program recognizes the new card and assigns the written specimen identification to the corresponding tray position. The program then directs the processing of the card (once each hour) until sufficient detector readings are made. The data then are processed, and the results are communicated to the operator.

Data processing methods differ with the type of test card used. In the identification cards, biochemical reaction patterns are compared to a probability table of known isolate reactions. The two organisms with the best pattern matches are reported along with their overall probabilities. In the susceptibility cards, organism growth rates in the presence of dilutions of antibiotics are compared with growth rate in the control well. The MIC values are calculated from these data.

If a bidirectional interface is installed, the Vitek® AMS can receive patient information directly from the laboratory information system and transmit microbiology data directly to it. A second Vitek® terminal and printer may be placed outside the laboratory to send susceptibility data to physicians or pharmacists. This allows for rapid adjustment of antibiotic therapy without the laboratory having to telephone results.

QUALITY CONTROL AND MAINTENANCE OF THE VITEK

Test card quality control functions are handled by the Vitek® AMS. The Vitek® needs little routine maintenance.

MicroScan Systems for Microorganism Identification and Susceptibility Testing

The MicroScan Division of Baxter Diagnostics (Sacramento, CA) historically has approached bacterial identification and susceptibility testing in several different ways with their partially and fully automated systems.[8]

The TouchScan®, introduced in the 1970s, incorporates turbidimetric and colorimetric detection in a microtiter plate system. Turbidimetry quantitates cloudiness resulting from bacterial growth in broth. Colorimetry detects color changes in conventional biochemical testing media caused by bacterial metabolic end-products. The TouchScan® system needs manual setup, incubation, and readout. The only automation is microcomputer-assisted bacterial identification.

The autoSCAN® is a more automated system. The three components of the autoSCAN®—tray reader, DMS, and printer—leave only plate inoculation and reagent additions for the operator to perform manually. The newer autoSCAN®-W/A ("walk away") system automates incubation, reagent dispensing, reading of biochemical reactions, and bacterial identifications and susceptibilities. Panel inoculation is still manual. This system uses a more rapid fluorometric panel as well as conventional dried plates.

BASIC PRINCIPLES OF MICROSCAN SYSTEMS

The TouchScan®, autoSCAN®, and autoSCAN®-W/A use 96-well microtiter plates. The wells of microorganism identification plates contain chromogenic or fluorogenic (autoSCAN®-W/A only) substrates. The wells of susceptibility plates contain multiple concentrations of antibiotics for MIC or breakpoint susceptibility testing. All plates have growth control wells to confirm organism viability. Each well is inoculated with $100\,\mu L$ of a 0.5 McFarland turbidity standard of the microorganism. A rehydrator-inoculator (RENOK™, provided by the manufacturer) aids in the manual setup of the plates. Plates are placed directly in the system (the autoSCAN®-W/A) for reagent dispensing and incubation, or they are placed in a non-CO_2 incubator. The microtiter plates are read after an appropriate incubation time (18–24 hours for chromogenic panels, 2–5 hours for rapid fluorogenic panels). As previously described, the MicroScan systems use both turbidimetry and colorimetry. Light is transmitted to the bottom of each well through fiber optics bundles after the plate is placed in the reader (Fig. 22-5). The reader optically scans all 96 wells simultaneously. The light

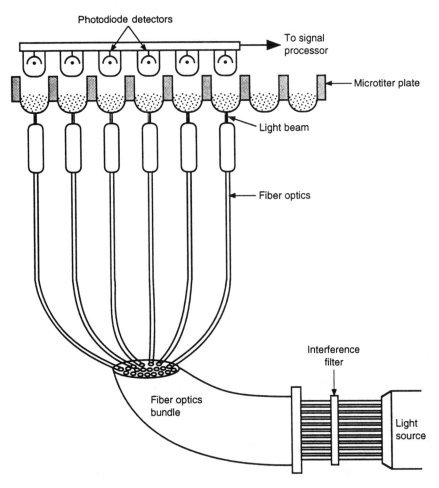

Figure 22-5. MicroScan reader and microtiter plate.

transmitted through the panels is measured by photodiodes from above. Transmittance is measured at six wavelengths (440, 470, 505, 560, 590, and 620 nm). The readings are processed by the onboard microcomputer and then are sent to the DMS microcomputer. An important feature of the MicroScan systems is that the panels can be read manually if any part of the system fails.

Fluorogenic substrates are used with the autoSCAN®-W/A to identify microorganisms in less than 5 hours. A special fluorometry unit lies above the colorimetry unit. Unlike the colorimetry unit, the fluorometry unit tests one well at a time. Computer-driven robotics align the microtiter plate and the fluorometry unit. Excitation light is shown down into the selected well. Light emitted upward passes through a cutoff filter to reach the detector. Fluorescence intensity results are transmitted to the DMS. These values are compared to those of known organisms.

MICROSCAN DATA MANAGEMENT SYSTEM

The DMS compares each test well's turbidity reading with a growth threshold value derived from the blank turbidity reading in the sterile well of the plate. The transmittance of light through the wells with chromogenic substrates allows quantitation of biochemical reactions. The DMS compares all the color intensities to stored values from more than 150 microorganisms. Identifications are accomplished in approximately 30 seconds. Results are displayed on a video panel and are sent to a printer.

The DMS can identify gram-negative rods, gram-positive cocci, anaerobes, and yeasts. The DMS also determines antibiotic susceptibility based on the simple principle that growth (turbidity) in a well with antibiotic indicates lack of susceptibility at that antibiotic concentration. The DMS stores and sorts test data and calculates various parameters from the patient data. This information can be used for laboratory or pharmacy studies and for preparing antibiograms.

QUALITY CONTROL AND MAINTENANCE OF MICROSCAN SYSTEMS

Daily quality control diagnostic tests are run each morning. The DMS checks the date each time a tray is placed in the reader, and it will not calibrate or read if the diagnostics are not completed.

For the two autoSCAN® systems, the operator selects "PERFORM DAILY QC DIAGNOSTICS" from the Main Menu. The autoSCAN® automatically performs self-diagnostic tests of its microcomputer, light source, and electromechanical systems. Diagnostic test results are displayed on the monitor and can be sent to the printer. If a problem is found, the diagnostic test name is highlighted on the monitor with the word "FAILED" in the RESULTS column. Operation will not continue until the problem is fixed.

Before reading MicroScan panels inoculated with patient isolates, quality control strains must be tested. This should be done weekly using American type culture collection (ATCC) strains of representative microorganisms. MicroScan provides detailed information on which strains to use with each type of panel. The expected biochemical reactions and MIC patterns are also given. These results should be stored to document good quality control practices.

Routine maintenance tasks include daily inspection of the diffuser plate for dirt or scratches and proper alignment and weekly inspection of the photodiode shield for dirt or scratches.

Other Systems for Microorganism Identification and Susceptibility Testing

ABBOTT LABORATORIES SYSTEMS

Abbott Laboratories (Irving, TX) has developed three bacterial identification systems since the early 1980s: the MS-2, the Quantum II, and the Abbott Avantage.[9] These systems use disposable plastic cartridges that contain lyophilized substrates with biochemical indicators. Cartridges are inoculated with a 0.5 McFarland turbidity standard of a microorganism culture. The cartridge is locked into place on the incubation tray. The cartridge's seal is perforated, and 200 μL of the bacterial suspension are delivered to each well. The cartridge is inserted into the analysis module for initial absorbance readings. The cartridge then is placed in an incubator for 4 hours. It is reinserted into the analysis module for the final absorbance readings. A microcomputer analyzes the results and identifies the microorganism.

The MS-2 and Avantage instruments can be used for susceptibility testing. Sealed, 11-well cuvette cartridges with upper and lower chambers are used. The upper chambers are filled with culture medium and inoculum. The same inoculum used for bacterial identification can also be used for susceptibility testing. The lower chambers contain antibiotic disks and are initially unfilled. Sample and antibiotic disk information is entered into the microcomputer, and the cuvette cartridge is placed into the analysis module. When the instrument detects turbidity changes that correspond with active log phase growth, it automatically transfers liquid into the lower cuvette chambers. One of the 11 chambers serves as a growth control. Growth within each lower chamber is monitored photometrically at 5-minute intervals. These readings are stored electronically. Algorithms stored in the microcomputer are used to compute the susceptibility results. Qualitative and quantitative results are printed out in 3 to 5 hours.

ALADIN SYSTEM

The Automated Laboratory Diagnostic Instrument, ALADIN (Analytab Products, Plainview, NY),[10] uses digital video imaging to detect biochemical reactions and microorganism growth. A microcomputer identifies the organism and interprets the susceptibility results. ALADIN is a consolidated, automated instrument composed of a reagent dispenser, incubator, digital video read station, disposal station, and two microcomputers.

After manual inoculation, UniScept® (API®) strips are placed in a labeled universal carrier. The carrier is a disposable plastic frame that keeps the strips correctly positioned in the reagent dispenser and reading stations. The carriers (as many as 60) are placed in the incubator module. At appropriate incubation intervals, carriers are transferred to the dispensing station for addition of reagents. Reagent reservoirs are monitored by the instrument. An alarm sounds if the reagent volume is insufficient.

After incubation, the carrier is transferred to an illuminated read station. A video camera is focused on the strips. The 5″-by-5″ viewing area of the camera contains 262,144 pixels. The color density of each pixel is represented digitally for computer processing. Four different color filters are used, yielding four different color densities for each pixel. Only the pixels corresponding to micro-cup (or well) positions on the API® strip are analyzed. The video image processor analyzes data from as many as 300 pixels per well. The image processor ignores air bubbles and particulates within a well.

A microcomputer analyzes the raw data and assigns positive and negative results to each well. This information is sent to a second microcomputer for interpretation. Identification and susceptibility results are printed.

When testing is completed, the universal carrier and the test strips are dumped into the disposal station. When the waste bag is full, a warning light is turned on.

Analytab Products require that specific ATCC strains of microorganisms be run with each test batch, as do most other bacterial identification systems.

The VIDAS® System for Antigen Detection and Serological Testing

The Vitek® ImmunoDiagnostic Assay System (VIDAS®), developed by bioMerieux Vitek®, Inc., performs common infectious disease immunoassays.[11] The VIDAS® expands Vitek®'s automated systems approach by integrating automated direct antigen and serological testing with microbial growth and susceptibility testing.

BASIC PRINCIPLES

The VIDAS® uses the enzyme linked fluorescent immunoassay (ELFA) method. The target analyte (antigen or specific antibody) is bound to solid-phase antibody or antigen molecules, and other specimen components are washed away. A second biotinylated antibody is added, and unbound components again are washed away. Streptavidin with an alkaline phosphatase conjugate is added, followed by the 4-methylumbelliferyl phosphate substrate. The substrate is hydrolized to 4-methylumbelliferone, a fluorescent compound. Fluorescence intensity is directly proportional to analyte concentration.

THE VIDAS® INSTRUMENT

The assay processor module executes all the procedures for up to 30 different immunoassays. The processor module is composed of five sections with six assay positions in each section. This multibatch design allows simultaneous performance of five assays, multiple start times, and stat testing capabilities. The VIDAS® can also be configured for single-batch runs with up to 30 samples. The assay processor controls pipetting, mixing, incubation, analytical steps, and quality control. The VIDAS® is easy to set up and run. The instrument and reagents are stable, and assay calibration is good for 2 weeks. Bar-coded reagent strips allow the VIDAS® to ascertain and record test types, lot numbers, and expiration dates. The detection system uses dual-beam optics with one beam as reference. The test beam passes through the sample in the reagent strip cuvette. Fluorescence is quantitated by a photomultiplier tube, and the results are sent to the microprocessor for analysis.

SPECIMEN TESTING

The following assays were available on the VIDAS® system in 1993: respiratory syncytial virus (RSV) antigen, anti-rubella IgG, anti-toxoplasma IgG, anti-cytomegalovirus IgG, Chlamydia antigen, *Herpes simplex* virus antigen, *Clostridium difficile* toxin A, and Lyme disease and Rubeola antibodies. The manufacturer plans to add assays for anti-mumps IgG, anti-rubella IgM, cytomegalovirus, *Varicella zoster,* rotavirus, and adenovirus.

Serology assays are run on serum specimens. Several antigen assays use heat-treated samples or samples with a processing reagent added. The assay for *C. difficile* toxin A needs sample centrifugation at $12,000 \times g$.

The VIDAS® uses a disposable solid-phase receptacle (SPR) as a pipetting device and solid-phase reaction container (Fig. 22-6).[11,12] The SPR is pre-coated with polyclonal antibodies or with a specific antigen. An analyte-specific reagent strip

Reagent Strip

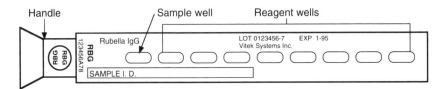

Solid Phase Receptacle

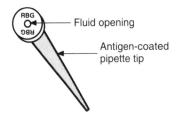

Figure 22-6.   VIDAS® reagent strip and solid-phase receptacle (SPR).

contains the diluent, biotinylated antibody, streptavidin alkaline phosphatase conjugate solution, wash solutions, and substrate solution (Fig. 22-6). Several of the antigen detection assays (those used to test complicated specimens such as stools or bronchial washings) need a dual reagent strip. The second strip, or reference strip, measures the nonspecific fluorescence generated by the specimen matrix.

Approximately 0.4 mL of sample is added manually to the reagent strip. The reagent strips and the SPRs are placed in the instrument. The assays are completed automatically by the VIDAS® module. The instrument scans the reagent strip bar code to confirm that it matches the assay requested. Sample from the reagent strip is added to the SPR, where antigens and antibodies bind. After an incubation period, wash solution is drawn into the SPR to remove unbound substances. The biotinylated antibody is drawn into the SPR, and there is another wash step after incubation. Next, the streptavidin conjugated to alkaline phosphatase is drawn into the SPR. After a final wash, the 4-methylumbelliferyl phosphate substrate is drawn into the SPR. After a brief incubation period, fluorescence intensity is quantitated. The results are analyzed by the computer. Fluorescence readings of the sample and reference strips are used to calculate a test value. Test values are compared to a set of thresholds, and the results are interpreted. A report is printed for each sample.

COMPUTER MODULE

The VIDAS® instrument contains six microprocessors. Each of the five assay-processing sections has a microprocessor that controls incubator and liquid-handling functions. The sixth microprocessor has overall control of the systems, interprets results, and generates reports. Additional VIDAS® modules can be linked to the main computer system to increase testing capacity.

CALIBRATION AND QUALITY CONTROL OF THE VIDAS®

All VIDAS® quantitative and qualitative serology assays and some of the antigen assays use standards. Quantitative serology assays use at least four standards. Qualitative serology and antigen assays use one standard. Those assays using a dual strip do not need standards. Standard values for a particular test kit lot are stored in the computer. Calibration is good for at least 2 weeks. Recalibration is necessary when control results are unacceptable or when a new kit lot is used. Controls should be run at least once each day the VIDAS® is in use.

Summary and Future Developments

Automated microbiology testing systems have improved microorganism detection, identification, and treatment. The new systems are easy to use and are faster than manual methods. However, except for direct antigen and serological tests, microorganism detection and identification can take days. Often, multiple broad-spectrum antibiotics must be administered until positive identification and antimicrobial susceptibility tests are completed. The future of microbiology testing lies in rapid detection and identification.

In the 1980s DNA probe testing to identify microorganisms appeared in some microbiology laboratories. Mycobacteria, chlamydia, *Neisseria gonorrhoeae, Staphylococcus aureus,* and other organisms can be identified with DNA probes. The probes are labeled segments of DNA that will bind to complementary DNA strands of the microorganism. Chemiluminescent labels are commonly used. As this technology gains wider acceptance, more advances will be made in automating the entire procedure.

Polymerase chain reaction (PCR) technology is in use in some microbiology laboratories. It is based on multiple cycles of DNA replication. An organism-specific sequence of DNA is selected for PCR amplification. This technique can detect and identify microorganisms in native samples, and no culturing is necessary. In PCR, a selected segment of DNA is replicated and other DNA is ignored. The original DNA and its copy are denatured by heat. The mixture is cooled and replication occurs again. Each cycle doubles the amount of the selected DNA sequence. A heat-stable form of DNA polymerase enables rapid cycling between replication and denaturation. Heating and cooling of the water bath are controlled by a microcomputer. The amplified DNA can be detected by a variety of methods.

Other molecular technologies being developed include ligase chain reaction (similar to PCR). GenProbe (San Diego, CA) is developing technologies for human papilloma virus detection. This should allow for more automation and decreased turnaround time for detection of this and other important infectious disease organisms.

Also being developed is an automated enzyme probe assay system that amplifies messenger RNA using a three-enzyme approach that does not need a thermocycler. Liquid-phase enzyme linked end products allow detection of amplified target mRNA in the same instrument now used for current antigen and antibody assays.

References

1. Daly JA, Eisenach KD. Instrumentation in clinical microbiology. ASM Workshop. American Society for Microbiology General Meeting, New Orleans, LA, May, 1992.
2. Henry MM. Automated microbiology systems. In: Hicks MR, Haven MC, Schenken JR, McWhorter CA, eds. Laboratory instrumentation, 3rd ed. Philadelphia: JB Lippincott, 1987:321-23.
3. Johnston Laboratories operation and maintenance manual for the BacTec 460. Cockeysville, MD: Johnston Laboratories, 1984.
4. Johnston Laboratories Bactec NR-660 operations and maintenance manual. Towson, MD: Johnston Laboratories, 1985.
5. Nolte FS, Williams JM, Jerris RC, Morello JA, Leitch CD, Matushek S, et al. Multicenter clinical evaluation of a continuous monitoring blood culture system using fluorescent-sensor technology (BACTEC 9240). J Clin Microbiol 1993, 31:552-57.
6. Thorpe TC, Wilson ML, Turner JE, Di Guiseppi JL, Willert M, Mirrett S, Reller LB. BacT/Alert: An automated colorimetric microbial detection system. J Clin Microbiol 1990, 28:1608-12.
7. Ibid., Henry MM, 312-17.
8. Baxter Healthcare Corp. MicroScan Operator's Manual. Sacramentro, CA: Baxter Healthcare Corp. MicroScan Division, 1986.
9. Ibid., Henry MM, 318-29.
10. Ibid., 324-25.
11. Rogers CH, Hoffman KL, Juris RM. An automated system for infectious disease diagnosis. Am Clin Products Review 1989, 8(5):35-37.

12. Sandin RL, Knapp CC, Hall GS, Washington JA, Rutherford I. Comparison of the Vitek® Immunodiagnostic Assay System with an indirect immunoassay (Toxostat Test Kit) for detection of immunoglobulin G antibodies to Toxoplasma gondii in clinical specimens. J Clin Microbiol 1991, 29:2763-67.

Suggested Readings

D'Amato RF, Isenberg HD, McKinley GA, Baron EJ, Tepper R, Shulman M. Novel application of video image processing to biochemical and antimicrobial susceptibility testing. J Clin Microbiol 1988, 26:1492-95.

Hopson DK, Niles AC, Murray PR. Comparison of the Vitek® Immunodiagnostic Assay System with three immunoassay systems for detection of cytomegalovirus-specific immunoglobulin G. J Clin Microbiol 1992, 30:2893-95.

Kelly MT, Leicester C. Evaluation of the AutoSCAN® Walkaway System for rapid identification and susceptibility testing of gram negative bacilli. J Clin Microbiol 1992, 30:1568-71.

O'Hara CM, Miller JM. Evaluation of the AutoSCAN® W/A System for Rapid Two Hour Identification of Members of the Family Enterobacteriaceae. J Clin Microbiol 1992, 30:1541-43.

23

AUTOMATED BLOOD BANKING SYSTEMS

James D. Landmark

Objectives

After completing this chapter, the reader will be able to:

1. Explain the need for automation in blood banks.
2. Describe hemagglutination by IgM and IgG antibodies.
3. List methods of detecting hemagglutination.
4. List and understand tests performed by transfusion services.
5. Describe liquid-suspension and solid-phase hemagglutination methods.
6. Explain the importance of standardized bar-code systems to blood banking.
7. Describe the component parts of blood serology analyzers.
8. Describe three automated microplate blood grouping analyzer systems.
9. List the component parts of cell washing centrifuges.
10. Describe maintenance and quality control procedures for blood typing systems and cell washing centrifuges.

Definitions

Allogeneic: Pertaining to different genetic makeup within the same species. Blood transfusions, unless from an identical twin or oneself, are allogeneic.

Antihuman Globulin: An antibody mixture from another species that reacts with human IgG antibodies. Some mixtures detect activated complement also.

Antigen Typing: Identification of specific antigens, particularly on the surface of red blood cells, by agglutination with specific antisera.

Automation: The use of technology to automate performance of an activity, especially tedious repetitive tasks or dangerous tasks, with the beneficial intent of increased efficiency and/or safety.

Bar Code: One of numerous (>50) incompatible systems of machine-readable symbols that use bars and spaces of differing widths to encode binary data. Bar-code data are translated by a reading device into numeric or alphanumeric information for electronic transmission to another device such as a data-logger or computer.

Blood Bank: An organization that collects blood from healthy volunteer donors for allogeneic use or from patients before surgery for autologous use and provides blood components to transfusion services.

Blood Component: A preparation of a functionally useful cellular or plasma protein concentrate from a whole-blood unit.

Checksum: A method of checking the accuracy of computer-written data stored on magnetic or optical media.

Forward Grouping: Use of reagent anti-A or anti-B mixed with red cells to detect A or B antigens by hemagglutination.

Hemagglutination: The visually or optically detectable formation of adherent red cell masses that result when antibodies combine in appropriate ratios with red cell surface antigens.

Irregular Antibody Screening: Detection of anti-erythrocyte antibodies formed subsequent to immunization by transfusion or pregnancy.

Reverse Grouping (back typing): Identifying the presence of isoagglutinins (anti-A or anti-B) in donor or recipient plasma by mixing with reagent A or B cells and observing hemagglutination.

Symbology: Any defined systems of symbols, particularly machine-readable symbols such as bar codes. The term does not refer to the study of symbols. The term *code* is synonymous and preferable.

Transfusion Service: The section of the hospital laboratory that (at a minimum) performs blood typing on inpatients and outpatients, tests whether blood is safe for transfusion, stores blood components, modifies components when needed, and maintains detailed records of these functions.

Zeta Potential: The potential difference between the negative charges on the surface of the red blood cell membrane and the cations in the aqueous medium. Cations are divided into two groups, those that always move with the red blood cell and those that can move freely in the medium. The zeta potential is measured from the boundary of these two cations to the negative charge on the membrane. A large zeta potential makes hemagglutination difficult.

Introduction

In 1901, Karl Landsteiner discovered human blood groups from his observation of red cell agglutination patterns in differing mixtures of red cells and serum. Ninety years later, the routine methods for pretransfusion testing have changed little. The simplicities of Landsteiner's methods allow widespread availability of allogeneic transfusion. These standard manual test methods are effective for preventing hemolytic transfusion reactions. The use of automation in transfusion services has been limited because of cost. The widest use of automation by hospital transfusion services is for cell washing with semiautomatic centrifuges. The most important use of automation by hospital transfusion services has been in maintaining blood donor and recipient records with a laboratory information system.

Automation in blood banks is far more advanced and widespread than in most hospital transfusion services. To grasp the importance of automation in blood banks, one must recognize the need for *zero defects* in donor selection, blood product testing, product labeling, and in the permanent documentation of the aforementioned activities. A mind-boggling quantity of permanent records are generated by blood banks. Blood banks range in size from small collection facilities within a hospital to large operations serving numerous hospitals over an extended geographic area. Without automation and electronic record processing, storage, and retrieval, operation of all but the smallest blood banks becomes a daunting endeavor. Moderate-size and large blood banks have adopted automation extensively to cope with increased testing and quality control. Over the past decade, the Food and Drug Administration (FDA) has required greater numbers of process control standards in blood bank operations. These process controls are the same as those in pharmaceutical manufacturing. Maintaining present standards would be impossible without machine-readable codes, computer control of labeling, high-speed on-line automation of blood typing and infectious disease testing, and electronic recordkeeping.

In this chapter we describe automated systems for red cell serology. Automated systems for infectious disease testing also are used extensively in blood collection centers, but these are discussed in Chapters 19 and 22.

Principles of Blood Bank and Transfusion Service Automation

Automated testing systems for red cell serology detect hemagglutination. The strength of the agglutination depends on (1) characteristics of the antigen and the antibody; (2) reaction conditions such as temperature and incubation time; and (3) the effective intercellular gap resulting from ions and water molecules creating a repulsive shear plane (zeta potential) between red cells.

Red cell antigens may be glycoproteins (such as A or B antigens) or proteins (such as Rh system antigens). IgM antibodies react with oligosaccharide chains on red cell glycoproteins. IgM antibodies produce agglutination of red cells because the 30-nm wide molecule spans the intercellular gap created by membrane effects. IgG molecules, with a maximum dimension of 14 nm, cannot span the gap. Agglutination does not occur even though the antibodies bind to red cell surface antigens. Hemagglutination by IgG occurs only after additional steps are performed such as:

1. Reducing the ionic strength of the solution in which the red cells and antibody are suspended to reduce the intercellular gap.
2. Using proteolytic enzymes to remove red cell surface glycoproteins which decreases the surface negative charge and reduces the intercellular gap.
3. Adding antihuman globulin (rabbit antibody to human IgG) to the washed suspension of sensitized red cells. Antihuman globulin will span the distance between two IgG molecules bound to separate red cells; the cross-links produce hemagglutination.
4. Centrifuging the sensitized cells with sufficient force to decrease the intercellular gap to less than 14 nn.

Hemagglutination is detected by a variety of means:

1. Particle size histograms generated by electrical impedance measurements or light scattering in blood cell counters.[1]

2. Fluorescence of stained, agglutinated red cells.[2]
3. Density gradient gel separation of agglutinated from nonagglutinated red cells.[3]
4. Photometry of a liquid red cell suspension. Most automated blood typing systems of the 1970s and 1980s used photometric detection in continuous flow, proprietary cuvette, or microtiter plate systems.
5. Image analysis.
6. Visual appearance of cells resuspended after centrifugation. Resuspension may be performed in test tubes (conventional manual technique) or in microtiter plate wells.

Tests performed by all transfusion services include forward and reverse ABO grouping, Rh typing (with testing for weak D antigen when appropriate), irregular antibody screening, and compatibility testing. Both forward and reverse ABO grouping are automated easily because the antigen-IgM antibody binding directly results in hemagglutination. Automation of testing for weak D antigen, for irregular antibodies, and for donor-recipient compatibility is difficult because antigen-IgG antibody binding does not produce hemagglutination. Therefore, successful automation for these procedures must include one or more of the IgG antibody hemagglutination steps listed. These constraints add considerable mechanical complexity to the process. The STS-A automated antiglobulin test device, developed by Gamma Biologicals, performed all steps in a special cuvette.[4-5] Hemagglutination was detected by image analysis. Available testing protocols included irregular antibody detection and compatibility testing. This device is no longer marketed, presumably because it was not profitable.

As an alternative to antihuman globulin, proteolytic enzyme treatment of red cells, often coupled with low ionic strength solution, can enhance hemagglutination by IgG. These techniques were used in continuous-flow devices originally derived from Technicon™ chemistry modules in the late 1960s. This equipment was available until the mid-1980s. Although enzyme treatment made automation of IgG antibody testing less complex than with centrifugation, a major limitation was found—proteolytic enzymes denature several red cell antigens (including M, N, Fy^a and Fy^b). Clinically significant antibodies were missed and, conversely, extremely weak antibodies of doubtful clinical significance were detected in these systems.[6] Continuous-flow blood typing systems are no longer marketed.

Currently available automation systems for red cell serological testing use *microplates* (microtiter plates). Most microplate systems detect agglutination photometrically. Some systems use computer analysis of a digitized image of the microplate wells. The advantages of microplate systems are reduced reagent consumption and increased sample throughput.

MICROPLATE HEMAGGLUTINATION SYSTEMS

Numerous semiautomated methods of red cell typing are available. Most use photometric detection of hemagglutination in microplates. The liquid-phase serological reactions are identical to traditional manual tube methods. Manual microplate hemagglutination methods initially used 96 well microplates with V-bottom wells.[7]

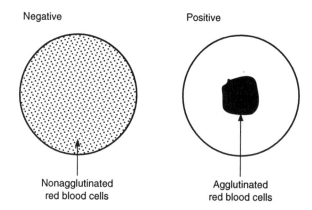

Negative   Positive

Nonagglutinated   Agglutinated
red blood cells   red blood cells

Figure 23-1. Hemagglutination test results in U-bottom microplate wells. No agglutination results in a nearly uniform distribution of red cells after resuspension. Hemagglutination results in a central button of clumped cells.

Very dilute cell suspensions were used. Positive reactions were detected by the lack of red cell "streaming" when the microplate was tilted after centrifugation. Later, trays with U-bottom wells were used with less dilute cell suspensions.[8]

Figure 23-1 illustrates the appearance of standard hemagglutination in a U-bottom microplate well. When the microplate contents are resuspended by agitation after centrifugation, the wells with negative reactions show a uniform suspension of red cells across the well diameter. Strong positive reactions show a central agglutinate surrounded by clear supernatant. Weaker positive reactions will show smaller agglutinates that are still in the center of the well. These different patterns can be distinguished by automated microplate readers programmed to measure photometric absorbance. The absorbances can be sent to a computer for interpretation. The results of ABO and Rh antigen testing for each specimen can be evaluated by the computer, which then can provide automated blood type results.[9-11]

SOLID-PHASE TECHNIQUES

In contrast to traditional liquid-suspension hemagglutination methods, alternate detection methods use an antibody or antigen bound to a solid surface. Indicator red cells adhere to a localized site on the solid surface because of the formation of immune complexes. This technique is the *solid-phase adherence assay.* Solid-phase techniques can detect both plasma antibodies and red cell antigens. To perform ABO typing, anti-A or anti-B antibodies are bound to U-bottom wells in a microplate. Suspensions of the red cells to be typed are added to the wells, and the microplate is centrifuged. The cells are *not* resuspended after centrifugation. Antigen-positive cells will adhere uniformly to the solid-phase antibodies attached to the well. Antigen-negative cells will flow freely "downhill" to the center of the well. Solid-phase

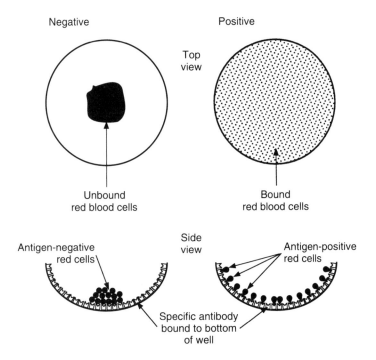

Figure 23-2.   Positive and negative reactions in solid-phase techniques. Antigen-negative red cells do not adhere to antibodies and settle to the bottom of the wells. Antigen-positive cells are caught by the solid-phase antibodies and are distributed evenly across the well.

techniques produce visible reaction patterns that are the *reverse* of standard hemagglutination patterns. Positive reactions show nearly uniform deposition of the red cells across the well bottom. Negative reactions show a central cell "button" surrounded by clear supernatant. Figure 23-2 illustrates the appearance of positive and negative reactions. The results can be read by an appropriately programmed automated microplate reader and then interpreted by computer software. This technique commonly is used for *forward ABO typing.* Reverse ABO typing can be done by binding red cell surface antigens to the solid-phase. The corresponding plasma antibody binds to the antigen. Then, antigen-positive, indicator red cells are added. Figure 23-3 illustrates this "sandwich" of antibody between antigen on the solid phase and antigen on the indicator red cells. If antibody is present in the plasma being tested, indicator cells will adhere to the entire bottom of the well. If antibody is absent, indicator cells will not adhere and will form a central cell button. As with other microplate methods, these reactions can be read by an automated microplate reader that can send the photometric readings to a microcomputer for interpretation.[12] Variations on this latter technique are used to detect irregular antibodies. Numerous publications report excellent agreement between hemagglutination and solid-phase methods for red cell antibody detection.[13-16]

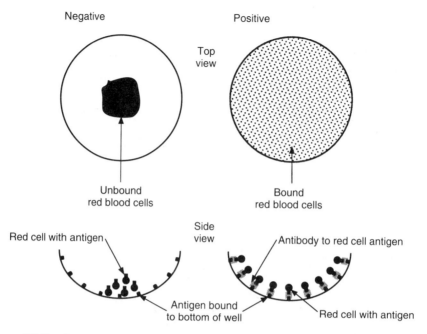

Figure 23-3. Reverse ABO typing using the "sandwich" technique. Presence of an antibody to the red cell antigen being tested results in a solid-phase antigen–antibody–red cell (with antigen) sandwich.

Component Parts of Blood Serology Analyzers

BAR-CODE READER

The usefulness of bar codes is evident to any person who has ever been in a store checkout line. The universal product code (UPC) symbol found on almost all commercial products has (almost) eliminated the need for manual price entry. The advantages to both the seller and customers are increased checkout speed and accuracy of the information entered into the cash register (assuming that the correct price has been assigned to each product code). This example demonstrates the benefits of using bar-code symbologies for data entry into laboratory information systems. Bar codes are also useful for tracking materials and for process control in manufacturing. Unfortunately, implementation of bar codes has been hampered by the independent development of multiple incompatible coding schemes.[17]

Bar-code standardization is not an easy effort because different bar code systems have features (and limitations) that make them attractive in different circumstances. The Health Industry Business Communications Council (HIBCC) has approved four (out of more than 50) bar-code systems for use in the hospitals and clinical laboratories.[18] The system known as Code 39 is used extensively in chemistry and hematology laboratories. However, blood banks and transfusion services use a different system.

The Committee for Commonality in Blood Banking Automation (CCBBA) was convened in 1974. Its goal was to reduce human errors in transfusion recordkeeping by establishing a standard label format for use by all blood bank establishments. A combination of human- and machine-readable label information was an essential element of the standard. Machine-coded identification of the donor unit and the test sample allows electronic linking of test data (needed for product labeling) with donor records. With a standardized bar code linking all information regarding the donor unit data, electronic control of unit labeling is possible. This greatly decreases the risk of erroneous release of potentially unsafe blood products. This same unit coding information can be used by hospital transfusion services to create electronic transfusion records.

The CCBBA adopted the *CODABAR* system as its standard. A CODABAR character is composed of four bars and the intervening three spaces, both of differing widths. The CODABAR system represents a seven-bit binary code with 128 possible combinations. Twenty-four of these combinations were selected for the CODABAR character set (10 for Arabic numerals and 14 symbols for start codes, stop codes, and other operational codes). These 24 bar-code characters were chosen to minimize the likelihood of character substitution if there is a misread by the scanning device. Two misreadings would have to occur within the same character image for the bar code reader to substitute one character for another. A single misreading (of a wide bar as a narrow bar, for example) will not result in a substitution but will be recognized as nonsense by the scanning device. This feature made CODABAR more reliable than other bar codes at the time, and incorporation of a binary checksum into the coded data was believed to be unnecessary. Brodheim and others documented that CODABAR had a reading error rate of less than one in 1.5 million characters read.[19] This is far superior to the one in 300 character error rate of manual data entry.

The final report of the CCBBA was accepted by the FDA's Bureau of Biologics (BoB) in 1979. CODABAR became the only FDA-approved machine-readable symbol system. The final report also included numerical blood product codes, blood group codes, container codes, anticoagulant and preservative codes, label layout formats, and printing specifications. Thatcher[20] described similar features in a proposed international uniform labeling system in 1981. The BoB issued proposed regulations and guidelines for voluntary use of the uniform label system in 1980.

The adoption of this uniform label by many blood banks in the 1980s increased reliability and speed of blood unit data entry into central data processing systems. A unit identifier linked component processing records and blood testing data with control processes for blood product labeling and product release and shipping records. Bar-coded identification decreased data errors in records and improved process control during a decade in which the number of tests performed on each donation increased from five to eleven. The limitations of a labeling system that did not provide completely unique product identifiers were demonstrated in the 1980s, especially for products that could be shipped nationwide or even worldwide.

In 1992, an international consortium proposed revisions to the uniform label guideline. These include an expanded donation identification number format to make each donation uniquely identifiable worldwide. Characters would be added to the seven-digit blood unit number to identify the collection center and the year of collection. To squeeze this additional information into approximately the same amount of bar code space, the denser Code 128 is recommended. Code 128 is also one of the four symbol systems approved by the HIBCC.[21]

Each Code 128 character is composed of three bars and three spaces of differing width. The maximum width of a character is 11 times that of the narrowest printable line or space. The recommended layout of the uniform label accommodates the increased amounts of bar-coded product information.

AUTOMATIC SAMPLE HANDLER

The front end of any modern automated blood typing system is a device for identifying and pipetting the test sample. Microprocessor-controlled, programmable Cartesian robots (able to move a sample pipetting probe in three perpendicular dimensions) are linked to a laser bar-code scanner in most automated systems. Some systems have liquid-level sensing capability to ensure proper sampling. Samples are loaded manually into holding racks or carousel trays. Each sample's bar-coded label is read as sample aliquots (plasma and red cells pipetted separately) are delivered to reaction cuvettes. U-bottom wells in a standard 96-well microplate are a common type of reaction cuvette. In some systems, the reaction cuvettes already contain the reagents. In others, the aliquots of reagents are delivered to the reaction wells along with the test samples. Automated sample handlers have a standard communications port for transmitting sample and test position information to a computer. This information is matched to the photometric readouts taken after all test reactions are completed.

INCUBATOR

Microplate ABO and Rh typing methods incubate at ambient temperature. Methods for detecting IgG antibodies need 37°C incubation. Dry-heat incubators commonly are used.

SEROLOGICAL ROTATOR/SHAKER

Standard microplate tests need resuspension of cells. This can be done using a variety of shakers or rotators.

AUTOMATED MICROPLATE READER

Automated microplate readers were used originally for microplate enzyme-linked immunosorbent assays, but can also be used to detect hemagglutination. Both red cell antigen typing (ABO and Rh) and serum antibody identification assays can be performed with automated microplate readers. The microplate reader positions each well over a photometer. The pattern of red cell distribution across the bottom of the well is measured photometrically. Early methods used a single measurement at one wavelength. The photometric beam was offset from the center of the well.[22] If the reaction was positive (as in Figure 23-1), absorbance would be low because the beam would miss the central button. A negative reaction would have increased absorbance due to the resuspended red cells. Modern microplate readers take overlapping readings across the bottom of each well. This decreases the number of indeterminate reactions.[23] Absorbance readings are compared to thresholds to determine whether the test result is clearly positive or negative. When the absorbance values fall *between* the positive and negative thresholds, as occurs with some weak positive reactions, the result is indeterminate. Indeterminate reactions can be interpreted visually or can undergo additional testing. The absorbance readings are linked to tray identification and well location. The readings are ultimately communicated to the microcomputer that merges them with sample identification. The test results are interpreted automatically. Antigen and antibody reports are generated for each sample. Discrepant results (such as disagreement between ABO front typing and reverse typing) or indeterminate results need on-line editing by the technologist. Sample identification and test result data can be transferred to a laboratory information system for incorporation into donor or patient files.

Some automated microplate readers use image analysis to assess hemagglutination. (See the description of the ALADIN system in Chapter 22.) A high-resolution digitized image of the entire microplate is made through a special camera. Each well image is analyzed on a pixel-by-pixel basis for recognition of agglutination patterns. Sophisticated image analysis software allows proper classification of weak reactions. Published data are not available about actual performance of these devices for blood bank tests.

Current Instrumentation for Red Cell Serology

The three blood group analyzer systems described below use microplates.

INVERNESS BLOOD GROUPING SYSTEM

This blood serology system, the Inverness Blood Group System[24] (IBG Systems, Inc., Laytonsville, MD 20882), does ABO and Rh typing and performs a solid-phase antibody screen using a test kit manufactured by Immucor, Inc. (Norcross, GA 30071). The system consists of separate modules that can all fit on 6 to 8 feet of counter space. The system is not fully automated: An operator must transfer microplates between modules, centrifuge microplates, and resuspend cells.

The modules are listed below.

1. Reagent dispenser for adding reagents to standard 96-well microplates. Testing configurations allow up to 8 tests on 12 samples per tray, or up to 12 tests on 8 samples per tray.
2. Robotic sampler with automated bar-code reader for sample identification. This is a modified Cartesian robot. The microplate moves beneath a row of twelve pipet tips that add blood samples to one microplate row at a time. Centrifuged

anticoagulated specimens are loaded into a carrier for sampling. Sample identification is linked to the well location.

3. Photometric microplate reader.
4. Microcomputer linked to the sampler and the reader to provide test interpretations for each sample. The microcomputer can be interfaced with a laboratory information system computer.
5. Microplate shaker.
6. A countertop centrifuge with carriers for microplates is needed, too.

The Inverness Blood Grouping System uses inexpensive reagents and disposable microplates. Throughput is 200 samples per hour. Initial results can be obtained within 20 minutes. It can be operated cost-effectively with as little as 70 samples per day.[25] It is used effectively in small blood banks and in large transfusion services.

GAMMA BIOLOGICALS STS-M™

This is an automated device for performing ABO and Rh typing.[26] It is a microprocessor-controlled countertop instrument that needs less than 3 feet of counter space. The STS-M™ is a unique system. Centrifuged, anticoagulated, barcoded specimens are loaded in a sample carousel. Reagents and sample aliquots are placed in 84 tear-shaped reaction cuvettes. The reaction cuvettes are attached side by side in a disposable polyvinyl chloride plastic belt. Twelve specimens can be tested per belt. The optical reader detects gravitational "streaming" of red cells from cell buttons in the reaction cuvettes. The optical imaging system focuses its array of 128 photodiodes on two separated areas of each reaction cuvette: the central button area and the sloped cuvette area below the button (Fig. 23-4). In a positive reaction, agglutination holds the red cells together, and no cells will be detected in the lower optical image region. In a negative reaction, nonagglutinated red cells flow "downhill," and they will be detected in the lower optical image region. Test results are linked to specimen identification, and interpretations of ABO and Rh types are made automatically.

Reagent antisera and cells are used undiluted and unmodified from the manufacturer's bottles. This has the advantage of eliminating manual reconstitution and the need to perform quality control studies on the reagent dilutions. The disadvantage is that reagent costs are greater than for other systems.

STS-M™ throughput is 60 specimens per hour. The STS-M™ is suitable for small-to medium-size blood banks and transfusion services.

OLYMPUS PK 7100® AND PK 7200™

The Olympus (Olympus Corp., Lake Success, NY 11042) systems are completely automated.[24] The operator loads appropriately diluted reagents and places centrifuged anticoagulated specimens and control samples into racklike cassettes. Both systems complete ABO and Rh blood typing automatically. The PK 7100™ needs 51 sq. ft. of floor space (about 5' by 10'). It is composed of a microplate-handling unit,

Positive test reaction

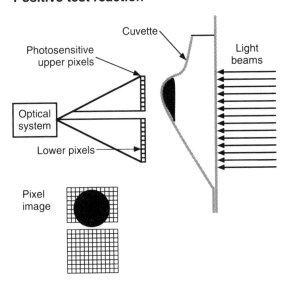

Negative test reaction

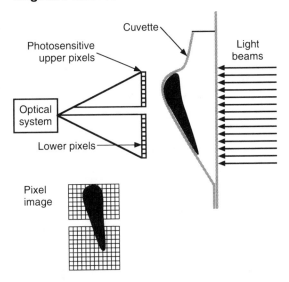

Figure 23-4.   Magnified schematic of positive and negative reactions detected by the Gamma Biologicals STS-M™ automated blood typing system digital imaging system. Agglutinated cells do not drift downward, and, therefore, they are only seen in the upper set of imaging pixels. Nonagglutinated cells drift downward and are seen by the lower set of imaging pixels.

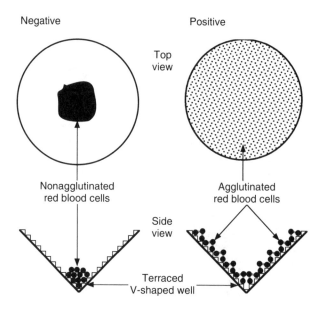

Negative   Positive

Top view

Nonagglutinated   Agglutinated
red blood cells   red blood cells

Side view

Terraced
V-shaped well

Figure 23-5.   Negative and positive reactions in terraced V-bottom wells used by the Olympus PK 7200™ automated blood typing system. Agglutinated cells become lodged on the terraces, resulting in a scattered distribution. Nonagglutinated cells settle to the bottom of the well.

a printer, and a computer module. Sample identification, sample and reagent pipetting, incubation, and microplate reading occur within the microplate-handling unit. Bar codes allow positive sample identification. Throughput for the microplate handling unit is 240 samples per hour. Both systems use a special proprietary V-bottom microplate. These specially fabricated 120-well (10 rows of 12 wells) microplates are expensive. However, they may be reused indefinitely if properly cleaned, rinsed, and dried. The microplate wells have microscopic concentric engraved "terraces" (Fig. 23-5). The terraces prevent agglutinated red cells from settling to the center of the well. Nonagglutinated cells will flow down and form a central button of cells. As with the solid-phase microplate techniques, the appearance of reactions in the terraced well is the reverse of standard microplate hemagglutination reactions. The advantage of the terraced well is that no centrifugation of the microplate is necessary. Gravitational settling of the cells or agglutinates occurs during a 1-hour incubation at 30°C. This eliminates the manual centrifugation step, allowing a fully automated test cycle.

A Cartesian pipetting apparatus delivers samples, diluted antisera, and cell suspensions. After pipetting is completed, the microplates move in sequence through the incubator and then to the detector.

Hemagglutination detection on the PK 7100® is photometric. Seventeen readings are taken across the bottom of each well (3 central and 14 peripheral). The central readings are averaged, as are the peripheral readings. The ratio of the peripheral average to the central average is calculated for each well. This ratio is compared to threshold values, and the microcomputer assigns a positive, negative, or indeterminate result. Samples with indeterminate results can be read visually, or additional manual testing can be done.

Hemagglutination detection on the newer PK 7200™ is performed by image analysis (see Automated Microplate Readers in the Component Parts section). The PK 7200™ has improved software which allows two microplate handling units to be connected to the computer module, doubling throughput to 480 samples per hour.

Microprocessor software controls all actions of the Olympus PK 7100® or PK 7200™. The software also interprets photometric or image analysis results and determines the samples' blood types. Reports can be printed, and they can be transmitted to a laboratory information system through a bidirectional interface.

The Olympus systems perform well in large blood banks, because of their high speed and reliability. Reiss et al.[27] found that 95% of samples were accurately typed on a single pass through the machine. Indeterminate specimens on the initial run were retested, and only 1.1% of specimens could not be typed automatically.

This equipment is designed for batch ABO and Rh testing of large numbers of samples. It is not cost-effective for small blood banks or for most transfusion services.

CELL WASHING CENTRIFUGES

The automated devices most widely used by transfusion services are *countertop centrifuges*. They are designed to wash, centrifuge, decant, and resuspend red cells multiple times in up to 12 test tubes simultaneously. Since most red cell tests need an antiglobulin addition as the final step to hemagglutination, automated washing centrifuges are almost essential equipment. The component parts of cell washing centrifuges are:

1. Centrifuge timer (analog or digital).
2. Centrifuge rotor to contain 12- by 75-mm test tubes.
3. Variable speed motor with speed controller.
4. Saline pump with volume delivery controls. These are typically small rotary pumps that deliver fluid by using rollers to squeeze flexible plastic tubing against a platen.
5. Saline stream splitter or distributor to fill multiple test tubes.
6. Saline decanting system.
7. Fused power supply.

Some of these devices have microprocessors that allow the operator to customize centrifuge speeds, duration of centrifugations, and the number of saline wash steps. All automated cell washing centrifuges have "standard" wash protocols for testing red cells with antihuman globulin. A few systems also have automated antihuman globulin dispensing.

Maintenance and Quality Control

AUTOMATED OR SEMIAUTOMATED BLOOD TYPING SYSTEMS

Many of these systems have self-diagnostic routines to verify proper function. Other quality control checks are performed by the operator. Quality control specimens are assayed with each analytical run. Specimens with A_1, A_2, B, D, and (when appropriate) weak D antigens are used. Control red cells are used to check forward typing; control plasma aliquots are used to check reverse typing. Controls commonly are placed at the start and end of each run. With large batch runs, controls are used at periodic intervals such as after every 100 samples. Control products must all be typed correctly before sample results are accepted.

Microprocessor software must be thoroughly evaluated after every revision, however minor. One validation method is to use a standard data set that will test all decision branches of the program. Again, results must be perfect before the revised software is accepted for use.

Microplate reader calibration can be performed (in some systems) by using a test plate with neutral density filters. This confirms proper alignment and photometric linearity.

New lots of antisera reagents must be tested to verify the proper working dilution. This can be done with appropriate positive target cells. Cells without the antigen of interest should also be tested as negative controls.

AUTOMATED CELL WASHING CENTRIFUGES

Maintenance and quality control tasks for these devices are:

1. Periodic verification of saline pump function and delivery volume accuracy and precision. Test tubes should be less than 80% full to avoid cross-contamination.
2. Periodic verification of centrifuge rotor speed. The actual speeds should be within 100 revolutions per minute of the selected speeds.
3. Periodic verification of the centrifuge timer against an accurate stop watch. The timer should deviate less than 2 seconds from the last calibration.
4. Recalibration of serological reactions (selection of appropriate centrifuge speed and time) needs to be done after centrifuge service or repair. Recalibration should also be done when centrifuge rotor speed or timer checks deviate from previously established limits.
5. Periodic verification of the saline decanter. The cell button should be dry.
6. Routine assessment of IgG-coated "check cells" in tested tubes with negative antiglobulin reactions. This verifies that antiglobulin activity is present in the tube. Hemagglutination should always occur.

Summary

Blood banks type and identify antibodies in scores to hundreds of blood samples daily. Automated equipment is essential for cost-effective testing. The use of universally standardized bar code labels on all blood samples and products has greatly reduced errors. Blood banks and transfusion centers strive for zero defects because a single mislabeled or incorrectly typed unit can be fatal to a recipient.

A number of automated devices are available to detect hemagglutination, the common endpoint of many blood tests. The linkage of bar code readers, samplers, and readers to microcomputers allows positive specimen identification and tracking. Microcomputer software also provides rapid, accurate interpretations of blood test results. These results can be printed and downloaded to laboratory information systems with essentially no reporting errors.

All equipment used in blood centers and transfusion services must be properly maintained. Stringent quality control procedures are used to minimize errors.

References

1. Tatsumi N, Tsuda I, Inoue K. Trial of ABO and Rh blood typing with an automated cell counter. Clin Lab Haemat 1989, 11:123-30.
2. Ellisor S. Automation of red cell testing. In: Selection of methods and instruments for blood banks. Arlington, VA: American Association of Blood Banks, 1987:47.
3. Lapierre Y, Rigal D, Adam J, Josef D, Meyer F, Greber S, Drot C. The gel test: A new way to detect red cell antigen-antibody reactions. Transfusion 1990, 30:109-13.
4. Ellisor S. Automation of red cell testing. In: Dixon M, Ellisor S, eds. Selection of methods and instruments for blood banks. Arlington, VA: American Association of Blood Banks, 1987:42-44.
5. Hatcher BF, Turner JL. An automated standardized test system for the antiglobulin procedure. Lab Med 1985, 16:779-82.
6. Taswell H, Grina J. Evaluation of single-channel hemagglutination AutoAnalyzer for antibody screening and quantitation. In: Automation in analytical chemistry. Technicon Symposium 1967. Tarrytown, NY: Mediad, 1968:165-68.
7. Wegmann TG, Smithies O. A simple hemagglutination system requiring small amounts of red cells and antibodies. Transfusion 1965, 6:67-73.
8. Crawford MN, Gottman FE, Gottman CA. Microplate system for routine use in blood bank laboratories. Transfusion 1970, 10:258-63.
9. Piccirilli RJ, Tomchick C, Williams R, Beckjord PA, Park FK. An automated microplate system for blood group serology. Lab Med 1985, 16:775-78.
10. Peoples JCA. A microplate system for semiautomated ABO and Rh testing. Lab Med 1985, 16:783-85.
11. Chung A, Birch P, Ilagan K. A microplate system for ABO and Rh(D) blood grouping. Transfusion 1993, 33:384-88.
12. Sinor LT, Rachel JM, Beck ML, Bayer WL, Coenen WM, Plapp FV. Solid-phase ABO grouping and Rh typing. Transfusion 1985, 25:21-23.
13. Plapp FV, Sinor LT, Rachel JM, Beck ML, Coenen WM, Bayer WL. A solid phase antibody screen. Am J Clin Pathol 1984, 82:719-21.
14. Rachel JM, Sinor LT, Beck ML, Plapp FV. A solid-phase antiglobulin test. Transfusion 1985, 25:24-26.
15. Rolih SD, Eisinger RW, Moheng MC, Dean WD, Eatz RA. Solid phase adherence assays: Alternatives to conventional blood bank tests. Lab Med 1985, 16:766-70.
16. Uthemann H, Poschmann A. Solid-phase antiglobulin test for screening and identification of red cell antibodies. Transfusion 1990, 30:114-16.
17. Burke HE. Handbook of bar coding systems. New York: Van Nostrand Reinhold Company, 1984:126.
18. Kasten BL, Schrand P, Disney M. Joining the bar code revolution. Medical Laboratory Observer. 1992, 24:22-25.
19. Brodheim E, Ying W, Hirsch RL. An evaluation of the CODABAR symbol in blood-banking automation. Vox Sang 1981, 40:175-80.

20. Thatcher RK. Recommendations of the task force on codes and machine-readable symbols. Vox Sang 1981, 40:144-55.
21. Sazama K, Aller R, Weilert M, Carey K. New bar-coding system in blood banks' future. CAP Today 1992, 7:66-71.
22. Severns ML, Schoeppner SL, Cozart MJ, Friedman LI, Schanfield MS. Automated determination of ABO/Rh in microplates. Vox Sang 1984, 47:293-303.
23. Severns ML, Kline LM. An improved method for detection of hemagglutination using an automated microplate reader. IEEE Trans Biomed Eng 1985, BME-32:349-52.
24. Blood grouping systems, automated. Product Comparison System, ECRI, May 1993.
25. According to a letter from JCA Peoples, Executive Vice President, IBG Systems, Inc., in April 1993.
26. Walker RW, ed. Technical manual, 10th ed. Arlington, VA: American Association of Blood Banks, 1990:527-37.
27. Reiss RF, Malavade V, Johnson CL, Hendricks E, Rabin BI, Marsh WL. Blood grouping with the Olympus PK7100 testing system. Clin Lab Haemat 1988, 10:385-90.

24

PHYSICIAN'S OFFICE LABORATORY INSTRUMENTATION

Diana Headley
Gregory A. Tetrault

Objectives

After completing this chapter, the reader will be able to:

1. Describe the unique instrumentation needs of a physician's office laboratory.
2. Explain the importance of instrument simplicity and reliability in physician's office laboratories.
3. Find information on instruments suitable for different test types, specimen fluids, and test volumes.
4. Describe the workings of the i-STAT™, VISION®, QBC® II, and Biotrack® 512 instruments.
5. List maintenance and quality assurance procedures for physician's office laboratories.

Definitions

Ion-Selective Electrodes (ISEs):   Electrodes with special membranes or glass that are permeable only to the ion being analyzed. Ion concentration is measured by comparing the test signal to a reference signal.

Microhematocrit: The percentage of blood volume occupied by red blood cells calculated from blood centrifuged while in a capillary tube.

Reagent Strips: Plastic or paper strips coated with reagents that change color after urine or other liquid sample containing the analyte of interest is applied. Reagent strips can have separate regions for multiple analytes.

Throughput: The number of specimens or test results an instrument can process per hour.

Introduction

Physician's office laboratories increased in number and complexity throughout the 1980s. In the past, a typical physician's office laboratory consisted of a microscope, urine reagent strips, and perhaps a microhematocrit centrifuge. The proliferation of small, easy-to-operate, low-cost analyzers enabled many physician's office laboratories to offer numerous chemistry, hematology, and coagulation tests. Another factor that contributed to the increase in physician's office laboratory testing was the proliferation of group practices. Instrumentation, equipment, space, and personnel too costly for solo practitioners were shared by groups of practitioners. Other factors that contributed to the growth of physician's office laboratories include the desire for shorter turnaround times, patient convenience, and profitability of laboratory testing.

The rapid growth of physician's office laboratories created problems. There was a shortage of adequately trained personnel. Many of the instruments had been designed for small hospital laboratories and were not well suited to a physician's office laboratory. Physician's office laboratory personnel often had insufficient training in quality assurance procedures and documentation. More recently, government regulations, requirements, and fees increased the operating expenses of physician's office laboratories. The number of physician's office laboratories is expected to decrease. However, tens of thousands of laboratories will continue to operate, and more may arise, especially in large multispecialty group practices.

In this chapter we describe the unique needs of physician's office laboratories and the principles that should apply to their instrumentation. Numerous tables list instruments that can be used in physician's office laboratories, and a number of instrument systems are described. We then conclude with a section on maintenance and quality assurance.

Factors Affecting Instrumentation for Physician's Office Laboratories

Physician's office laboratories differ significantly from hospital or large private laboratories. Physician's office laboratories generally have fewer specimens and employ personnel with less training in medical laboratory testing. Low test volume makes high-throughput or large-batch instruments impractical. Physician's office laboratories rarely can afford duplicate instruments. Reagents with short shelf lives are also impractical because they won't be used before their expiration date. Bulky reagents or reagents that require manual preparation are ill-suited to physician's office laboratories because of the lack of space or lack of volumetric flasks, pipettes, and reagent grade water.

Instruments for physician's office laboratories should be easy to operate. Operators should need only a brief training period. In addition, instruments should be easy to calibrate and maintain. Quality control and quality assurance procedures should be easy to perform and document, understandable, and described clearly by the manufacturer. Ideally, a troubleshooting plan to handle control outliers or quality assurance problems should also be provided. The instrument manufacturer or service agency should be able to repair or replace broken instruments quickly.

Technological advances have led to the production of numerous easy-to-use, cost-effective instruments suitable for the physician office setting. These are usually smaller and less expensive that those designed for hospital or independent laboratories. They usually have a limited test selection or lower sample throughput. Continued development of smaller instruments will increase the diagnostic capabilities of physician's office laboratories.

Instrumentation for Physician's Office Laboratories

Tables 24-1 through 24-11, in an appendix at the back of the chapter, are organized by type of instrument. Each table lists instrument manufacturers, models, and the method(s) used by each model. A few noteworthy instruments are described in the following sections.

Manual chemistry analyzers analyze one sample (and sometimes only one test) at a time. Few steps are automated. Centrifugal clinical chemistry analyzers perform one test at a time on batches of samples. They cannot perform quickly multiple tests on a single sample. Discrete automated clinical chemistry analyzers perform numerous tests on one or more samples. They are the most versatile chemistry analyzers. Automated chemistry analyzers are described in Chapter 18.

Blood glucose monitors report glucose concentrations by using small quantities of blood. Results often are available in less than 2 minutes. Electrolyte analyzers quantitate sodium, potassium, and often chloride and bicarbonate in whole blood, serum, or plasma. (Some analyzers will accept urine or other body fluids.) Urine analyzers automatically read multitest reagent strips.

Immunoassay analyzers are manual or semiautomated. Hundreds of compounds can be measured by immunoassay methods. Numerous immunoassay analyzers are described in Chapter 19.

Semiautomated hematology analyzers need manual specimen loading. They count erythrocytes and leukocytes, measure hemoglobin or hematocrit, and calculate red cell indices. Automated hematology analyzers do all these tasks, and some can perform partial white blood cell differential counts. Hematology analyzers are described in Chapter 20.

Coagulation analyzers measure prothrombin time (PT), activated partial thromboplastin time (aPTT or just PTT), and perhaps other tests such as thrombin time (TT), fibrinogen, fibrin degradation products (FDP), and factor assays. These instruments use plasma or whole-blood samples. Coagulation analyzers are described in Chapter 21.

i-STAT™ PORTABLE CLINICAL ANALYZER

The i-STAT™ (i-STAT Corp., Princeton, NJ 08540) system is composed of a portable hand-held analyzer, disposable test cartridges, and a portable printer.[1] The analyzer measures $20 \times 6.5 \times 5.0$ cm and weighs 540 g. It is powered by two 9-V batteries. The analyzer has a slot at the base to insert cartridges, a mechanical system that controls the flow of sample and calibration fluid in the cartridges, an electronic system that connects with the biosensors on the cartridges, a keypad for entering sample information, a liquid crystal display screen, and a light emitting diode (LED)

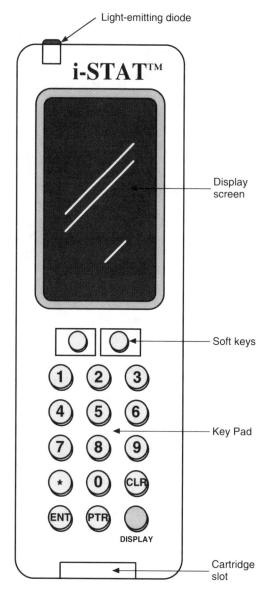

Figure 24-1.   Portable i-STAT™ analyzer unit.

for transmitting data (Fig. 24-1). The analyzer never comes into contact with samples or calibration fluids.

The disposable cartridges contain a sample port, sample chamber, sample fluid channel, waste chamber, calibration fluid reservoir, biosensors embedded in a silicon chip, and contact pads (Fig. 24-2). Whole blood (approximately 65 μL) is put into the

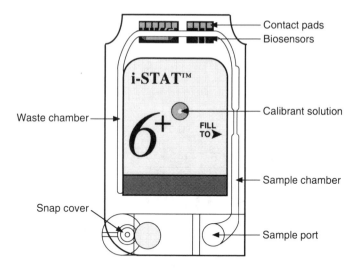

Figure 24-2. i-STAT™ disposable test cartridge. Sample is introduced at the sample port. Calibration fluid and sample are sequentially directed to the biosensors by the analyzer unit.

sample well with a capillary tube or a syringe. The analyzer ruptures the calibration fluid reservoir. The calibration fluid covers the biosensors, and voltage readings are transmitted to the analyzer through the contact pads. The calibration fluid then is sent to the waste chamber, and the sample is sent to the biosensors. The sample's voltage signals are compared to the calibration fluid's. Results are displayed numerically and as bar graphs. This entire process takes only 90 seconds. The results also can be sent to a portable printer that uses rolls of heat-sensitive paper. The analyzer can store 50 sets of results that include patient identification numbers and dates and times of analysis. The data can be downloaded to a microcomputer through an infrared LED. The microcomputer can transmit the results to a laboratory information systems computer.

The cartridges have different combinations of tests. The most comprehensive cartridge measures sodium, potassium, chloride, urea, glucose, and hematocrit. The electrolytes are measured by ion-selective electrodes (ISEs). Urea is enzymatically hydrolyzed to ammonia, which is also measured by an ISE. Glucose oxidase reacts with glucose and produces hydrogen peroxide, which is measured amperometrically. Hematocrit is determined by conductivity, and hemoglobin is calculated using a mathematical formula. Other tests (blood gases, ionized calcium, creatinine, leukocytes) are under development.

The i-STAT™ is a unique instrument suitable for physician's office and point-of-care testing. Accuracy and precision are excellent. Maintenance is minimal because fluids never come in contact with the analyzer. The use of a calibration fluid with each sample ensures cartridge viability and proper instrument function. The i-STAT™ is an excellent example of nearly foolproof instrument design.

Front View

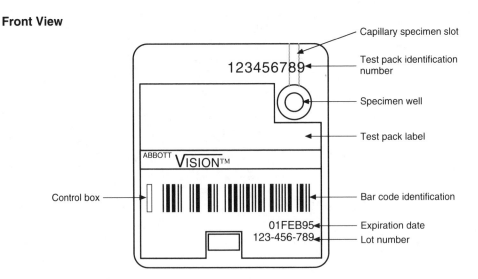

Back View

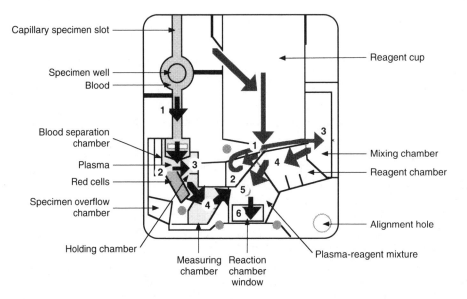

Figure 24-3. Front and back of an Abbott VISION® test pack. Sequential centrifugation and 90° reorientation steps move specimen and reagents through numerous channels and chambers. (After specimen addition, centrifugation drives the reagent(s) into the measuring chamber and the blood into the blood separation chamber [Step 1]. Blood and plasma are separated [Step 2]. The pack rotates 90° counterclockwise, which dumps reagents into the mixing chamber and plasma into a holding chamber [Step 3]. The pack rotates 90° clockwise, which sends reagents into the reagent chamber and plasma into a measuring chamber [Step 4]. The pack rotates 90° counterclockwise, which dumps plasma and reagents into a mixing chamber [Step 5]. A final 90° clockwise rotation dumps the reaction mixture into the reaction chamber where transmittance is measured.)

ABBOTT VISION® CHEMISTRY ANALYZER

The Abbott VISION® Analyzer (Abbott Laboratories, Abbott Park, IL 60064) consists of an enclosed centrifuge, a spectrophotometer, a potentiometer, a microprocessor, and a display.[2] The centrifuge processes 1 to 10 samples in individual test packs simultaneously. Whole blood, plasma, or serum is placed into the specimen well or capillary slot on the test pack, which is loaded on to the test pack holder on the centrifuge platform.

The analyzer uses a unique two-dimensional centrifugation process to separate plasma from red cells and to deliver and mix fluids in the test packs (Fig. 24-3). Upon initiation of an assay, the centrifuge platform spins. The centrifugal force moves test pack reagents into one or more measuring chambers. At the same time, the specimen moves into the blood separation chamber. If the specimen is anticoagulated whole blood, the centrifugal force separates red cells from plasma. Next, the test pack holder rotates counterclockwise 90°. This transfers reagents into the mixing chamber and the upper portion of the specimen into a holding chamber.

The test pack holder then rotates back to its original position. This transfers the reagents into the reaction chamber and the specimen into a measuring chamber. Again, the test pack holder rotates counterclockwise 90°. This transfers the measured specimen and the reagents into the mixing chamber.

A final rotation brings the test pack holder to its original position. (Some analytes require additional rotations of the test pack.) The specimen-reagent mixture moves to the reaction chamber. The spectrophotometer measures transmittance of monochromatic light through the reaction chamber. The Abbot VISION® spectrophotometric system can perform endpoint, linear rate, and timed turbidimetric (for clot detection) assays.

Potentiometric reactions are measured with a VISION® LYTE™ Pack. Two undiluted calibrators and the specimen react with paired ion-selective and reference electrodes. Analyte concentration is calculated from a two-point calibration curve.

Results are shown on a liquid-crystal display and are printed to a paper tape. Results can also be downloaded to a computer. The operator uses a touch pad to enter date, time, and specimen identification number.

The Abbott VISION® is suited to laboratories that process less than 100 tests per hour. It is easy to operate and generates results in less than 15 minutes for most analytes. Samples and reagents never come into contact with the analyzer, which minimizes cleaning and maintenance tasks. Analyzer function is easily verified with self-check packs. Over 25 chemistry tests are available.

BECKTON DICKINSON QBC®-II PLUS HEMATOLOGY ANALYZER

QBC® Hematology Analyzers (Becton Dickinson Diagnostic Instrument Systems, Sparks, MD 21152) consist of a high-speed microcentrifuge and a tube reader.[3] The reader makes electrooptical measurements of the discrete layers of packed blood cells in a special capillary tube. High-speed centrifugation of blood produces layering because of cell density gradients. The instrument measures or calculates hematocrit, hemoglobin, mean corpuscular hemoglobin concentration (MCHC), and leukocyte,

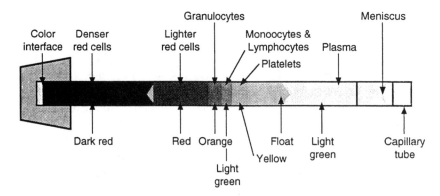

Figure 24-4.   Special capillary tube and internal float for the QBC® II Centrifugal Hematology System. Cells are stained with acridine orange. The float displaces platelets, leukocytes, less dense erythrocytes, and some of the plasma. The length of the cell zones is proportional to cell counts.

granulocyte, lymphocyte plus monocyte, and platelet counts. Results are compared to stored hematologic data, and the microcomputer generates diagnostic reports.

Blood is collected in precision-bore glass tubes coated with potassium oxalate, the fluorochrome stain Acridine Orange, and agglutinating agent. Potassium oxalate increases the density of red cells by osmotically drawing water out of the cells. This allows better separation of granulocytes and young red cells (including reticulocytes). Tubes are supplied with an insertable plastic float and a plastic cover. The float is added to the tube before centrifugation. Its purpose is to displace fluid and increase the length of the white cell and platelet layers.

During high-speed centrifugation, the float moves into the region occupied by leukocytes and platelets (the buffy coat). Displacement by the float lengthens the stained white cell and platelet layers by a factor of 10 (Fig. 24-4). The centrifuged tube is inserted into the QBC Autoreader where it is illuminated by blue-violet light. An optical scanner automatically makes absorbance and fluorescence measurements along the tube. These measurements allow the lengths of the layers to be determined. A microprocessor converts the layer lengths to common units. Hemoglobin is estimated from red blood cell density factors. The MCHC is calculated from the hematocrit and hemoglobin values. The results are displayed and printed, and interpretations are provided.

The QBC® II Hematology Analyzers work well in small physician's office laboratories. Capillary tube collection of finger-puncture blood provides sufficient sample for a complete blood count and partial white blood cell differentiation. Manual processing steps are uncomplicated. Results are available with 10 minutes of collection.

THE BIOTRACK® 512 COAGULATION MONITOR

The Biotrack® 512 Coagulation Monitor (Biotrack, Mountain View, CA 94043) determines prothrombin and activated partial thromplastin times (PT and aPTT,

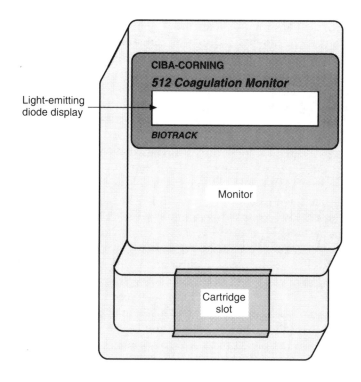

Light-emitting
diode display

CIBA-CORNING
512 Coagulation Monitor

BIOTRACK

Monitor

Cartridge
slot

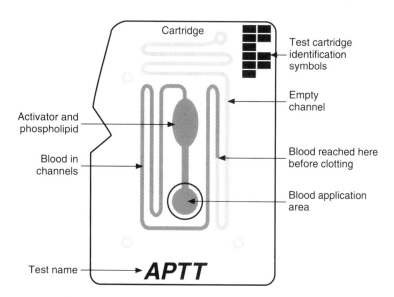

Cartridge

Test cartridge
identification
symbols

Empty
channel

Activator and
phospholipid

Blood reached here
before clotting

Blood in
channels

Blood application
area

Test name

APTT

Figure 24-5.   Biotrack® 512 Coagulation Monitor and prothrombin time (PT) cartridge.
Movement of whole blood and then of the blood-reagent mixture is by capillary action.
Migration distance is detected by a laser optical system in the monitor.

respectively) on capillary blood specimens.[4-7] The small (approximately $5 \times 9 \times 17$cm), battery-powered monitor consists of a heater, a laser optical system, and a microprocessor that checks for errors while guiding the user through the test. Disposable plastic cartridges for PT or aPTT testing are inserted into a slot at the base of the monitor.

The Biotrack® system uses a unique method for measuring PT or aPTT (See Chapter 21). Clot formation in most analyzers is detected optically (increased turbidity) or mechanically (increased viscosity). The Biotrack® detects clotting by measuring time taken for the whole blood to stop moving through a capillary channel.

To perform a test, a reagent cartridge is inserted into the monitor (Fig. 24-5). The cartridge bar code is read to identity the test. The cartridge is heated to 37°C, and calibration and self-diagnostic tests are performed. If all is well, the monitor display prompts the operator to apply a finger-puncture whole-blood sample to the cartridge's application well. The blood is drawn by capillary action and mixes with activator and phospholipid in the reagent chamber. The blood then flows out through another capillary channel. The coagulation process begins as soon as blood mixes with the reagents. Capillary flow ceases when clotting occurs. The laser photometer continuously monitors the capillary channel and detects cessation of blood flow. The time from activation to clotting is converted mathematically to a plasma-equivalent PT or aPTT. This result is shown on the liquid crystal display. Results are also displayed as a ratio of sample clotting time to normal control clotting time. For PT tests, the International Normalized Ration (INR) and percent activity also are displayed.

The Biotrack® 512 Coagulation Monitor works well in physician's office and bedside or point-of-care testing. It is completely portable (battery-powered) and produces results in a few minutes or less.

Maintenance and Quality Assurance in Physician's Office Laboratories

Good maintenance begins with the arrival of the instrument in the laboratory.[8] The operator's manual should be read and understood before the instrument is unpacked. Some instruments can be set up by the operator, but complicated and expensive equipment may need to be set up by specially trained outside personnel. Ideally, physician's office laboratory instruments should need little routine maintenance. Maintenance tasks can be organized by frequency: daily, weekly, monthly, and so on. The maintenance needs should be clearly specified in the operator's manual. A record sheet can be prepared for each instrument that lists all maintenance tasks. The person completing each maintenance task should record the date and her/his name or initials. Records should also be kept of service calls and repairs.

Quality assurance must cover all components of laboratory testing from ordering tests through reporting results. Procedures need to be developed and written for all aspects of testing: transmittance of test orders; patient preparation; specimen collection, labeling, transport, storage, and processing; specimen rejection criteria; analytical procedures including maintenance and calibration; interferences; quality control criteria and procedures for dealing with out-of-control values; test validation; and reporting results. The best way to ensure good quality is to adhere to thorough, well-written procedures. Quality assurance processes must be documented. Simple forms, log sheets, and charts work well. More information on quality assurance in physician's office laboratories can be found in *The Physician's Office Laboratory.*[9]

Summary

Physician's office laboratories differ greatly from hospital and independent clinical laboratories. Instruments need to be smaller, less expensive, and easy to operate and maintain. Rapid turnaround time is often essential, because the physician may need results while the patient is in the office.

A wide variety of chemistry, serology, hematology, and coagulation testing instruments are available for physician's office laboratories. We described a few of those instruments in this chapter. The medical and technical directors of physician's office laboratories must ensure good quality throughout the testing process. Many instruments are designed to be nearly foolproof, which lessens the burden of assuring quality.

References

1. Erickson KA, Wilding P. Evaluation of a novel point-of-care system, the i-STAT portable clinical analyzer. Clin Chem 1993, 39:283-87.
2. Abbott Laboratories. Abbott VISION® instrument manual. Abbott Park, IL. Abbott Laboratories, Diagnostics Division, 1991.
3. Becton Dickinson Primary Care Diagnostics. QBC® Autoread hematology system operators manual. Sparks, MD. Becton Dickinson Primary Care Diagnostics, 1991.
4. Mungall DR, Wright J. Summary report-performance evaluation of the Biotrack protime test system. Mountain View, CA. Biotrack, Inc., 1989.
5. Summary report-performance evaluation of the Ciba Corning 512 coagulation system for determination of activated partial thromboplastin time. Medfield, MA: Ciba Corning Diagnostics, 1990.
6. De Marzi-Jeye D. Near-patient coagulation testing laser-based accuracy. American Clinical Lab 1993, 12:12.
7. Jensen R, Ens G. Whole blood coagulation monitoring. Clinical Hemostasis Rev 1992, 6:4.
8. Belsey RE, Baer DM, Statland BE, Sewell DL. The physician's office laboratory. Oradell, NJ: Medical Economics Books, 1986:263-66.
9. Ibid.

Suggested Readings

Baer DM, Belsey RE. Limitations of quality control in physician's offices and other decentralized testing situations: The challenge to develop new methods of test validation. Clin Chem 1993, 39:9-12.
Commission on Laboratory Accreditation. 1993 Inspection Checklist. Limited Service Laboratory. Section XXV. Northfield, IL: College of American Pathologists, 1993.

Appendix

Table 24-1
Manual Chemistry Analyzers*

Manufacturer	Model	Method
Abbott Laboratories, Abbott Park, IL 60064	VISION®	Photometry, ISE
Bio-Analytics, Palm City, FL 34990	Smart Alex® III; Stat-Fax 1904 Plus®	Filter photometry
Boehringer Mannheim, Indianapolis, IN 46250	Reflotron®, Reflotron® Plus	Reflectance photometry
DataChem, Indianapolis, IN 46268	DC-100	Photometry, grating monochromator spectrophotometer
Eastman Kodak, Rochester, NY 14650	Ektachem DT-60 II	Reflectance photometry
i-STAT, Princeton, NJ 08540	i-STAT™ System	ISE, amperometry, conductivity
Labsystems, Helsinki, Finland	FP900	Filter photometry
Miles, Inc., Tarrytown, NY 10591	Clinimate®-TDA; Seralyzer®; Clinistat®	Reflectance photometry
Roche Diagnostic Systems, Branchburg, NJ 08876	COBAS® READY™	Reflectance photometry
Romark Diagnostics, Hillsdale, NJ	Discovery f2 Models 2101, 2102	Photometry, ISE
Schiapparelli Biosystems, Fairfield, NJ 07004	Gemstar® II	Filter photometry
Seradyn, Indianapolis, IN 46206	QUICK-CHEM™ II	Filter photometry
Texas International, Houston, TX 77036	Chema 1; CH-16; CH-100; Screenmaster	Filter photometry

*Clinical chemistry analyzers, manual. ECRI product comparison system. 1993, Feb:1-23.

Table 24-2
Clinical Chemistry Analyzers, Automated, Centrifugal*

Manufacturer	Model	Method
Du Pont Medical Products, Wilmington, DE 19880	Analyst®	Endpoint, kinetic
Instrumentation Laboratory, Lexington, MA 02173	Monarch Plus	Endpoint, kinetic, bichromatic, rate, ISE
Microgenics Instruments, Concord, CA 94520	ASCA with ASCA; LDM autoloader	Endpoint, kinetic, immunoassay, bichromatic
Roche Diagnostic Systems, Branchburg, NJ 08876	COBAS Bio-FP	Kinetic, enzyme multiplied immunoessay technique (EMIT), fluorescence polarization, ISE, absorbance
	COBAS FARA®	Absorbance, kinetic, endpoint, ISE, turbidimetry, EMIT, particle enhanced turbidimetric inhibition immunoassay (PETINIA)
	COBAS FARA II®	Absorbance, kinetic, endpoint, ISE, nephelometry, EMIT, fluorescence polarization
Schiapparelli Biosystems, Fairfield, NJ 07004	Gem*Profiler™	Kinetic, endpoint

*Clinical chemistry analyzers, automated, centrifugal. ECRI product comparison system. 1992: July:1-11.

Table 24-3
Clinical Chemistry Analyzers, Automated, Discrete*

Manufacturer	Model	Method
Abbott Laboratories, Abbott Park, IL 60064	Spectrum® CCx™	Endpoint, ISE, kinetic
Beckman Instruments, Brea, CA 92621	SYNCHRON ASX®	Endpoint, indirect ISE, kinetic, rate
	SYNCHRON CX®3	Bichromatic, endpoint, indirect ISE, rate
Bio-Chem Laboratory Systems, Lakewood, NJ 08701	ATAC® 6000	EIA, endpoint, kinetic, rate
Boehringer Mannheim, Indianapolis, IN 46250	Hitachi 704	Endpoint, kinetic, optional ISE
Ciba-Corning Diagnostics, Medfield, MA 02052	Express™ Plus	Endpoint, kinetic, rate
Coulter, Miami, FL 33116	OptiChem Models 120, 180	Endpoint, initial rate, ISE, kinetic
Dupont, Wilmington, DE 19880	aca® IV	Endpoint, rate, turbidimetry
Instrumentation Laboratory, Lexington, MA 02173	Phoenix™	ISE, polarographic electrodes, rate
	Monarch Plus	Bichromatic, endpoint, ISE, kinetic, rate
Miles, Inc., Tarrytown, NY 10591	Technicon RA-XT™;	Endpoint, kinetic, rate, optional ISE
	Technicon RA-2000™	
NOVA Biomedical, Waltham, MA 02254	Nucleus	Absorbance, ISE, endpoint, rate, polarographic electrode
Precision Systems, Natrick, MA 01760	Analette 120, 180	Bichromatic, endpoint, kinetic
Roche Diagnostic Systems, Branchburg, NJ 08876	COBAS MIRA® Plus;	Endpoint, kinetic
	COBAS MIRA Plus® CC	
Schiapparelli Biosystems, Fairfield, NJ 07004	Gem*Profiler™	Endpoint, kinetic, optional potentiometric, bichromatic
	Gemstar® II	Bichromatic, endpoint, kinetic
Texas International, Houston, TX 77036	H-16	Endpoint, kinetic, multipoint kinetic
Wako Diagnostics, Richmond, VA 23237	WAKO-20R; WAKO-30R	Endpoint, optional ISE, rate

*Clinical chemistry analyzers, automated, discrete. ECRI product comparison system. 1993, Jan:1–41.

Table 24-4
Blood Glucose Monitors, Portable*

Manufacturer	Model	Method
Boehringer Mannheim, Indianapolis, IN 46250	Accu-Chek II Freedom; Accu-Chek III; Tracer II	Reflectance photometry
Cascade Medical, Eden Prairie, MN 55344	Checkmate	Reflectance photometry
Home Diagnostics, Eatontown, NJ 07724	DIASCAN-S; ULTRA	Reflectance photometry
Hypoguard/British American Medical, Laguna Hills, CA 92653	Supreme bG; Vision bG	Reflectance photometry
Lifescan, Milpitas, CA 95035	ONE TOUCH® BASIC™; ONE TOUCH® II; ONE TOUCH® II Hospital	Reflectance photometry
Medisense, Waltham, MA 02154	ExacTech Pen Exactech Companion; Medisense Pen 2 Sensor and Companion 2 Sensor; Satellite G	Electrochemical
Metertech, Taipei, Taiwan	Model 5000	Reflectance photometry
Miles, Inc., Tarrytown, NY 10591	Glucometer® 3; Glucometer® M+; Glucometer® ENCORE™ QA	Reflectance photometry

*Blood glucose monitors, portable. ECRI product comparison system. 1992, Dec:1-21.

Table 24-5
Electrolyte Analyzers*

Manufacturer	Model	Method
AVL Scientific, Roswell, GA 30077	AVL Models: 982-S, 983-S, 984-S, 985-S, 985-S1, 986-S, 987-S, 988-3, 988-4, 9120, 9130, 9140	ISE
Bacharach, Pittsburgh, PA 15238	Bacharach® Coleman 51Ca	Flame photometry
Baxter Lytening Systems, Danvers, MA 01923	AMDEV® LYTENING Systems: Models 1, 2, 5 and 6	ISE
Beckman Instruments, Brea, CA 92621	LABLYTE® Systems: 800: 810: 820: 830	ISE
	SYNCHRON CX® 3	ISE, bichromatic endpoint, rate
	SYNCHRON EL-ISE®	ISE
Bio-Chem Laboratory Systems, Lakewood, NJ 08701	ATAC® ISE+	ISE
Buck Scientific, East Norwalk, CT 06855	PFP-7	Flame photometry
Ciba-Corning, Medfield, MA 20252	664 Fast 4	ISE, thermal conductivity detection
	480	Flame photometry
	614; 644; 654	ISE
	925	Coulometric
Coulter, Hialeah, FL 33010	Flexlyte 3; Flexlyte 6	ISE
Dupont Medical Products, Wilmington, DE 19880	Na+, K+ Analyzer; Na+, K+, Li+ Analyzer	ISE
Instrumentation Laboratories, Lexington, MA 02173	IL 943™	Flame photometry
Ionetics, Costa Mesa, CA 92626	Electrolyte Analyzers Models 310, 400, 450	ISE
Kone Instruments, Espoo, Finland 358	Microlyte 3 + 2; Microlyte 6	ISE
Liston Scientific, Irvine, CA 92715	ECS™ 2000	ISE
Medica, Bedford, MA 01730	EasyLyte Na/K; EasyLyte PLUS Na/K/Cl; EasyLyte Lithium Na/K/Li	ISE
NOVA Biomedical, Waltham, MA 02254	NOVA Models: 1, 4, 5, 8, 10, 11, 12, 13, 14; Stat Profile®	ISE
Radiometer America, Westlake, OH 44145	CMT 10 Chloride Titrator	Coulometric
	FLM™ 3	Flame photometry
Romark Diagnostics, Hillsdale, NJ 07642	Models KNA1 and KNA2	
	Discovery Models: 2301, 2302, 2304, and 2305	ISE
Schiapparelli Biosystems, Fairfield, NJ 07004	Starlyte™ II; Starlyte™ III	ISE

*Electrolyte analyzers. ECRI product comparison system. 1993, April:1-41.

Table 24-6
Urine Analyzers, Automated*

Manufacturer	Model	Method
Behring, Sommerville, NJ 08876	Rapimat® II/T	Reflectance
IRIS, Chatsworth, CA 91311	Yellow IRIS® Model 250	Reflectance, automated intelligent microscopy (AIM)
Miles Diagnostic, Tarrytown, NY 10591	CLINITEK® 100; CLINITEK® 200+	Reflectance

*Urine analyzers, automated: semiautomated. ECRI product comparison system. 1993. Oct:1-10.

Table 24-7
Enzyme Immunoassay (EIA), Fluorescence Immunoassay (FIA), and Chemiluminescence Immunoassay (CLIA) Analyzers*

Manufacturer	Model	Method
Abbott Laboratories, Abbott Park, IL 60064	ADx®	FPIA
	IMx®	FPIA, microparticle EIA with fluorescence detection (MEIA)
	TDx®	FPIA, radiative energy attenuation, nephelometry
Baxter Diagnostics, Miami, FL 33152	Stratus® Systems	Solid-phase, FIA, EIA, kinetics
bioMerieux Vitek, Hazelwood, MO 63042	VIDAS®	Enzyme-linked FIA
Biotrol, Exton, PA 19341	System 7000®	Magnetic microparticles EIA
BioWhittaker, Walkersville, MD 21793	FIAX 400	Solid-phase FIA
Boehringer Mannheim, Indianapolis, IN 46250	ES 300	EIA (coated tube)
Ciba-Corning Diag., East Wampole, MA 02032	ACS:180™	Chemiluminescence immunoassay (CLIA) (direct)
Diagnostics Products, Los Angeles, CA 90045	IMMULITE®	CLIA
Diamedix, Miami, FL 33127	Fluid FSH	ELISA
Hybritech, San Diego, CA 92121	Photon ERA®-QA	ELISA
Laboratory Technologies, Roselle, IL 60172	Acculyte	CLIA
Labsystems, Helsinki, Finland	Auto-EIA II	EIA
PB Diagnostic Systems, Westwood, MA 02090	OPUS®; OPUS® Plus	Fluorogenic ELISA and thin dry-film technology
Roche Diagnostic Systems, Branchburg, NJ 08876	COBAS FARA II®	FIA
Serono-Baker Diagnostics, Allentown, PA 18103	SR1	EIA, magnetic solid-phase separation
Tosoh Medics, South San Francisco, CA 94080	AIA-600®; AIA-1200®	Magnetic, microbead, rate fluorescence EIA
Wallac, Gaithersburg, MD 20877	DELFIA	Time-resolved fluorescence immunoassay

*Enzyme immunoassay analyzers, fluorescence immunoassay analyzers, chemiluminescence immunoassay analyzers. ECRI product comparison system. 1993. March:1-28.

Table 24-8
Hematology Analyzers, Semiautomated*

Manufacturer	Model	Method
Abbott Laboratories, Abbott Park, IL 60064	Cell-Dyn® Models: 400, 500, 610, 700, 900, and 1500	Volumetric impedance
Becton Dickinson, Sparks, MD 21152	QBC®-II Plus	Density
Coulter, Hialeah, FL 33010	CBC5; M430 and M430 System; ZM	Volumetric impedance
Danam Electronics, Dallas, TX 75237	HC 510; HC 820; HC 1020	Volumetric impedance
Diagnostic Technology, Hauppauge, NY 11788	PS-4; PS-5	Volumetric impedance
Mexxem Diagnostics, Dusseldorf, Germany	BC-1A; MC-1A Multi-4; BC-1A Multi-5; BC 1A Multi-7; BC-2; BC2 Multi-5; BC-2 Multi-6; BC-2 Multi-8	All Mexxem analyzers use electronic imped-ance for RBC, WBC, and platelets and microprocessors for hematocrits, mean cell volume, mean cell hemoglobin (MCH), and MCH concentration
Moelab, Hilden, Germany	Models: 8700, 8700A, 8701, 8702, 8503, 8602	Volumetric impedance
Texas International Laboratories, Houston, TX 77036	H3/HCT; H5-M; H-10	Volumetric impedance
TOA Medical Electronics, Distributed by, Baxter Scientific Products, McGaw Park, IL 60085	Sysmex™ Models: F300, F500 and F800	Volumetric impedance

*Hematology analyzers, semiautomated. ECRI product comparison system. 1993, Jan:1-25.

Table 24-9
Hematology Analyzers, Automated*

Manufacturer	Model	Method
Abbott Laboratories, Abbott Park, Il 60064	Cell-Dyn® 1400; Cell-Dyn® 1600	Volumetric impedance
Becton Dickinson, Sparks, MD 21152	QBC®-II; QBC® Reference; Autoread	Density
Coulter, Hialeah, FL 33010	JT, JT2, JT3	Volumetric impedance
	MAXM and MAXM with Autoloader	Volume, conductivity, and light scatter (VCS) technology, i.e., volumetric impedance, high-frequency conductivity, and light scatter
Danam Electronics, Dallas TX 75237	MD8 and MD16; T540; T660; T890	Volumetric impedance
	Datacell 16CP; Datacell 18	Volumetric impedance
Nova Celltrak, Waltham, MA 02254	Celltrak 11; Celltrak 12	Volumetric impedance
Roche Diagnostic, Branchburg, NJ 08876	COBAS MINOS® Models: STE, STEL, and STX	Volumetric impedance
Serono-Baker, Allentown, PA 18103	System Models: 9000RX™, 9018™, 9020 CAP™, and 9020AS™	Volumetric impedance
Texas International, Houston, TX 77036	H-8; H-12	Volumetric impedance
TOA Medical Electronics, Distributed by Baxter Scientific Products, McGaw Park, IL 60085	Sysmex™ K-1000; Sysmex™ NE-Alpha	Volumetric impedance
Toni Diagnostics, Wichita Falls, TX 76308	Micro-Count Diff	Volumetric impedance

*Hematology analyzers, automated. ECRI product comparison. 1993, Jan:1-37.

Table 24-10
Coagulation Analyzers, Automated*

Manufacturer	Model	Method
Becton Dickinson Microbiology System, Cockeysville, MD 21030	Fibrometer	
Bio/Data Corporation, Horsham, PA 19044	MCA 210	
Helena Laboratories, Beaumont, TX 77704	Cascade® 480	
Instrumentation Laboratory, Lexington, MA 02173	ACL® Models: 100, 200, 1000, 2000, 3000, 3000+	LED nephelometer
Medical Laboratory Automation, Pleasantville, NY 10570	ELECTRA 700™, 800D™, 900™, 900C™; 1000C™	
Organon Teknika, Durham, NC 27704	Coag-A-Mate® Instruments: X2 with Data-Mate; RA4; MDA-180; Coag-A-Mate RA4; MDA-180	
Teco, Ergoldsbach, Germany	Coatron II	

*Coagulation analyzers, automated: semiautomated. ECRI product comparison service. 1993, Feb:1-15.

Table 24-11
Coagulation Analyzers, Whole Blood*

Manufacturer	Model	Method
Biotrack, Mountain View, CA 94043	Coumatrak™; Biotrak® 512	Laser photometric
Haemoscope, Morton Grove, IL 60053	CTEG®	Electromagnetic
International Technidyne, Edison, NJ 08820	Hemochron® Models: 401, 801, and 8000	Electromagnetic
Logos Scientific, Henderson, NV 89015	ELVI Biclot 816	Electromagnetic
Medtronic Hemotec, Englewood, CO 80112	Medtronic Hemotec Automated Coagulation Timer Hepcon® System HMS	Mechanical and photometric Mechanical impedance
Sienco, Morrison, CO 80465	DP-154 Sonoclot®, Coagulation Analyzer; DP-2951 Sonoclot® II; Surgical Analyzer	Mechanical impedance

*Coagulation analyzers, whole blood. ECRI product comparison system. 1992, Dec:1-10.

ANSWERS TO QUESTIONS AND PROBLEMS

Chapter 1

1-1. a. $i = E/R = 5\ V/200\ \Omega = 0.025$ A.
   b. ΔE between a and b = 0 V.
1-2. a. $R_T = 200\ \Omega + 200\ \Omega = 400\ \Omega$.
   b. $i_1 = 5\ V/400\ \Omega = 0.0125$ A.
   c. $i_2 = i_1 = 0.0125$ A.
   d. ΔE across first resistor $= iR = 0.0123A * 200\ \Omega = 2.5$ V.

   Starting voltage $- \Delta E$ across first resistor $= E_b = 5\ V - 2.5\ V = 2.5$ V

1-3. See section on the photomultiplier tube.
1-4. $1/R_T = 1/R_1 + 1/R_2 = 1/100 + 1/300 = 4/300 = 1/75$. Therefore, $R_T = 75\ \Omega$.
1-5. $i = E/R = 5\ V/75\ \Omega = 0.066$ A.
1-6. See Safety section.

Chapter 2

2-1. $RCF = 1.12 \times 10^{-5}\ (20.0)\ (2500)^2$. $RCF = 1400 \times g$.
2-2. $1500 = 1.12 \times 10^{-5}\ (25.0)\ (rmp)^2$. rpm = 2315.
2-3. Time $= \dfrac{(8)\ (3000)}{2400}$. Time = 10 minutes.
2-4. The relative centrifugal force is not specified; with the centrifuge's rotating radius unknown, proper centrifugation cannot be reliably achieved.

Chapter 3

3-1. See sections on mechanical and electronic balances.
3-2. The 100-g weight is outside specifications. You might try reweighing. If the result is still outside specifications, call the factory service or a qualified service representative to check the linearity of the balance.

3-3. Check the accuracy, precision, warm-up period, and whether there are variations in location on the balance pan. Calibrate according to the manufacturer's directions, check the Class S/ASTM Class 1 weights for accuracy, use two or three standard weights for the precision check, and check these weights when the balance is turned on, and at 15-minute intervals until the weight results are stable. Check a calibrated weight (a weight at least 60% of the balance's total capacity) at different locations on the balance pan.

3-4. See the Maintenance and Quality Assurance section.

3-5. There is no problem at any of these locations.

Chapter 4

4-1. Osmotic pressure, boiling point elevation, freezing-point depression, vapor pressure reduction.

4-2. The osmotic pressure of a 1 osm/kg aqueous solution is 17,000 mm Hg. An osmol/L is approximately equal to an osm/kg. Therefore,

$$1200\,\text{mOsmol/L} * \frac{1\,\text{osmol/L}}{1000\,\text{mOsmol/L}} * \frac{17{,}000\,\text{mm Hg}}{1\,\text{osmol/L}} * \frac{1\,\text{atm}}{760\,\text{mm Hg}} = 26.8\,\text{atm}$$

4.3 Freezing-point depression of a 1 osm/kg solution is $-1.858°C$. Again, an osmol/L is approximately equal to an osm/kg. Therefore,

$$\frac{-1.858°C}{1\,\text{osmol/L}} * \frac{1\,\text{osmol/L}}{1000\,\text{mOsmol/L}} * 2\,\text{mOsmol/L} = 0.00372°C$$

4-4. The response of a vapor pressure osmometer is nonlinear below 200 mOsmol/L. This is partly caused by variations in thermocouple response.

4-5. See Figure 4-6.

4-6. Osmolality = fnc, where f is 0.93 for NaCl and n is 2. First, solve for c, the concentration of NaCL:

$$\frac{0.300\,\text{osmol/L}}{0.93\,\text{osmol/mol} * 2} = 0.161\,\text{mmol/L}$$

The molecular weight of NaCl is 58.44 (22.99 + 35.45). Therefore,

$$\frac{58.44\,\text{g NaCl}}{1\,\text{mol NaCl}} * \frac{0.161\,\text{mol NaCl}}{1\,\text{L}} * 0.5\,\text{L} = 4.70\,\text{g NaCl}$$

Chapter 5

5-1. 1.3347.

5-2. 1.3673.

5-3. See Figures 5-5, 5-7, 5-8, and 5-9.

5-4. Amici compensators correct for dispersion of polychromatic (white) light. Compensation is complete at the sodium D line wavelength.

5-5. The refractive index of a substance is affected by its temperature. Liquids are more affected by solids. Accurate measurements of refractive index can only be made if temperature is constant.

5-6. See the Maintenance and Quality Assurance section.

Chapter 6

6-1. Dissolve 40 g $NiSO_4$ in 100 mL 1% HCl.

6-2. Green, purple.

6-3. Too wide a slit width, stray radiation, error in dilution of solution, instrument problem.

6-4. Linear, semilog, % T graph would be a curve on linear paper but is a straight line on semilog paper because of the logarithmic relationship.

6-5. Absorbance is inversely proportional to % T.

6-6. See Component Parts of Photometric Instruments section.

6-7. In order to ensure compliance with the conditions in Beer's law, to keep absorbances in the linear range.

6-8. Yellow-green, yellow, purple, blue, green-blue, blue-green.

6-9. a. 0.25; b. 0.09; c. 0.43; d. 0.02.

6-10. a. 10.5; b. 74.1; c. 21.9; d. 3.2.

6-11. Control 1 = 7.5 gm/dL; control 2 = 5.5 gm/dL; patient sample = 4.2 gm/dL.

6-12. Control = 4.3 gm/dL; patient sample = 2.9 gm/dL.

6-13. $A = abc$; $A = 0.656$, $a = 10.6$, $b = 1$, $c = A/ab = 0.656/(10.6) = 0.062$ M.

6-14. $m\lambda = d(\sin \theta)$; $m = 1$, $\lambda = 340$ nm, $d = (1 \times 10^6)/600 = 1666.7$ nm^{-1}, $340 = (1666.7)(\sin \theta)$; $\theta = \sin^{-1}(340/1666.7) = 11.8°$.

6-15. $m\lambda = d(\sin i + \sin \theta)$; $m = 1$, $\lambda = 340$ nm, $d = (1 \times 10^6)/600 = 1666.7$ nm^{-1}, $i = -15°$, $340 = (1666.7)[\sin(-15°) + \sin \theta] = (1666.7)[-0.2588 + \sin \theta] = -431.4 + 1666.7 \sin \theta$ $771.4/1666.7 = \sin \theta$; $\theta = \sin^{-1}(0.463) = 27.6°$.

6-16. $m\lambda = 2dN(\sin \theta)$; $m = 1$, $d = 250$ nm^{-1}, $N = 138$, $\theta = 90°$, $\lambda = 2 (250) (1.38)\sin 90° = 690$ nm.

Chapter 7

7-1. See Principles section.

7-2. See Principles section.

7-3. There would be a viscosity effect because increasing concentration of proteins would cause the specimen to be less readily aspirated. This would be much more apparent in automatic sample dilutions. Manually diluting the specimen, with TC (to contain) pipets and repetitive rinses, would compensate for the viscosity effect.

7-4. Draw the standard curve by plotting standard concentration on the x-axis, absorbance on the y-axis. Determine the least squares regression line of the standard curve: y = 0.09x + 0.026. For control I, y (absorbance) = 0.077; therefore 0.077 = 0.09x + 0.026, solve for x. Control I = 0.6 μg/mL; Patient 1 = 1.7 μg/mL; Patient 2 = 1.4 μg/mL; Control II = 1.8 μg/mL.

7-5. See Internal Standards in the Instrumentation section.

7-6. The sample analyzed by flame photometry is falsely decreased because there is decreased sample water in which the analyte can be found. Less sodium is contained in the aliquot of sample taken for flame photometric analysis because of the high triglyceride content. Direct measurement by a specific ion electrode circumvents this problem.

Chapter 8

8-1. Equation 8-2 describes the relationship between intensity of scattered light and angle of detection for very small particles. To compare $30°$ light scatter intensity to $60°$, the ratio of i_{s30} to i_{s60} is calculated. As all other terms are the same, $i_{s30}/i_{s60} = \sin^2(90° - 30°)/\sin^2(90° - 60°) = 0.866^2/0.5^2 = 0.75/0.25 = 3.0$.

8-2. The relationship between concentration and transmittance for a turbidimetric assay is given in Equation 8-4. Linear regression of standard concentrations versus $-\log(T)$ gives the following result: $-\log(T) = 0.399x + 0.003$. This can be rearranged to: $x = (-\log(T) - 0.003)/0.399$. For the sample, $T = 0.735$, therefore, $x = 0.328$ mol/L.

8-3. See the last paragraph of Types of Turbidimetric and Nephelometric Reactions in the Principles section.

8-4. See Figure 8-6.

8-5. See the Maintenance and Quality Assurance section and also the Maintenance and Quality Assurance in Spectrophotometry section in Chapter 6.

Chapter 9

9-1. a. See Chapters 6 and 9. Instrumentation is very similar except in fluorometry detector where measurements are usually at $90°$ angle from incident beam; detector wavelength is different from incident wavelength.

      b. See Reflectance in Chapter 6. Both detectors set at angles, but detection wavelength is different from incident in fluorometry. In reflectance the same wavelength is detected.

9-2. See Fluorescence Polarization Analyzers section.

9-3. Draw the standard curve by plotting standard concentration on the *x*-axis, fluorescent intensity on the *y* axis. Determine the least squares regression line of the standard curve: $y = 24.8x + 3.0$. For Sample #1, y (fluorescent intensity) $= 57.1$; therefore $57.1 = 24.8x + 3.0$, solve for x. Sample #1 $= 2.2$ mg/dL; Sample #2 $= 3.3$ mg/dL.

9-4. Theophylline on the TDx® analyzer is an immunoassay technique and the degree of polarization depends on the amount of labeled compound bound to antibody. The standard curve is similar to other immunoassay curves (see explanation following Eq. 9-3). In the phenylalanine assay, the fluorescent intensity versus solute concentration is linear (see Eq. 9-2).

9-5. See Advantages in Routine Operation section.

9-6. See Disadvantages in Routine Operation section.

Chapter 10

10-1. Use Equation 10-1, where A = original activity of 115,000 dpm, time elapsed of 2.25 years, and half-life of the isotope is 12.43 years. $A = 115,000\ e^{-0.683(2.25)/12.43}$, $A = 115,000\ e^{-0.125}$ [look up e^{-x} in math tables or some calculators have the function], $A = 115,000\ (0.88)$, $A = 101,200$ dpm. The activity left is 101,200 dpm.

10-2. Determine % efficiency for each standard. Plot external standard ratio on the x axis versus % efficiency on the y axis. Draw straight line between points. Determine slope and intercept of this line. The slope is 54.13 and the intercept is −4.95.

10-3. First determine the efficiency from the standard curve constructed above. The linear least squares regression line is $y = 54.13x - 4.95$. If the external standard ratio is 0.75, then $y = 54.13\ (0.75) - 4.95$ and the efficiency is 35.6%. To convert cpm to dpm, divide cpm by the efficiency; 30000 cpm/0.356 = 84270 dpm.

10-4. No, the eighth well is not performing satisfactorily. Possible contamination or the high voltage supply has drifted. Disable the well so the rest of the wells can be used, and call a service engineer to check out the problem.

10-5. No, the light-emitting diode housing could be dirty, clean it if possible. Or the high voltage supply to the photomultiplier tube has drifted. Or there is a problem in the current source to the light emitting diode. Call the service engineer.

10-6. See Figure 10-13.

10-7. A pulse-height analyzer is necessary to discriminate pulses of differing energies. In bioluminescence the light emitted is all of the same energy and discrimination is not necessary.

Chapter 11

11-1. $pH = -\log [H^+]$; therefore, $5.5 = -\log [H^+]$, and $[H^+] = 3.162 \times 10^{-6}$.

11-2. Modify the diagram for a pH meter, use a Na^+ ion-selective electrode instead.

11-3. 104 mEq/L.

11-4. See discussion on Clark oxygen sensor under Voltammetry.

11-5. See Potentiometry and Voltammetry.

11-6. See Glucose Electrode under Voltammetry.

11-7. Electrolyte methods that measure the chemical activity of analyte are not affected by increased amounts of lipids in plasma. Ion-specific electrode assays and most potentiometric assays will give valid results in spite of severe hyperlipidemia.

11-8. If the collection tube is not completely filled, excess heparin will bind to ionized calcium and will cause falsely decreased values. That is the reason that the specimen must be redrawn—it was not completely filled the first time.

Chapter 12

12-1. $\mu = d/Et$. Distance of travel (d) is 4 cm. Electrical field strength (E) is 150 V/10 cm (15 V/cm). Time of electrophoresis (t) is 1800 sec. Therefore, μ is 1.48 $\times$ 10^{-4} cm/V-sec.

12-2. $H = (E)(i)(t) = 120 \times 0.06 \times 1200 = 8,640$ J.

12-3. One calorie (cal) raises the temperature of 1 g of water 1°C.

$$\Delta T = 1°\text{C-g/cal} \times 1/50 \text{ g} \times 1 \text{ cal}/4.184 \text{ J} \times 8640 \text{ J} = 41.3°\text{C}.$$

Obviously, this much heating does not occur. Much of the heat is dissipated to the buffer chambers, sample holder, and surrounding air.

12-4. See the subsection Isoelectric Points and Electroendosmosis under Principles.

12-5. Serum protein electrophoresis.

12-6. Power supply, electrodes, buffer chamber, support medium, dryer, staining apparatus, and densitometer.

12-7. Capillary electrophoresis can only separate one sample at a time.

12-8. Isoelectric focusing: agarose gel with polyamino-polycarboxylic acids. Rocket immunoelectrophoresis: agarose gel with specific antibody. PAGE: polyacrylamide gel at three densities for loading, stacking, and separating sample macromolecules.

12-9. The most likely causes are shortened electrophoresis time, decreased voltage, or decreased current.

Chapter 13

13-1. (b).

13-2. (b).

13-3. (c).

13-4. See Figure 13-13.

13-5. (d).

Chapter 14

14-1. Fig. 14-4, component parts.

14-2. Partition, absorption, ion-exchange, and size exclusion. Reverse-phase partition LC is the most commonly used method.

14-3. See Figure 14-5.

14-4. A UV/VIS variable wavelength detector.

14-5. A C18 reverse phase column.

Chapter 15

15-1. See discussion of GLC and bonded-phase chromatography under Mobile and Stationary phases.

15-2. See discussion on columns under Instrumentation.

15-3. Assuming that sufficient quantities of solute are present, the following detectors may be used: (a) TCD, FID, GC/MS; (b) TCD, FID, ECD, GC/MS; (c) TCD, FID, NPD, GC/MS.

15-4. See discussions on detectors under Instrumentation.

15-5. See discussion on injectors under Instrumentation.

15-6. Solute A: $t_r' = 5.50$, $I = 370$; Solute B: $t_r' = 9.35$, $I = 485$.

Chapter 16

16-1. An ion source, a mass analyzer, a detector, and a recording device.

16-2. Electron impact ionization produces many fragmentation ions but few parent ions. Chemical ionization is gentler and produces mostly parent ions.

16-3. See the following figure.

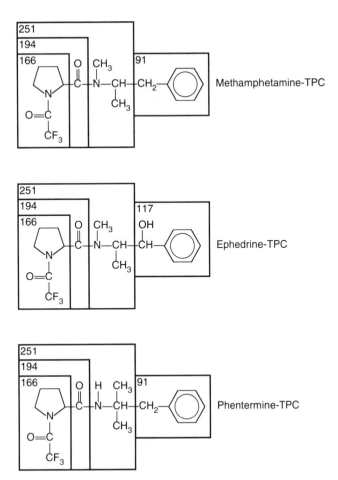

Methamphetamine-TPC

Ephedrine-TPC

Phentermine-TPC

16-4. The isotope abundance is equal to the frequency with which that isotope occurs in nature. Thus, for caffeine ($C_8N_4O_2H_{10}$):

$M^+ + 1$ (%)	$M^+ + 2$ (%)
$^{13}C = 1.100\% \times 8 = 8.8$	$^{18}O = 0.200\% \times 2 = 0.40$
$^{15}N = 0.370\% \times 4 = 1.5$	$^{13}C + ^{15}N = 8.8\% \times 1.5\% = 0.13$
$^{17}O = 0.400\% \times 2 = 0.8$	$^{13}C + ^{17}O = 8.8\% \times 0.8\% = 0.07$
$^{2}H = 0.015\% \times 10 = 0.2$	$^{13}C + ^{2}H = 8.8\% \times 0.2\% = 0.02$
Total $\qquad = 11.3$	$^{15}N + ^{17}O = 1.5\% \times 0.8\% = 0.01$
	$^{15}N + ^{2}H = 1.5\% \times 0.2\% = 0.003$
	$^{17}O + ^{2}H = 0.8\% \times 0.2\% = 0.001$
	Total $\qquad = 0.634$

These figures agree with the spectrum in Figure 16-4.

16-5. a. Notice that heroin (diacetylmorphine) has two acetyl groups, monoacetyl-morphine has one, and morphine has none. As acetic ahydride acetylates free hydroxyl groups, heroin is synthesized from morphine and MAM during the derivatization reaction. The use of acetic anhydride will not allow differentiation of these compounds. Either deuterated acetic anhy-dride or *N*-methyl-bistrifluoroacetamide (MBTFA) can be used to distin-guish between the number of hydroxyl groups in the original compound. Derivatization reagents and their reaction products always need to be considered during assay development.

   b. MBTFA replaces hydroxyl groups with trifluoroacetyl groups (CF_3COO^-), adding 97 to the mass of the analyte for each added trifluoroacetyl group. These groups are most susceptible to fragmentation:

   Morphine $477 = M^+$
   $\qquad\qquad 380 = -97\ (CF_3CO)$
   $\qquad\qquad 364 = -113\ (CF_3COO)$
   MAM $\qquad 423 = M^+$
   $\qquad\qquad 380 = -43\ (CH_3CO)$
   $\qquad\qquad 364 = -59\ (CH_3COO)$
   $\qquad\qquad 267 = -156\ (CH_3COO + CF_3CO)$
   Heroin $\quad 369 = M^+$
   $\qquad\qquad 310 = -59\ (CH_3COO)$

   c. Optimally one would like a deuterated standard for each analyte, but because of their similarity the use of (^2H) morphine alone will suffice.

16-6. See Figures 16-9 and 16-10.

16-7. See the Microcomputer subsection under Recorders in the Instrumentation section.

Chapter 17

17-1. Resolution is decreased because there is a greater likelihood of more than one cell reaching the flow chamber at one time. Sensitivity is enhanced because the cells take four times as long to pass through the flow chamber and because the optic properties of the quartz chamber are better than the jet-in-air system.

17-2. Intense, monochromatic, coherent light; simplified optics; steady power output; ability to select different emission wavelengths.

17-3. See Figure 17-4 and the subsection on lasers under Light Source in the Principles and Component Parts section.

17-4. Forward angle light scatter: related to particle size. 90° light scatter: related to particle granularity. Fluorescence: fluorochrome dyes bind to cell components such as nuclei, chromosomes, organelles, cytoplasm, cell membranes. Fluorochrome-tagged antibodies can bind to specific receptors, proteins, or nucleic acids.

17-5. See Figure 17-5.

17-6. 0.1, ~18, and ~70 FITC fluorescence intensity units.

17-7. Fluorosphere solutions are used to align flow cytometer optics and sample stream, to adjust amplification and gain settings of fluorescence detectors, and to determine instrument linearity.

INDEX